DATE DUE

NO			
DE 0 8 '80			
DE 1 2 '80 DE 3 1984			
AP 0 2 85			
MAR 29 1988			
MAY 0 4 '88			
MAR 0 8 '90			
MAR 0 8 '90			
MAY 2 6 '94			
RT'D MAY 0 6 94			
RECEIVED JUN 0 2 2009			
MAY 0 5 2009			
GAYLORD			PRINTED IN U.S.A.

National Priorities
for Health:

Past, Present, and Projected

WILEY SERIES IN HEALTH SERVICES
Stephen J. Williams, Sc.D., *Series Editor*

Health Care Economics
Paul J. Feldstein

Issues in Health Services
Stephen J. Williams

Introduction to Health Services
Stephen J. Williams and Paul R. Torrens

National Priorities for Health:
  Past, Present, and Projected
Robert F. Rushmer

National Priorities for Health:

Past, Present, and Projected

ROBERT F. RUSHMER, M.D.

Director, Center for Advanced Studies
   in Biomedical Sciences
Professor of Bioengineering
School of Medicine, College of Engineering
University of Washington

A WILEY MEDICAL PUBLICATION
JOHN WILEY & SONS
New York · Chichester · Brisbane · Toronto

This publication was supported in part by NIH Grant LM 00010 National Library of Medicine, Bethesda, Maryland.

Library of Congress Cataloging in Publication Data

Rushmer, Robert Frazer, 1914-
  National priorities for health.

  (Wiley series in health services)
  Includes index.
  1. Medical Policy—United States. 2. Medical
research—United States. 3. Medical care—
United States. I. Title. II. Series.

RA395.A3R88   362.1'0973   79-25313
ISBN 0-471-06472-6

Printed in the United States of America

10 9 8 7 6 5 4 3 2 1

This book is dedicated to academic faculties and students of medicine, nursing, public health, pharmacy and other dedicated health professions engaged in research and practice during a rapid transition to a new era.

Preface

Pervasive and profound changes are occurring in the national health enterprise that urgently require rational responses by all health professionals, from biomedical scientists to practitioners at the bedside. These alterations stem from shifts in the priorities for health-related research and practices that have occurred during the rapid evolution of the biomedical sciences since World War II. Unfortunately, health professionals, researchers, and faculty do not fully recognize the nature and extent of these changes, and they are neither equipped nor fully prepared to make the comprehensive adjustments that new policies, priorities, and operational approaches by government agencies will require. The objective of this book is to explore the past, present, and projected priorities for health-related research and practices in the United States during the past thirty years and their impact on the biomedical community and our health care system.

Powerful public pressures are challenging politicians, health professionals, and academic faculty to function more responsibly in the public interest. An accent on *accountability* defines a newly emerging era in Washington, Bethesda, and the medical community as a whole. This emerging era of increased accountability is the third phase of the explosive evolution of our massive health-related research, development, and delivery system. It was founded and flourished during a period of unbridled enthusiasm and exorbitant expectations that science and technology could resolve the major ills of the world if sufficient resources could be mobilized. The biomedical research effort experienced growth rates far in excess of the capacity of a budding bureaucracy to efficiently and responsibly channel the deluge of dollars over a period of about a dozen years. Inevitable criticism and skepticism ushered in a period of uncertainty and frustration with mounting pressures for payoffs for lavish investments in health-related research. Support of biomedical research wavered, but the performance and prospects of modern medicine never really lost their luster in the eyes of the general public and their representatives in government. The creation of agencies to support health research and health care has been a direct response to public and political pressures to attack the dramatic "killer diseases" and has originated largely from a highly effective lay lobby (Chapter 1).

New forward planning processes represent significant transfer of initiative from individual investigators to the Institutes of Health and entails the development of more explicit statements of goals, guidelines, strategies, and programs. The biomedical research community needs to be aware of the contemporary status of these forward plans to intelligently adapt individual research programs to the altering availability of research funds for various topics supported by the institutes. Chapter 2 summarizes some recent versions of forward plans of each Institute. Many of these forward plans have not been formally published, and their citations may appear incomplete. However, an effort was made to supply in the cited references sufficient information to permit the interested reader to request the material from the individual Institutes.

The requirements for basic and applied research have always been obscured by a widespread failure to develop definitions that distinguish between them. Even more fundamental is general ambiguity regarding the distinctions between theoretical problems and technical problems, which require very different approaches. Finally, the priorities for allocation of resources have generally been based predominantly on certain vital statistics and particularly on mortality rates. Rationalization of research resources can be rendered more realistic by careful consideration of these issues as indicated in Chapter 3.

The masses of information emerging from biomedical research laboratories have greatly enhanced our understanding of the structure, function, control, and effects of stresses and diseases on various organ systems. Notable advances in elucidating causes and eliminating diseases have been made for some ailments but not for a very large number of persistent problems. It seems time to encourage a resurgence of targeted research into the specific causes and cures of crucial conditions that are currently being managed primarily by symptomatic management methods, by supplemental drugs or devices, or by pseudosolutions in accordance with some principles enunciated in Chapter 4.

The practice of medicine has been transformed by the development of increasingly complex and costly health technologies. The predominant thrust has been toward development of diagnostic technologies, while progress in the cure, control, and prevention of diseases has lagged far beyond our ability to recognize or to monitor them. Enhanced sophistication of health techniques and technologies has resulted in expansion of professional and support personnel; the average physician is supported by some 13 other persons with widely varied responsibilities. The escalating costs of health care have not produced commensurate improvement in health status because of deficiencies in effective therapeutic methods (Chapter 5).

Health services have been so highly regarded and revered throughout history that, until very recently, they have never been subjected to critical evaluation or to considerations of contributions, costs, consequences, and outcome. The newly developing methods for program evaluation are still extremely primitive, and the effects of their application are largely untested.

However, the underlying issues are so compelling that methods and materials for data collection, analysis, and interpretation must surely emerge. Examples of some of the many opportunities and options are presented in Chapter 6.

Health professionals are increasingly confronted by dilemmas resulting from the need to assume new roles for which they are ill-equipped or unprepared. As one consequence, the numbers and diversity of health professionals and practitioners have greatly expanded during the past decade. A recent pronouncement by Joseph Califano, former Secretary for Health, Education and Welfare, indicated that there are too many doctors and that the size of medical student classes should be reduced. Such a reversal of views suggests a time of transition for medical education and provides a new opportunity to adapt academic health science centers toward the realities of the nation's needs for a new mix of health professionals with support personnel having increased responsibilities. Even more important would be active programs of health team development as implied by examples in Chapter 7.

The average citizen has become increasingly dependent on physicians for management of many common conditions formerly managed by home remedies and common sense. The soaring costs of health care coupled with the relatively slight benefits derived by encounters with physicians for trivial problems are sufficient motivation for defining and developing mechanisms for enhancing self-reliance and reducing unnecessary and unrewarding use of health services. This problem looms ever larger with progressive approach to some form of national health insurance. Some of the opportunities and approaches to increased self-reliance are presented in Chapter 8.

The problems encountered in the evolution of modern medicine have been approached by many different means in the various developed countries of the world. This world laboratory contains a wealth of experience and experiment with organization, operational and financial mechanisms for providing health services to populations under widely varying conditions. In Chapter 9 some specific examples of potentially valuable or undesirable approaches to health care are briefly summarized from three very different countries, namely Britain, Sweden, and Canada. The prototypes that have evolved in these countries contain valuable information that we cannot afford to neglect or to ignore.

Throughout this book a conscious effort has been made to offer specific suggestions or examples of mechanisms that might be used to resolve the problems under discussion. These suggestions are represented as intuitively attractive alternatives rather than definitive answers.

Robert F. Rushmer, M.D.

Acknowledgments

The support of the National Library of Medicine is most gratefully acknowledged for the award of a Special Scientific Project that made possible the two-year period of study leading to the preparation of this manuscript. The cooperation and courtesy extended by Dr. Roger Dahlen and the staff of the National Library of Medicine during a month of intensive study is especially appreciated. I am also grateful to Drs. Donald Fredrickson, Hans Stettin, James Dickson, John Sherman, and my many other friends and colleagues among the dedicated administrators at NIII, NSF, and other agencies in Washington, who so graciously devoted their precious time to convey to me their perceptions of the programs and problems faced by the biomedical research community in general and the National Institutes of Health in particular. Dr. John Sherman and Dr. Ernest Allen were kind enough to review the chapters dealing with the history of NIII.

A three-month period of intensive exploration was spent in Great Britain to gain additional perspective of both biomedical research and health care delivery in a very different setting. Space does not permit my acknowledgment of the valuable insight gained through countless conferences with dedicated and talented health professionals from the tip of Cornwall to northern Scotland and from Wales to Norfolk. I cannot resist a special word of thanks to Sir Harold Himsworth, Dr. James Gowan, Dr. Rosemary Rue, Dr. Alwyn Smith, Gordon McLachlin, Sir John Brotherston, Sir Andrew Watt Kay, Dr. Sandy Cavenaugh, Professor Robbie Kenedi, Heinz Wolf, Christopher Freeman, Geoffrey Dawes, Nurse Marion McCarthy, Denis Leslie, and a host of others too numerous to mention.

The preparation of the manuscript would have been impossible without the patience, dedication, and skill of Carla O'Reilly in typing and Hedi Nurk in drawing illustrations and charts. Some illustrative caricatures by Hal Street are included to add some spice to serious subjects. The cordial cooperation of Cathy Somer, Scott Klein, and the editorial staff of John Wiley & Sons is also greatly appreciated.

Contents

PART ONE: RESEARCH PRIORITIES: PAST AND PRESENT   1

CHAPTER 1: The Evolution of Biomedical Sciences   3

 Health Benefits from Technical Accomplishments   6
 Delayed Development of Biomedical Sciences   6
 Turning Points in Recent Times   10
 · Origins of the National Institutes of Health   13
 Sources of Research Support   17
 · Expansion of the National Institutes of Health   21
 Stages in Development of the National Institutes of
  Health   25
 Timeliness of a Comprehensive Reappraisal   37
 Summary   39
 References   39

CHAPTER 2: Forward Planning of Health-Related Research   41

 Crisis in Credibility   42
 Pressures for Accelerated Progress   43
 The National Cancer Program: Prototype for Planning   47
 Forward Planning at the National Cancer Institute: Processes
  and Procedures   47
 Rationalizing Research Support: The New Dimensions   54
 Organizational Obstacles to Rational Forward Planning   56
 Forward-Planning Process: NIH Directorate   61
 Forward-Planning Programs in the Individual Institutes of
  Health   65
 Forward-Planning Priorities in "Disease-Oriented" Institutes
  65
 Organ-System Oriented Institutes   69
 Composite or Age-Oriented Institutes   75
 Territorial Boundaries: The Need for Clarification   79

Summary 82
References 83

PART TWO: RESEARCH REQUIREMENTS 85

CHAPTER 3: Priorities and Strategies for Forward Planning 87

Strategic Misconceptions 88
Indistinct Definitions of Basic vs Applied Research and
    Development 93
Rationalizing Basic and Applied Research Requirements 94
Developmental Processes: Ultimate Output of Research and
    Development 100
Criteria for Categorical Balance 106
Assessing Research Progress and Status: Reducing Redun-
    dancy 110
Mechanisms for Monitoring Research Progress 112
Summary 124
References 125

CHAPTER 4: Targeted Research: Quest for Causes and Cures 126

Perspectives from Earlier Progress 127
Epidemiological Etiologies 130
Stages or Steps Toward Cure and Control (Idealized) 132
Cancer and Neoplastic Diseases: Current Status 138
Atherosclerosis 144
Other Leading Causes of Death, Disease, Disability, and
    Discomfort 154
Summary 160
References 161

PART   ASSESSMENT OF HEALTH TECHNOLOGIES AND
THREE: SERVICES 163

CHAPTER 5: Impact of Health Technologies: Contributions and
            Consequences 165

Conversion of Research Technologies into Diagnostic
    Devices 166
Metamorphosis of Clinical Laboratories 169
Therapeutic Progress 176
Complications of Technological Triumphs: Direct and
    Indirect 180
Soaring Costs of Health Care 188
Comparative Return on Investment 190
Health Technology Assessment 192
Summary 196
References 197

CHAPTER 6:   Appraisal of Health Services   199

The National Center for Health Services Research   200
The Evaluation Process   206
Conceptual Considerations in Health Services Research   211
Outcome Assessment: Value Added   217
Evaluating Effectiveness: Clinical Trials   222
Choosing Targets for Program Evaluation   223
Appropriate Utilization of Available Technologies   232
Sources of Standards for Evaluation of Health Care   236
Surveys by the National Center for Health Statistics   239
Needs for New Mechanisms for Clinical Assessment   241
Summary   246
References   247

PART FOUR: ATTRACTIVE ALTERNATIVES FOR THE FUTURE   251

CHAPTER 7:   Professional Pathways: Evaluation of Education   253

Metamorphosis of Medical Schools   254
Career Options from Common Curricula   258
Family Medicine and Primary Care   263
Roles and Responsibilities of Physicians   270
Underutilized Professional Personnel   275
Preparation for Diverse Professional Careers   287
Competence and Creativity: Their Roles in Research   291
Summary   296
References   296

CHAPTER 8:   Self-Care as a Health Service: Opportunities for Participative
Partnerships   298

Deepening Dependence on Professionals   302
Opportunities for Participative Partnership   308
Health Advocates: A Prototype   311
Health Counseling and Supportive Self-Care   317
Health Information Center Concept   318
Summary   324
References   325

CHAPTER 9:   Alternatives From Abroad: Prototypes in the World Laboratory   327

Characteristics of Health Services in Selected Countries   328
British Biomedical Research   330
Prototype: A National Health Service (Britain)   337
Comprehensive and Compassionate Primary Care (Britain)
347
An Integrated Health Team (Wales)   352

A Hospital Specifically Planned for Primary Care
  (Oxfordshire) 354
Health Services Research 355
Long-Range Planning Priorities 356
Contrasting Characteristics: United States and United
  Kingdom 359
An Integrated Regional Hospital System (Sweden) 361
A Fee-For-Service, Insurance-Based National Health Program
  (Canada) 368
Summary 373
References 374

INDEX   377

Part One

Research Priorities: Past and Present

The profound changes in all elements of the American health enterprise since World War II were initiated by a major national commitment to biomedical research. The current conditions in both biomedical sciences and in health care delivery have evolved in response to a combination of public, political, and professional pressures over a period of three decades. The significance of present national policies and priorities can best be understood on the basis of historical perspectives and present trends. Biomedical investigators and clinicians in the health care system are all finding it necessary to plan ever farther in the future and to adapt to rather rapid changes in goals and guidelines from Washington and Bethesda. The first two chapters included in Part 1 are intended to provide insight into evolution of modern biomedical sciences and clinical practices with particular attention to underlying factors that influenced the evolution to their present state.

The biomedical metamorphosis during the past 30 years represents a valiant effort to accomplish, in that time, a process that required some 300 years in the fields of physics and engineering (Chapter 1). The major supporting mechanism was the development of the National Institutes of Health (NIH), occurring through three distinct phases: (1) a mobilization phase, marked by exuberant expansion; (2) a fall from favor phase, with mounting pressures for payoff; and (3) the forward-planning phase, involving a transition from bursar toward manager for the national research effort.

The National Institutes of Health, in company with most other governmental agencies, are now caught up in a drive for greater accountability. A key component is the development of forward-planning processes to develop five-year programmatic plans, which are updated annually. To an increasing degree, funding by all the Institutes is being made available in accordance with planned priorities through invitations to appropriate investigators to submit applications in specified categories. The stability and continuity of many academic research programs will require that the responsible investigators keep abreast of the changing policies and priorities evolving through this forward-planning effort. It is now incumbent on the scientific community not only to be as fully informed as possible but also to take an active part in the identification of those topical areas that can derive the greatest progress from intensified investigation. Part of our present problem derives from a failure of the scientific leadership to exert sufficient influence in the development of goals, guidelines, policies, and priorities in the past.

CHAPTER 1

The Evolution of
Biomedical Sciences

The progress in health-related research during the past 30 years has been prodigious and productive. Huge investments in support of basic and applied research have paid handsome dividends in the form of information and insight into basic biological phenomena. Enormous arrays of new research and clinical technologies have become widely available for investigation and application to scientific and practical pursuits. Health-related research occupied a preeminent position in the minds of the public in the period following World War II. The prospects of overcoming disease and disability were so enticing and exciting that they obscured a fundamental and generally unrecognized deficiency. It was quite generally assumed that the state of biomedical knowledge was sufficiently firm and well founded for the mounting of large-scale assaults on the many diseases. Only a few key persons recognized that the enormous progress in science and technologies had not been accompanied by corresponding advances in the basic medical sciences. One appealing concept was that disease and disability could be attacked and overpowered by the same process that brought victory in the war against the Axis powers: namely, the mobilization of overwhelming manpower, facilities, and hardware. In retrospect, it is now abundantly clear that the advances in biomedical research had failed to keep pace with those in the physical sciences and engineering during the past several centuries (Fig. 1-1).

The mathematical sciences descended from a long tradition that extends from prehistoric times in many cultures. The Egyptians, the Mayans, and the Greeks had developed both practical and theoretical approaches to mathematics, largely oriented toward measurements on the land or in the skies. Thus, mathematical methods had become a rigorous intellectual discipline during eras when human understanding of the natural world was based on strange and wondrous mythologies. Major advances occurred during the

3

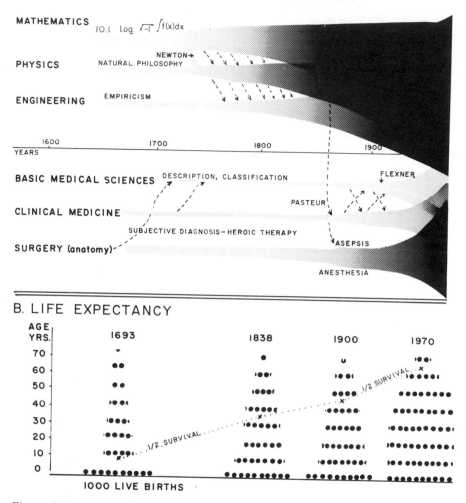

Figure 1-1. (*a*) During the past three centuries, science and technology have evolved at accelerating rates through progressive integration of mathematics and engineering physics. The Age of Rationalization was introduced by the development of natural laws described in quantitative terms. Progressive amalgamation of physics and chemistry into engineering was responsible for the industrial revolution. Biology and medicine persisted as largely subjective and empirical endeavors into the present century. Only recently have physics, engineering, and basic medical sciences entered into strong interactions between laboratory research and clinical practice. (*b*) The life expectancy (in terms of 50% survival of 1,000 live births) increased from about 18 years in 1693, to more than 70 years by 1970. Clearly, there was considerable improvement in health status occurring long before the modern age of "medical science" beginning after World War II (Data from McKeown and Lowe [1]).

4

seventeenth century, including the acceptance of the decimal system, the use of logarithms, and the development of the calculus by Newton and Leibnitz. At the turn of the eighteenth century, the Age of Rationalization emerged through the development of natural laws so concisely conceived that they could be expressed in terms of mathematical formulas. The adoption of mathematics as the language of science produced a continuous fertilization of physics (and later chemistry). Quantitative concepts were transferred from physics to engineering. Empiricism was converted into quantitative and later into analytical approaches to engineering. During the latter part of the nineteenth century, a period of intensive innovation and invention developed. From a relatively brief span of years emerged the fundamental conceptions in agriculture, mechanization, transportation, and communication, which have literally transformed the human condition through engineering exploitation in this century.

A hallmark of our present era has been the merging of mathematics, physics, chemistry at the molecular level, and accelerating applications of the innermost secrets of nature into powerful capabilities. As one result, industrial exploitation has succeeded to a remarkable degree in substituting mechanical energy for human exertion. Mechanization and automation have largely taken the place of human skills in production of materials, goods, and even services. Computers are increasingly serving as substitutes for both brain power and judgment.

While physical phenomena were being described by increasingly sophisticated quantitative expression, the biomedical disciplines were largely preoccupied with subjective descriptions of structure and function. The generally accepted concepts regarding the inner workings of living things continued to combine mythology, intuitive expressions, and authoritarian dogma. Advocates for the concept of spontaneous generation of life were still visible and vocal while atomic structure was being explored and analyzed quantitatively.

Surgery and gross anatomy were coupled by strong and mutually supportive ties, which brought these disciplines much farther along toward their ultimate attainments. Before the advent of anesthesia and asepsis, surgery was heroic, but it was relatively effective and based on accumulated knowledge of anatomy. Otherwise, basic biomedical science and clinical practice were intellectually and functionally separate. Pasteur's demonstration that diseases could be caused by microorganisms initiated the beginning coupling of basic biomedical research to clinical medicine and surgery (Fig. 1-1).

A fledgling Age of Rationalization for biomedical research began with the recognition of the microbial origin of diseases, initiating a trickle of information and technology from basic research efforts into clinical practice, largely informal and expedient. Organizational channels for the transfer of concepts and techniques from basic research into clinical practice awaited the restructuring of medical institutions following the Flexner report, published in 1911. As a consequence of these factors, biomedical concepts and research were largely subjective, empirical, intuitive, and qualitative right up to the end of World War II.

HEALTH BENEFITS FROM TECHNICAL ACCOMPLISHMENTS

By the end of World War II, the triumphs of science and technology appeared to promise the prospect of ultimate affluence in the form of wealth and health for all people. The remarkable improvement in the health status of the people in developed countries, so frequently ascribed to advances in medicine, is now increasingly recognized as having resulted primarily from improvements in living conditions through technical progress.

The first objective estimates of life expectancy were developed at Breslow in 1693, with results illustrated in Figure 1-1B. At that time, from 1,000 live births, only 500 people were expected to survive to the age of 18. Some persons survived to ages of 60 and 70, but these were the hardy ones. Substantial improvement was noted in the first vital statistics obtained in Britain in 1838. At this time, half of 1,000 live births were expected to survive to age 42. By 1900, the average life expectancy increased further to about 53 or 54 years of age. By 1970, 80% of 1,000 live births would be alive at 60, and half would still be alive at 72.

Thomas McKeown (1,2) has provided a different perspective by presenting evidence that declines in death rates began well before 1875. Death rates from noninfectious diseases remained quite steady over the entire century under discussion. The spectacular decline of mortality was associated primarily with a reduction in the fatality rate from infectious diseases. The death rate from tuberculosis was demonstrably declining before the tubercle bacillus was identified, and nearly a century before effective chemotherapy was developed (Fig. 1–2). Similar phenomena are identifiable for scarlet fever and whooping cough, where a progressive decline in death rates was clearly demonstrable before the causal organisms were identified, and long before effective therapy or immunization had been perfected. The evidence suggests that improved longevity was based largely on improved nutrition through advances in agriculture as well as the effects of hygiene, housing conditions, and public health measures. The common tendency to ascribe to medical progress the greatly improved health status and extended life expectancy is obviously not justified by these data. Improved environmental conditions apparently enhanced the resistance to infections, even before measures for their control had been developed.

DELAYED DEVELOPMENT OF BIOMEDICAL SCIENCES

For many reasons, the knowledge base for biomedical sciences was in a very primitive state at the beginning of World War II. The research community was small and intimate, and various viewpoints were debated rather than clarified by quantitative data. Sophisticated instruments, which had long held an important place in physical science, were rarely adopted or adapted in biomedical laboratories. Furthermore, the preparation for profes-

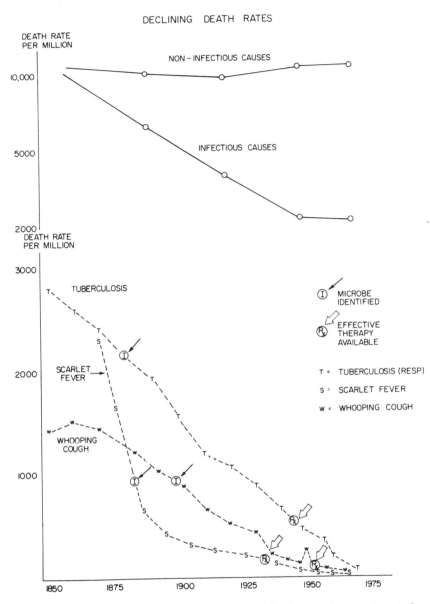

Figure 1-2. A precipitous fall in age adjusted death rates from various infections was clearly visible beginning by the mid-1800s, and persisting into present times. The death rates from noninfectious causes did not decline significantly during this period. The death rates from some of the most prevalent and serious of infectious diseases (i.e., tuberculosis, scarlet fever, whooping cough, diphtheria, etc.) were declining years before the causal microbes were identified and decades before effective therapy or immunization was available. This phenomenon is now ascribed to substantial improvement in nutrition and living conditions (Data from McKeown and Lowe [1]).

sional careers in either medicine or in basic medical sciences placed little premium on a background in mathematics and physics. While many of the definitions and concepts of physics could be expressed in mathematical terms, the nomenclature of biology remained purely descriptive. The isolation of biomedical sciences from the quantitative sciences is indicated by definitions in standard medical dictionaries (Table 1-1). Mathematical and physical terms in standard medical dictionaries of the prewar era often failed to emphasize their quantitative implications. The insulation of biomedical sciences and medicine from the physical sciences and engineering may be attributable to the mystery and complexity of living organisms. Similarly, investigative approaches to living systems were characterized by reliance on subjective observation coupled with a lack of rigor in interpreting descriptive data and a lack of quantitative or dynamic analysis in exploration of function and control. These deficiencies were partially obscured by imaginative explanations of most observed phenomena.

OBSERVATION-EXPLANATION COUPLING

When confronted with any new and interesting natural phenomenon, the normal human reaction is to devise or seek some explanation as to its cause. This might be regarded as an "itch to postulate," which is an exceedingly powerful stimulus. As an extreme example, the Greeks were a pragmatic people, but the imaginative explanations they devised for natural phenomena included outlandish fables of interplay between panoplies of gods and goddesses.

There appears to be a common sequence initiated by experiencing or observing some natural phenomenon. A first response is to confirm its existence by repeated observations. Almost immediately, some kind of an explanation is devised. In scientific circles, such an observation may be reported to colleagues, who in turn would attempt to repeat the observation and perhaps come up with still other explanations. If the phenomenon is of sufficient interest, there will come a time when it will qualify for inclusion into some kind of a textbook. At that time, a decision must be made regarding the most likely explanations among those which have been advanced. As soon as selected explanations have been indelibly inscribed in print, a degree of permanence is suddenly attained, not guaranteed by the preceding process. If this whimsical version bears any resemblance to the truth, then it is virtually assured that every conceivable observation will be coupled to one or more explanations, many supported by the "weight of authority." A misleading impression of a solid body of knowledge is thereby created in both the minds of the casual observer, and even the professionals in the field (Fig. 1-3). It leads to the mistaken impression that all the important problems have been solved, and only the details need be inserted in the chinks between established concepts.

Most concepts, based on subjective observation, tend to be incorrect in whole or in part. The errors can be eradicated only by more precise measurement and more rigorous analysis. Before World War II, the body of biomedi-

TABLE 1-1. Medical Dictionary Definitions of Scientific Terms[a]

CALCULUS: An abnormal concretion occurring within the animal body and usually composed of mineral salts.

INTEGRATION: 1. Assimilation; anabolic action or activity.
2. The combination of different acts so that they cooperate toward a common end.

DIFFERENTIATION: 1. The distinguishing of one thing or disease from another.
2. The act or process of acquiring distinction or individual characters.

ANALYSIS: Separation into component parts or elements; the act of determining the component parts of a substance.

TENSOR: Any muscle that stretches or makes tense.

MASS: 1. A body made up of cohering particles
2. A cohesive mixture suitable for being made up into pills.
3. A characteristic of matter which gives it inertia.

ENERGY: Ability to operate or work; power to produce motion, to overcome resistance and to effect physical change.

FORCE: That which originates or arrests motion.

TEMPERATURE: The degree of sensible heat or cold.
Absolute t.: That which is reckoned from absolute zero, $-273°C$.

FLUID: A liquid or a gas

FLOW: 1. To menstruate copiously
2. A free liquid discharge
3. The menses

PRESSURE: Stress or strain, whether by compression pull, thrust, or shear.

TENSION: 1. The act of stretching
2. The condition of being stretched or strained; the amount to which anything is stretched or strained.
3. Voltage

POTENTIAL: 1. Existing and ready for action, but not yet active.
2. Electric tension or pressure as measured by the capacity of producing electric effects in bodies of a different state of electrization.

RESISTANCE: 1. The opposition by a conductor to the passage of an electric current.
2. In psychoanalysis, opposition to the coming into consciousness of repressed material.

[a]From Dorland, W.A.N., *The American Illustrated Medical Dictionary*, 17th Edition, 1934.

cal knowledge was largely lacking in both quantitative stability and conceptual substance. The outward appearance of a solid, immutable structure appeared to belie the flimsy facade that obscured large voids in understanding.

The remarkably primitive state of the basic medical sciences at the time of World War II was not fully recognized, even by most of the leadership.

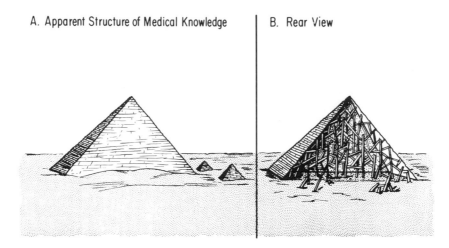

A. Apparent Structure of Medical Knowledge   B. Rear View

Figure 1-3. At the end of World War II, the state of biomedical knowledge was widely regarded as being advanced and poised for rapid technical progress—like physics and engineering. Deficiencies in fundamental concepts were obscured by an illusion of a massive and stable edifice, largely complete except for details to fill the chinks. Just beneath the thin veneer of contemporary concepts resided a veritable void representing the vast number of unexplained or unexplored biological and medical problems.

During the past quarter century, a massive effort has been mounted to gain the scientific status in the biomedical enterprise that had been reached over the preceding centuries in the physical sciences and engineering. During this century, a number of critical events have greatly influenced the progress of the biomedical research effort.

TURNING POINTS IN RECENT TIMES

At the turn of this century, medical education in America was in a dreadful state. A large majority of the medical schools were turning out "physicians," largely through apprenticeship-type training, with little didactic or formal background. Quality medical education was obtainable in a relatively few prestigious institutions, epitomized by Johns Hopkins University. Research activities were essentially limited to those few really academic institutions. This dismal picture was changed dramatically in a relatively few years after a notable study by Abraham Flexner.

FLEXNER REPORT

Critical evaluation of medical education was commissioned by the Carnegie Institute, and Abraham Flexner (3) was chosen to conduct it. With boundless energy, he visited virtually all medical schools and assembled a report that pulled no punches. It identified those institutions of quality, and equally clearly designated those that were obviously deficient. This report might not have had much impact without some external support. The Rockefeller Foundation was induced to provide generous funding for some of the more prestigious medical schools, and at the same time, those showing serious deficiencies were encouraged to dwindle and disappear. In the 10 years after 1910, the number of medical schools in the United States was reduced by approximately half.

Included in the Flexner report (3) were specific recommendations regarding mechanisms for upgrading the standards of medical education, the design of didactic curricula, the incorporation of basic medical sciences in medical school education, and a recognition of the importance of research. Flexner's fundamental philosophy is indicated in the following quotation.

> Thus medicine, moving as rapidly as may be towards scientific status, recognizes no difference in intellectual attitude between laboratory and clinic. Neither can—nor should—any distinction in intellectual attitude be drawn between investigator and practitioner. For centuries, the question was not even raised. From Hippocrates down, those who contributed their successive bits of precious knowledge to the growing structure were practitioners, using their keen wits at the bedside. The more systematic and self-conscious promoters of scientific medicine in modern times did not for a moment suppose that the spirit of scientific inquiry belonged to them as investigators, while, as physicians or teachers, a merely practical, empirical, or technological method was appropriate . . . The mental attitude of the investigator seeking to disentangle an unsolved problem does not in essence differ from that of the physician who has been summoned to see a patient.

This quotation vividly displays the traditional view that distinctions should not be drawn between the pursuit of information by practicing physicians and by investigators in laboratories. The mutual dependence of research in biomedical sciences and the medical practice was confirmed at this time and incorporated into the process of medical education.

ASCENDANCE OF SCIENCE
AND TECHNOLOGY
DURING WORLD WAR II

Pearl Harbor ushered in a complete national mobilization for the war effort and endowed science and technology with very high priorities. The Office of Scientific Research and Development had parallel committees in medicine and in weaponry, under the direction of Dr. Vannevar Bush. Expansion and improvements in weaponry exposed men in uniform to a wide variety of stresses, including exposures to blistering heat and shivering cold, to dehydration, and to malnutrition. Scuba diving exposed man to high pressures, and aircraft exposed him to low pressures. High-speed aircraft induced high rates of acceleration and blackout during rapid turns. Such gross changes in environmental circumstances confronted basic medical scientists with overriding incentives to provide adequate protection. In addition to these challenging environmental problems, the armed forces were subject to higher incidence of trauma under extremely difficult conditions of transport and the need for greatly enhanced rehabilitation. Furthermore, the crowding and congestion of large numbers of men subjected them to a greater danger of epidemics. All these conditions presented the biomedical community with problems that were clearly defined with high priority, for which solutions were desperately needed. The National Research Council of the National Academy of Science organized 51 committees and panels. They dispensed contracts involving 1,700 doctors of medicine and 3,800 scientists and technologists. They spent about $25 million between 1941 and 1947 for medicine ($3.8 million), surgery ($2.8 million), aviation medicine ($2.4 million), physiology ($3.9 million), and chemistry ($2.3 million) (4). Impressive results were achieved during this active, coordinated medical research effort. Protection for members of the armed services against the exposures to severe stresses was greatly improved. Furthermore, progress was evident in the control of epidemics such as rheumatic fever during the wartime period. In addition, the development and industrial production of penicillin, sulfanilomides, gamma globulin, adrenal steroids, cortisone, and other drugs and techniques appeared in rapid sequence. The general public and Congress were impressed, correctly attributing this magnificent progress to adequate financing, coordination, and teamwork.

POSTWAR PRIORITIES

When the attention of the public and their representatives in government was diverted from a massive wartime effort to problems on the domestic front, the deficiencies in health and health care emerged as a prime target. Some 30% of the draftees had been rejected from military duty because of health-related deficiencies. Many of them came from small communities or from remote and rural areas that were lacking in either hospitals or physicians. There was widespread and unwarranted fear of a postwar depression. The impressive progress attained during the press of wartime research encouraged the belief that the time was ripe to mount a major campaign for the conquest of disease in this country. Confidence was widespread that the diseases that beset mankind could be overcome by the same processes of massive mobilization that had so successfully overcome the Axis powers through the enormous industrial capacity of this country. Continued collaboration between government and the private sector was appealing to President Roosevelt, who asked Vannevar Bush for recommendations regarding the mechanisms for mounting "a war of science against disease," and cited a concern that the annual death rates from one or two diseases were higher than those encountered on the battlefield. It seemed timely to consider the transfer of health-related research from a wartime basis into a civilian agency. A National Institute of Health was chosen for this role.

ORIGINS OF THE NATIONAL INSTITUTES
OF HEALTH

The political process by which the National Institutes of Health emerged
in the immediate post-war period is extremely involved and complicated.
This tangled web was meticulously explored and described by Stephen
Strickland (4). In brief, the story begins with the impassioned appeal by
Senator Matthew M. Neely, Democrat from West Virginia. On May 18,
1928, Senator Neely addressed the Senate about the monster that feeds and
feasts on the flesh and blood of men and women and children in every land:

> The tears that it has wrung from weeping womens' eyes would make
> an ocean; the blood that it has shed would redden every wave that
> rolls on every sea; the name of this loathsome, deadly, and insatiate
> monster is "cancer."

Senator Neely introduced a bill that would authorize the National
Academy of Sciences to investigate cancer and report on mechanisms by
which the federal government could assist in coordinating cancer research
and in conquering this destructive disease. This was an early step in efforts
to awaken interest among congressmen in the prospects of overcoming
cancer. The House of Representatives failed to act on the Neely Bill, and he
lost his bid for reelection that fall. Coincidentally, a bill introduced by
Senator Ransdell, drafted by officials of the Public Health Service, authorized the establishment and operation of a National Institute of Health. The
Ransdell Act was signed into law in 1930 and included provision for a
complex of buildings dedicated to research activities of the Public Health
Service. Although the Public Health Service proposed an attack on disease
along many lines, it was really cancer that worried people most, and it was
cancer that gave the peoples' elected representatives in Congress a target that
was deeply dreaded. Senator Hugh Bone, Democrat from Washington, introduced a bill to establish a Cancer Institute, having secured the signatures of
all his Senate colleagues. Representative Warren Magnuson from Washington
enthusiastically introduced in the House a bill identical to the Senate version. A great deal of publicity had created the equivalent of a major "cancer
crusade." Public pressure was sufficient to stimulate rapid action by Congress; indeed, a joint Senate/House hearing was held on the bills that had
been introduced and a compromise was enacted that same month. The
National Cancer Institute was authorized by a statute with the following
mandate:

> To conduct and foster research and studies relating to the cause, pre-
> vention, and methods of diagnosis and treatment of cancer; to pro-
> mote the coordination of cancer research; to provide fellowships in
> the Institute; to secure counsel and advice from cancer experts from
> the United States and abroad; and to cooperate with state health
> agencies in the prevention, control, and eradication of cancer.

The establishment of the National Cancer Institute evoked little evidence of enthusiasm from the medical community. Basic medical scientists

were quite generally convinced that the time was not right for a major attack against that specific disease entity. The medical profession was generally suspicious that this might be regarded as a first step toward socialized medicine. These concerns might have been dispelled by the very favorable experience during World War II, when government-supported research made such notable progress. It is very doubtful that the National Institutes of Health would ever have attained anything resembling their present status and size if the impetus had been provided solely by the health professions. Our greatly expanded research capability was achieved in very large measure through the persistent and persuasive promotion by a most effective group of concerned private citizens. This "lay lobby" provided the initial stimulus and continues to exert enormous influence over the expansion and directions of the medical research enterprise.

THE LAY LOBBY FOR MEDICAL RESEARCH

If there was ever a question that a single concerned citizen could have influence on governmental activities, the successes enjoyed by Mary Lasker should erase all doubts. Mary Lasker had spent several years working with voluntary organizations and had become increasingly convinced that the state of the health of American people was poor and not improving fast enough. She was impelled by a conviction that something must be done by government, since the private sector alone could never make sufficient headway through philanthropic sources of funding. Albert Lasker, her husband, had made a modest fortune as a pioneer in modern advertising and lent his counsel and guidance to an effort, which began in 1944. She was determined to stimulate government involvement in medical research on a large scale and joined forces with Florence Mahoney, whose husband owned an interest in the Cox chain of newspapers published in Florida, Georgia, and Ohio. These two dedicated women, determined to enlist the help of Senator Claude Pepper, Democrat of Florida, by actively supporting his reelection bid with money and favorable publicity. From such simple beginnings began a saga of legislative accomplishment that is unique in American history.

During 1945, Mary Lasker initiated a special fund-raising effort for the American Society for the Control of Cancer, and raised over $100,000, largely through an article in the *Reader's Digest*. With help from her husband, a number of influential citizens were recruited, and the promotional skills typical of Madison Avenue were used by this small group to raise $4 million for the Cancer Society in 1945 (more than four times the donations of the previous year). The campaign the following year raised $10 million, and the new board of directors changed the name to The American Cancer Society. That same year, Congressman Percy Priest introduced a bill designed to attack the problem of mental health by providing funds for training psychiatrists. Florence Mahoney was joined by Mrs. Lasker in seeking the support of Senator Pepper to introduce a measure in the Senate. Recognizing the need for continuous and coordinated efforts to carry legislation through the tangled maze of legislation, Mrs. Lasker put up money for a full-time lobbyist. The National Mental Health Act was signed by President Truman in 1946. Such notable success in the legislative field brought about widespread recognition and support by key governmental officials in the White House in the Congressional committees.

The Lasker/Mahoney team became convinced that the Cancer Institute was an appropriate prototype for the national medical research enterprise. They were actively involved in the development of legislation that created the National Heart Institute. By this time, a small, cohesive, and effective lay lobby had been formed, commonly called the Lasker Lobby. The statute which authorized development of the National Heart Institute contained provisions for lay representation on the council of the Institute, a feature which spread to all other Institutes. Mary Lasker was the first lay council member in the National Heart Institute, and subsequently, members of the Lasker team were generously represented on councils of the other Institutes.

The success enjoyed by these legislative efforts stemmed in part from discovery of ways to parlay a few thousand dollars of private funds into millions of dollars of federal funds appropriated for health research. A consistent program of supporting key legislators with campaign funds provided entry for the discussion of the health needs of the country. The hiring of full-time lobbyists also was an extremely effective measure. A series of annual Lasker awards became extremely prestigious, and the first recipients were Senator Lister Hill and Representative John Fogarty. This was in recognition of their effective and continued support of health research legislation through their positions as Chairmen of the appropriate congressional committees. Public support for bills and for congressional initiatives was obtained through publications and newspaper coverage. The power and prestige of large voluntary health agencies like the American Cancer Society and American Heart Association were effectively involved. The members of the Lasker Lobby became familiar on a first-name basis with very large numbers of key officials in both executive and legislative branches of government. On many occasions, Mary Lasker and her colleagues had easier access to the ears of presidents and to key congressional leaders than of respective Cabinet members or other elected officials.

COALITION FOR HEALTH LEGISLATION

Although many other groups and individuals made large contributions to the growth and prestige of the health research enterprise, a large amount of credit must go to the persistence and persuasion of Mary Lasker, the political skills of Lister Hill and John Fogarty, coupled with the professional prestige of James Shannon, Director of NIH. Lister Hill, John Fogarty, and James Shannon assumed their respective posts in the years 1954-1955. Aided by the unremitting support of the Lasker Lobby, this coalition, individually and collectively, exerted great influence over direction and growth of the health-related research effort of the federal government.

Senator Lister Hill, son of a physician who had pioneered heart surgery, sponsored the Hill-Burton Hospital Construction Act in 1946. His profound interest and concerns with medical matters made him a most appropriate choice for chairing a committee dealing with health education appropriations. His dedication to health services and medical research was complete. As a legislator he was so persuasive, charming, and effective, that his colleagues rarely had occasion to take exception to his ambitions for the medical research activities. John Fogarty, Chairman of Health Appropriations in the House, was elected on a campaign strongly supporting medical research. His knowledge was respected by his colleagues in the House, because he did his homework and succeeded in marshalling overwhelming evidence in support of measures and budgets which flowed smoothly through the legislative process. He was personally convinced of the importance of health research and fully dedicated to its support.

Dr. James Shannon was handpicked by Surgeon General Leonard Scheele to serve as the Director of NIH. Dr. Shannon had received the Presidential Medal of Merit for research work in malaria during WW II and had directed the Squibb Institute of Medical Research before becoming Director of NIH August 1, 1955. He was equally interested in finding cures for the diseases and disabilities that affect mankind; however, he was far more conservative in his approach. He was unusually perceptive in recognizing that there was "no broad general theory, such as exists in the physical sciences," to serve as a foundation for launching major attacks on specific diseases. He undertook to develop a growing biomedical science enterprise, with primary emphasis on basic medical sciences and a broad inquiry into basic studies of structure, function, and control, as well as disease. In contrast to this point of view, there was a wide-scale conviction on the part of the vigorous supporters of expanding health research, that the scientists and medical community were far too conservative, and that the answers to their problems could be achieved much more quickly by a large and burgeoning effort. Because of these fundamental differences, Mary Lasker and James Shannon rarely communicated with each other. Indeed, the four key players in the drama played individual roles, but the net result was a concerted and apparently orchestrated collaborative effort.

The lobbyists insisted on bold and expansive approaches to the problems of health. The Congress as a whole was generally more cautious but were still more daring than the scientists and medical community, who consistently displayed a conservative attitude about targeted research.

The net result of these countervailing forces was an accelerating rate of growth that was stimulated by lay public, modulated by Congress and accepted with increasing enthusiasm by the biomedical research community. The objectives of research were identified on the basis of categories which had broad public appeal rather than a solid base of scientific knowledge from which to launch an attack. The intent of Congress was to support research that would contribute rather directly to improved diagnosis, management, cure, or prevention of the various diseases under attack. Dr. Shannon was able to persuade Congress that a large-scale development of basic medical sciences was an essential step toward the ultimate goal of curing or controlling pathological processes. The result has been a broad scale frontal attack on selected disease categories with simultaneous scientific intrusions from the most fundamental to the most applied research and development. The successive addition of categorical Institues of Health have represented the principle thrust of the effort, but there exist other important sources of research support that supplement the programs of the NIH.

SOURCES OF RESEARCH SUPPORT

The magnitude and diversity of concerns for health and safety are manifest in the many health-related research programs supported by a wide variety of governmental agencies. This dissemination of research and development on health-related issues inevitably produces severe problems of overview and evaluation of total health research effort and of its component parts. There is a common tendency to focus attention on the programs supported by the National Institutes of Health as the prime source of contributions and progress. Such a restricted view tends to grossly underestimate the full scope of health-related research and development on the national scale. The enthusiasm with which the nation adopted threats to life and health as the prime target for a massive national research enterprise affected many of the nation's private and public institutions. It is difficult to acquire dependable data reflecting the magnitude of this effort other than that afforded by the financial outlays which suggest the size and scope of various components.

The total biomedical research and development effort in 1975 was about $4.4 billion—of which federal funds made up about two-thirds. The relative distribution in Figure 1-4 is probably not very different today. Private research support is supplied by industry (mainly pharmaceutical, instrument, and hospital supply companies) with a relatively small contribution from private nonprofit organizations and institutions. Recall that before World War II, most biomedical research support stemmed from a relatively few philanthropic foundations at levels that appear miniscule today. Despite their smaller financial contributions, a great deal of influence is still wielded by the voluntary health organizations such as the National Cancer Society and the American Heart Association. Other private agencies strongly encourage research on favored topics such as arthritis, cystic fibrosis, multiple sclerosis, birth defects, and so forth. The financial contributions by voluntary agencies are often compounded by the influence exerted on the federal government through such organizations.

HEALTH-RELATED RESEARCH AMONG
GOVERNMENTAL AGENCIES

The scope of health-related research has been broadly extended beyond the problems of disease and disability to encompass an extremely wide spectrum of issues scattered throughout the whole of modern society. As a consequence of these trends, health research has become progressively easier to justify in widely different contexts by the various agencies of government interested in expanding the size and scope of their missions.

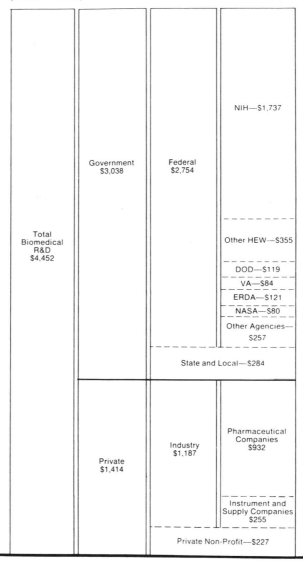

Sources of Support for Biomedical R&D in the United States

(Millions of Dollars)

			NIH—$1,737
	Government $3,038	Federal $2,754	
			Other HEW—$355
Total Biomedical R&D $4,452			DOD—$119
			VA—$84
			ERDA—$121
			NASA—$80
			Other Agencies— $257
			State and Local—$284
	Private $1,414	Industry $1,187	Pharmaceutical Companies $932
			Instrument and Supply Companies $255
			Private Non-Profit—$227

Figure 1-4. Biomedical research and development had financial support of about $4.4 billion in 1974, of which about $3 billion stemmed from governmental agencies and the remainder from private sources. The contribution by NIH ($1.7 billion) was large in comparison with other federal and state appropriations. The pharmaceutical companies accounted for most of the private industrial funding. The absolute quantities of funding increased in subsequent years, but the distribution probably remained about the same (From Basic Data relating to the NIH, Washington, D.C., 1976).

18

The actual size, composition, and distribution of "health-related" research has attained a wide scope and complexity that defies precise definition (see Fig. 1-5).

The Department of Defense (DOD) has long been the undisputed leader as the recipient of the largest allocations of grants and contracts for research and development. Most any innovative investigator can phrase a proposal for fundamental research in terms that render the anticipated results relevant to missions as inherently practical as those of the DOD, VA, or NASA. As a consequence, very basic research is still supported by those agencies in substantial amounts within academic institutions. The biomedical research and development programs in the various governmental agencies tend to have many features in common with those of NIH and other health-oriented organizations. Liberal interpretation of their missions has allowed penetration of health research and development into most aspects of science and technology. An attempt to reverse this tendency was embodied in the Mansfield Amendment (1970), directed at military research and development.

> None of the funds authorized to be appropriated by this Act may be used to carry out any research project or study unless such a project or study has direct or apparent relationship to a specific military function or operation. (Section 203, Public Law 91–121, 1969.)

Indiscriminate curtailment or elimination of "basic" research supported by DOD or other agencies could have a destructive impact on academic institutions and disrupt projects that are vital to crucial social problems.

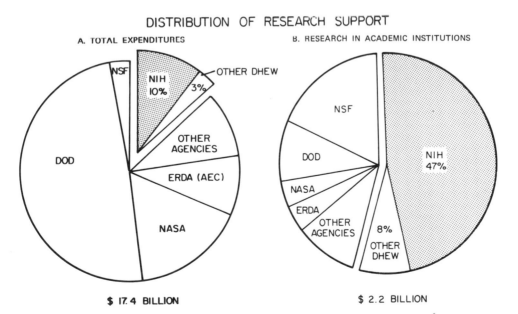

Figure 1-5. (a) Research budgets for NIH appear modest in relation to support of research and development by the Department of Defense (DOD) or NASA but (b) NIH support accounted for almost half of investigative efforts in universities (1974). The Department of Energy (DOE) has now replaced ERDA (see also Fig. 2-1).

Discriminative mechanisms are urgently required to provide and present to Congressional Committees reliable and balanced evaluations of research and development programs (see also Chapters 2, 3).

The Manned Spacecraft Program of NASA necessarily involved a major commitment to the development of life support systems to protect astronauts in extremely hostile environments. A conscientious effort was made to disseminate and transfer the technologies for use by research institutions and industry with only modest success in biomedical applications. Monitoring of man in space was developed using mostly modifications of traditional equipment to transmit and record standard vital signs, with few contributions of substance that could be applied to patients (Fig. 1-5).

The National Science Foundation (NSF) shares with NIH prime responsibility for *basic* biological and biomedical research activities. Expanded roles for NSF have encompassed programs designed to encourage the transfer of technology from basic research into commercial production with limited success.

The Veterans' Administration (VA) provides a broad spectrum of health care for former military personnel and their families. The VA hospitals are closely affiliated with medical schools and have active research programs that involve both basic medical research and clinical investigation.

The Department of Agriculture has implicit responsibility for nutrition—an obvious requirement for human health. Health-related research is actively pursued in agricultural-technical programs of state universities. Agricultural extension programs are effective mechanisms for technology transfer from basic research to practical applications.

The Department of the Interior has responsibility for the health of Native Americans through the Bureau of Indian Affairs.

Agencies involved in transportation (DOT), Housing (HUD), Occupational Health (OSHA), Environmental Protection (DPA), and Energy (ERDA, now DOE), all have recognizable commitments to environmental and occupational health and safety of the public (Fig. 1-5).

Federal funding for biomedical research stems largely from the National Institutes of Health, which are responsibile for basic, clinical, and applied research and development. Other agencies in DHEW account for a smaller increment along with substantial investments by Department of Defense (DOD), Veterans' Administration (VA), DOE, NASA, and other agencies. The contributions of state and local governments to biomedical research remain relatively unimpressive in comparison with other sources.

The commitment of various federal agencies to health-related research is most commonly indicated by budgetary allocations. The National Institutes of Health have received the largest investments by the federal government in biomedical research. In 1974 it accounted for about 10% of the total federal expenditure for research and development, placing third behind DOD (48%) and NASA (17%). Even more impressive is the fact that nearly half (47%) of federally sponsored research in academic institutions was supported by NIH with an additional 8% provided by other components of DHEW (Fig. 1-5). The federal outlays for health-related research in 1975 included $1.6 billion by NIH and support at lower levels from other components of HEW and a variety of other agencies.

EXPANSION OF THE NATIONAL
INSTITUTES OF HEALTH

When confronted by a challenge, the traditional American approach is to mobilize support, money, and resources and mount a campaign to proceed full speed ahead, with supreme confidence that obstacles can be overcome. It is generally accepted that unexpected complications will arise but that they can be overcome or circumvented through a sustained effort. Elements of such an approach are recognizable in the fascinating saga of the National Institutes of Health. At the outset, many key people in NIH were deeply concerned and often opposed to the exuberant expansion of the Institutes of Health toward missions specifically focused on the care and curing of diseases (5). Overwhelming public enthusiasm prevailed over such objections, and the medical community soon joined the ranks of the avid supporters of the campaign. As time went on, concern that the targets might be overly ambitious or out of reach was soothed by periodic surges of progress and technical triumphs.

A campaign against death and disease is much more complicated than merely building new governmental research laboratories or providing money for expanding research in academic and industrial institutions. At an early stage it was decided to accomplish NIH missions primarily by expanding the research capability of academic institutions, rather than through industrial or governmental facilities. Before World War II, biomedical research had been supported in medical schools at low levels of funding, primarily from scanty departmental research budgets supplemented for some by grants from a few philanthropic foundations. The basic science faculties were relatively few in number, heavily engaged in teaching. Biomedical research was commonly regarded as an interesting intellectual avocation. Full-time clinical faculty were in the minority and largely lacking in training for research during traditional medical education. The mounting of a massive attack on disease and disability required more than an expansion of existing personnel, facilities, and services. A major mobilization of essential national resources involved a crash program of recruiting and training of biomedical research talent.

The nationwide campaign against the multitude of threats to life and health of the American public has certain features in common with a major conflict or war. In this case, the enemies were numerous, diverse, and ubiquitous. Furthermore, they were cloaked in mystery; their origins were largely unknown and strategies for their downfall were only vaguely conceived. Clearly, massive research, development, and operational campaigns against such formidable foes required a nationwide effort that must be sustained for the many years of frustration and disappointment. From the beginning, the campaigns against categorical diseases were mounted with much fanfare, lofty objectives, and propaganda. Long experience had demonstrated that large-scale and expensive programs, financed by federal funds, can be continued only so long as overwhelming public support can be sustained. Fortunately, public and political support was periodically reinforced by notable successes sometimes supplemented by premature promises.

PUBLIC AND POLITICAL SUPPORT
FOR THE NATIONAL GOALS

Most large research and development efforts require many years of unremitting and widespread activity for their full development. Promises of rich rewards are required to develop the necessary high priorities for adequate funding. The continued viability of major public works is commonly dependent on the reaching of stated goals within the time span of popular support. Diminishing public interest can have drastic effects even on programs which have demonstrated great achievements. A recent example was the highly successful Apollo program with its spectacular mmon landings. The excitement of space exploration was brought into the living room through the miracle of mass communication. The post-Apollo program was extremely ambitious and carefully drawn, but was greatly curtailed as a result of waning public interest. The breathless anticipation and waves of enthusiasm during the first human landing on the moon were dissipated to ripples of interest by the third lunar landing. Similarly, the Mohole project was discontinued for lack of public interest and support when this oceanic drilling operation had penetrated only partway through the earth's mantle. The biomedical research community has been unusually successful in maintaining both public and congressional enthusiasm for its programs over the past 30 years.

Health-related research was favored by overwhelming public support because of its universal appeal. Natural interest in health and concerns about disease were effectively utilized to sustain public interest and assure Congressional support. Mobilization of political support resulted in sequential establishment of the Institutes of Health generally representing dread diseases most feared by the population as a whole.

THE LEGISLATIVE HISTORY
OF THE NIH

The processes by which Congress expanded health-related research were initiated by the conversion of the Hygienic Laboratory of the Public Health Service into the National Institute of Health (Ransdell Act of 1930). The National Cancer Act (1937) established the National Cancer Institute just before the outbreak of World War II (6). More than 10 years later, the National Heart Institute was created (1948), followed closely by the National Dental Research Act. An Omnibus Medical Research Act (1950) authorized Institutes dedicated to Neurological Diseases and Blindness (NINDB), Arthritis and Metabolic Diseases (NIAMD), and a broad scale program was launched. Interdisciplinary and fundamental areas of responsibility were awarded more official status by the designation of a General Medical Sciences Institute in 1962. The same year, the National Institute of Child Health and Human Development was authorized for research and training related to maternal and child health. This small sample of congressional legislation will serve to illustrate the exuberant growth of a large health-related enterprise, stimulated by unbridled enthusiasm in all quarters (Table 1-2).

TABLE 1-2. Chronology of Major Health Legislation

May 26, 1930. The Ransdell Act called for reorganization, expansion, and redesignation of the Hygienic Laboratory of the Public Health Service into the National Institute of Health.

August 5, 1937. The National Cancer Act established the National Cancer Institute to conduct and support research related to the cause, diagnosis, and treatment of cancer.

July 3, 1946. The National Mental Health Act was intended to improve the mental health of the American people through research into the causes, diagnosis, and treatment of psychiatric disorders. (The National Institute of Mental Health was subsequently formed on the authority of this law in 1949).

August 13, 1946. The Hospital Survey and Construction Act (Hill-Burton Act) authorized grants to states for construction of hospitals and public health centers, for planning of additional facilities and for survey of existing hospitals and other facilities.

June 16, 1948. The National Heart Act authorized the National Heart Institute to conduct, assist, and foster research and studies related to the cause, prevention, and methods of diagnosis and treatment of diseases of the heart and circulation to provide training and to assist the states in prevention, diagnosis, and treatment of heart disease. The National Institute of Health became the National Institutes of Health.

June 24, 1948. The National Dental Research Act authorized the National Institute of Dental Research to conduct, assist, and foster dental research; provide training and cooperate with the states in prevention and control of dental diseases.

August 15, 1950. The Omnibus Medical Research Act authorized the establishment of: National Institute of Neurological Diseases and Blindness, National Institute of Arthritis and Metabolic Diseases, and additional Institutes to conduct and support research and training relating to other diseases and groups of diseases.

July 30, 1956. The Health Research Facilities Act authorized federal matching grants to public and nonprofit institutions for the construction of health research facilities.

August 3, 1956. The National Library of Medicine was created by transferring the Armed Forces Medical Library under the Public Health Service.

October 17, 1962. The National Institute of General Medical Sciences was authorized to conduct and support research in basic medical sciences and related behavioral sciences which have significance to two or more Institutes or which are outside their areas of responsibility. (Established in 1963). The same act also authorized the development of the National Institute of Child Health and Human Development for research and training relating to maternal health and child health and development.

Health was so politically appealing that congressmen vied with each other in demonstrating their strong endorsement of health-related research. The chairmen of the House and Senate Appropriations Committee, (John Fogarty and Lister Hill) were instrumental in assuring sustained and unremitting growth. Financial support flowed from federal coffers in a swelling flood. During a period of 20 years (1948 to 1968) the annual budget requests for NIH were expanded by substantial amounts in all but four years (5) (three of the four were war years). As a specific example, the mechanisms by which the congressional appropriations for the National Heart

Institute exceeded by varying amounts the budget requested by the Executive Branch are illustrated in Figure 1–6.

Beginning in 1952, the normal sequence began with submission of a budget by the Executive Branch which was slightly increased by the House and greatly increased by the Senate. The final appropriation was a compromise between the House and Senate versions (Fig. 1–6). Appropriation of budgets far in excess of the Institute requests placed a heavy responsibility on the organization. A large and experienced staff would be required to assure that the funds were allocated only to projects of very high quality and that funds were disbursed with appropriate responsibility. The budgets for administrative staff of the NIH were totally inadequate for such a momentous task. A major responsibility for the quality of research and financial

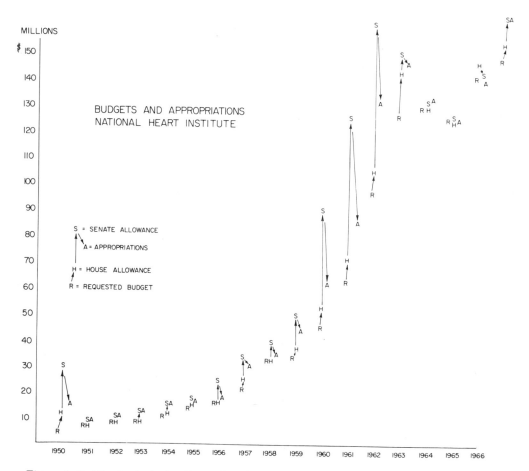

Figure 1–6. The budgets for the various Institutes of Health expanded gradually at first and then explosively in the early 1960s. For example, the basic budget request of the National Heart Institute was increased by the House, increased still further by the Senate, with a final compromise reached at an intermediate level. These "golden years" of NIH expansion were suddenly interrupted by criticisms leveled by the Fountain Committee (1962-3) (Data from Fact Book for Fiscal Year 1976, NHLBI, DHEW Pub. No. NIH 77-1172).

accountability was necessarily transferred to the investigators initiating requests, engaging in research, and reporting results in the scientific literature. The resulting appropriations were so generous that the National Heart Institute awarded virtually all the projects pronounced scientifically sound by study sections, over a period of many years. In retrospect it was inevitable that allegations of waste and loose management would stem from congressmen concerned for the public purse.

An abrupt discontinuity in escalating NIH budgets appeared in 1963, when the exuberant additions by House and Senate transiently disappeared. The underlying causes will be explored in a subsequent section.

STAGES IN DEVELOPMENT OF THE NATIONAL INSTITUTES OF HEALTH

The National Institutes of Health have attained their present stature through several recognizable stages of growth. The "golden" years of exuberant expansion persisted for more than a decade and were rather abruptly arrested in 1963. The unbridled enthusiasm for health-related research came under increasing scrutiny by critics in the Congress and outside. The break in stride temporarily threatened to arrest progress and the next decade was characterized by elements of ambivalence and uncertainty. The programs of research and development continued to be supported but the rate of growth was greatly slowed. The budgetary appropriations continued to grow but at rates sufficiently slow that the buying power began to diminish in the late 1960s. A major shift in both emphasis and operational mechanisms in support of health-related research is clearly evident beginning in 1971 and continuing to the present. This scenario can be viewed as a sequence of three successive stages:

1. Mobilization phase: Period of exuberant expansion.
2. Fall from favor: Pressures for payoff.
3. Forward-planning phase: Transition from bursar toward manager (see also Chapter 2).

The precise time intervals occupied by the individual stages are subject to some disagreement, but their distinguishing features facilitate consideration of the factors that have led to the current status of health-related research. The successive phases are summarized briefly here. Their implications become increasingly apparent in all subsequent chapters.

MOBILIZATION PHASE: PERIOD OF EXUBERANT EXPANSION

At the close of World War II, the power and prestige of science and technology had captured the imagination of the people. In the flush of victory, many firmly believed that problems of virtually any type or size could be solved if sufficient resources were mobilized. The development of an atomic bomb in six short years through the Manhattan Project appeared to demonstrate that mobilization of scientific competence, fully supplied with necessary resources, could penetrate to the innermost secrets of nature with resounding success. The nucleus of living cells appeared no more inaccessible than the nucleus of the atom. Mounting a crusade against disease by marshalling the necessary research and development programs caught and kept the public attention. Desire for health and dread of disease have always been sufficiently universal that it behooves any politican to be strongly and visibly supportive of measures identified with biomedical research and the provision of appropriate health services. Politicians and their families are all too familiar with disease and disability from personal experience. The series of legislative acts in Table 1-2 focused on readily identifiable diseases as targets the citizenry could recognize.

Congressional Strategies. The common congressional mode of action is to identify an appealing target and mount a major spearheaded attack by appropriating generous budgets. The allocation of funds is the most readily available mechanism by which the government can initiate action to meet public needs. The legislation generally contains the "intent of Congress" in rather explicit terms and the agencies of government are expected to carry out the mandate. If the fundamental knowledge required to mount the attack is well in hand, technical obstacles can be clearly defined along with the specifications of the desired result and acceptable criteria of success. In contrast, the ultimate causes and approaches to cure of most common illnesses remain largely mysterious so the obstacles are largely theoretical. Such problems cannot be clearly defined and the nature of the results cannot be specified in advance. As a consequence, the research and development efforts tend to be broad frontal attacks, with both fundamental and applied research being carried on simultaneously instead of sequentially. The essential differences between technical and theoretical obstacles are described in more detail in Chapters 3 and 4 (See Fig. 3-2).

Recruitment of Research Personnel. The NIH offered unique opportunities through which faculty members of medical schools could become entrepreneurs on their own initiative. Individuals in the medical community could request and receive grant support, assuming responsibility for the funds with remarkably few restrictions. By this means, virtually any qualified member of a medical school faculty could become an independent investigator and a potential empire builder, freed from former dependence on the parent insituation or department as sole source of the necessary resources. The initially cautious requests of medical faculty for research support rapidly swelled from a trickle into a flood. Attractions were great among the basic medical scientists whose departments were generally small and poorly funded. Their numbers multiplied as this rather elite and scholarly community responded to the glowing opportunities proferred by NIH. Research productivity soon became the crucial criterion for professional advancement of medical faculties. Clinical faculties were equally attracted to submit proposals and initiate research projects. The traditional medical education of physicians contained no requirements for mathematics, minimal requirements for physics or quantitative sciences, and virtually no experience with the conduct of laboratory research. The widely accepted concept that the process of diagnosis and therapy was roughly equivalent to engaging in research had been enunciated by Flexner but proved to be somewhat less than optimal as a basis for embarking on scientific investigations.

The swelling ranks of investigators engaged in health-related research rapidly absorbed the available manpower pool so new training programs were instituted to expand the supply of biomedical investigators. In the past 30 years, the research capability has been developed or improved in more than 90,000 trainees. Physicians with traditional medical education accounted for a large proportion of the recipients of such training. The surge toward research in medical schools produced profound changes in these remarkably adaptable institutions (see Chapter 7).

Laboratory Facilities. Research facilities in medical schools and other academic institutions were expanded and equipped to accommodate the growing research programs. The NIH occasionally contributed partial funding the renovation and capital construction, but most of the burden of building and maintaining of facilities was borne by the sponsoring medical schools, hospitals, and other institutions involved in health-related research.

Equipment. The expanding research enterprise provided a market for industrial production of new and necessary research tools and instrumentation for clinical medicine (see Fig. 5-1). First, the needs had to be recognized and the specifications defined by close collaboration between biomedical investigators and engineers. The resulting emergence of biomedical engineering promoted a progressively increasing supply of sophisticated research and clinical equipment. The consequences of this development are considered in more detail in Chapters 5 and 6.

Support Services. Institutions sponsoring and housing ambitious medical research programs assume extremely large financial and operational obligations. Provision of laboratory and office space is only the most obvious drain on institutional budgets. As research enterprises expanded, they generated pressures for support services like any "big business." Provision of light, heat, power, furnishings, involves capital expenditures to enlarge facilities and utilities. Requirements for central stores, purchasing, and other administrative services progressively expanded, and the need for cost accounting for responsibly managing large sums of money became increasingly urgent.

Peer Review of Investigator-Initiated Proposals. From the early days of NIH, a surprisingly democratic mechanism was devised to allow input from individual investigators in establishing strategies. The Institutes of Health were organized to receive and process spontaneously generated proposals for health-related research from the scientific community at large. The scientific quality of the projects was reviewed by study sections composed of scientists selected from among the leaders in the various fields. Each proposal was rated on the basis of the quality of the proposal, keeping in mind the qualifications of the investigators and their research environments (7).

Advisory councils were organized for each Institute and for the NIH directorate to establish broad policies, to assure balance, and to provide direction and oversight for the various programs. On these councils the biomedical community was represented predominantly by the clinical specialties with lesser participation by the basic medical scientists or the general public.

In marked contrast to most governmental bureaucracies, the Institutes of Health intentionally suppressed the natural tendency to manage and control the programs. Instead, the staff deferred to advisory bodies comprised of selected representatives of the medical community for decisions regarding broad policies, scientific evaluation, and priority of research projects. Displaying extraordinary restraint, the administration and staff of the Institutes of Health served as *bursars* of public moneys. They assumed responsibility for the distribution of funds but exerted little influence on the directions of research emphasis. The targets for research were generally identified by individual investigators through their research proposals.

The guidelines for study section review of scientific merit emphasized critical evaluation of the aims, approach, feasibility, and significance of the proposals along with the apparent competence of the investigator(s) and the research environment. Reviewers are asked to evaluate the prospects of obtaining "new data and concepts or confirming existing hypotheses." During the rapid mobilization phase, most applications that were regarded as scientifically "adequate" were approved for funding. Repetitive research efforts were often justified as valuable for confirmation of previous work. An implied assumption was that the review process by experts would identify excessively redundant research and avoid undesirable duplication of effort. The peer review system has successfully withstood critical review as a key component of the grant award system (8).

Self-governance and peer review proved to be extremely effective mechanisms for mobilizing and expanding resources for research. Initial concerns regarding potential governmental influence over academic institutions were rather rapidly dispelled by these mechanisms. The approach also attracted involvement in medical research by persons who could never have been identified by a talent search conducted by governmental agencies. Opportunities to expand research capabilities were extremely attractive to individual faculty members of medical schools and to the administrators of these institutions.

SUPPORT OF RESEARCH: GRANTS VS CONTRACTS

Agencies of government traditionally activate programs involving research and development in the scientific community by means of contract mechanisms. For this purpose, requests for proposals (RFPs) are distributed to competing organizations, describing in rather concise detail the nature and types of results that are required. Potential contractors respond with specific and detailed descriptions of their capabilities and approaches to the problem, and awards are made on the basis of competitive bids, taking into consideration quality, prospects, and relative costs. The contracts include clearly stated objectives, approved procedures, performance standards and specifications for desired results. Progress is monitored by contract officers, who regularly receive reports (monthly or quarterly) and give specific approval for any deviation from the contract or the budgetary provisions. Permission may be required before the responsible contractor can expend amounts as little as $100 for purposes other than those expressed in the contract. The contracts are normally commitments for one year, renewable with appropriate demonstration of progress or performance. The high level of specificity and accountability of contracts is obviously appealing to public servants or agencies responsible for the expenditure of public funds. Industrial organizations are accustomed to functioning under the restrictions imposed by contracts with government or other industries. Academic faculty are traditionally resistant to such restrictions in their "academic freedom" and gravitate toward acquisition of research grants for very obvious and tangible reasons.

Research grants are commonly directed toward rather general objectives and permit considerable latitude in shifting directions and emphasis as the work progresses. Such decisions are the prerogative of the principal investigator, who is rarely asked to defend such moves until the next request for grant funding. Commitments extend for periods of three to five years and departure from the original objectives and from the budgetary allocations are quite common. This latitude permits investigators to follow promising leads that might emerge in the course of the research. The number of grants mushroomed so rapidly that the agencies' staffs were not equipped to engage in either monitoring of progress or budgetary allocations, or to assess the outcome of the research efforts as the flow of research reports in the literature swelled from a trickle to a flood. In lieu of extensive reports of progress, the investigators were expected to exchange and utilize the results of their efforts through publications and scientific meetings. The responsibility for scientific performance and accountability for appropriate expenditures of grant moneys was delegated by the granting agencies to the members of the scientific community. The extreme latitude afforded by research grants is clearly attractive to academic investigators but a source of uncertainty on the part of public servants assigned responsibility for the appropriate utilization of public funds.

FALL FROM FAVOR: PRESSURES FOR PAYOFF

As long as unremitting popular support persisted, the overwhelming confidence of the public in the scientific community was not shaken by doubts or criticisms. For more than a decade, the health-related research enterprise prospered and grew at a prodigious rate. Its burgeoning growth rates rendered the entire program vulnerable to allegations of waste, inefficiency or questionable management methods.

Allegations: The Fountain Committee Report. The National Institutes of Health have thrived as an exceptional example of self-governance by a profession entrusted to a remarkable degree with the distribution of public resources to itself for the purpose of engaging in research and development for the public good. During the Mobilization Period the biomedical research effort was regarded generally as a most successful example of a Congressional initiative, but there was growing nervousness that it might have grown too rapidly.

During the massive expansion of the NIH budget, which soared from $52 million to $430 million in just 10 years (1950–1960), the bulk of the funds were earmarked for research grants with very limited provision for an administrative staff adequate to effectively monitor such a diverse and expanding enterprise. In 1964, the small staff of NIH was responsible for 14,000 research grants and 3,500 training grants in addition to intramural research and large center grants or program projects. Many of the Institutes were able to award funds to most of the applications that were judged as scientifically "adequate" by peer review. There was justifiable suspicion that some projects might not conform to uniformly high standards. The prestige of the NIH and the promise of health-related research were enough to muffle criticism for a decade, but the issue of fiscal responsibility and proper management of public funds is also an unassailable argument to Congressmen.

In view of the exuberant expansion of the biomedical research enterprise, it was inevitable that problems of management and administration would ultimately emerge. There was neither time nor administrative budgets sufficient to develop the sophisticated machinery for efficient allocation of such huge sums and maintenance of oversight on their expenditure in such widely diverse and dispersed laboratories and clinical facilities. In 1969, Representative L. H. Fountain, Democrat from North Carolina, began to probe the "potential weak spots" in his position as Chairman of the House Subcommittee on Intergovernmental Relations. The stated objectives were to help the agency discover and remedy management deficiencies. The initial motivation may have been to gently probe irregularities in management, but the ultimate outcome was an overt attempt to apply the brakes to the escalating appropriations to NIH by Congress. The report of the committee represented a bitter attack, charging "irresponsible administrative procedures, ineffectual central management, favoritism in distribution of money, and support of research of poor quality" (9). The impact of this report is clearly visible in the abrupt arrest of the soaring NIH appropriations in 1962 (see Fig. 1-6). The same activities that were so widely acclaimed by enthusiastic congressional committees suddenly became much more difficult to defend before a more critical and unsympathetic audience.

The officials at NIH acknowledged that their follow-up on grant projects was quite limited. However, they defended the policy of picking good people with good projects and giving them the freedom to carry them out. The grants were regarded essentially as a trust awarded to carefully selected investigators who assumed the responsibility for appropriate use of the funds and the performance of the proposed line of research.

A comprehensive review of NIH policies and practices was initiated by President Johnson in 1965 with the appointment of a "blue ribbon" committee, Dean F. Wooldridge, Chairman (10). After extensive review, the committee gave NIH very high marks for the quality of the research being supported but called for closer administrative overview of the investigators and the supporting institutions. At that moment in history, the budget for NIH had been soaring toward $1 billion per year and the basic question was whether the nation's capital investment in health through biomedical research was being spent wisely and with full accountability. A central question was the appropriate level of funding at which NIH would approach "maturity." An extra effort was deemed necessary to establish priorities and to maintain the "quality of its operations." The committee questioned the balance of programs and recommended that a Policy and Planning Council be formed to assist the Office of the Director of NIH in formulation of NIH programs and participate in Congressional hearings.

These recommendations were not followed and the process of establishing policies and priorities by NIH was left unchanged. During the decade between 1963 and 1973, the "most favored position" of health-related research in the halls and chambers of government was progressively undermined by growing concerns, uneasiness, and discontent. Major differences in perceptions have produced growing gaps in confidence and mutual regard among the biomedical community, the general public, and their elected representatives in government. Clearly, the biomedical community had accepted responsibilities for solving problems and creating cures for which they were decidedly unprepared. Normal function and control of tissues and organs were inadequately understood. The problems implicit in the various categories of disease are not only technical but profoundly theoretical. The causes of most of the disease categories were either unknown or extremely controversial. Mounting a major attack under such conditions is roughly equivalent to conducting a military campaign against an unknown enemy in unfamiliar terrain without maps. A vast amount of very fundamental information was required before major advances could be made toward the targets that had been selected on the basis of popular appeal.

The need for large investments in basic medical research was advanced by leaders of the scientific community and accepted by the public and their elected representatives. Implied or explicit promises of major breakthroughs provided repeated reassurance that both skirmishes and battles were being won. Sustained support by the public was recognized as essential to maintain the large and growing biomedical research effort. Despite recurrent announcements of major advances and technical triumphs, signs of impatience and "pressures for payoff" were signaled by reminders that enabling legislation for *each* of the National Institutes of Health indicated the intent of Congress to improve the health of the American people—not to develop greater "understanding of diseases." The public and Congress have become increasingly restive and insistent on demonstrated progress toward the curing, controlling, preventing, or eliminating of the diseases as reasonable responses to generous financial support over several decades. A common manifestation of this controversy is the recurring debate regarding the relative priorities that should be assigned to "basic" as contrasted with "applied" research (see also Chapter 3).

Causes of Controversy: Differences in Perspectives. The apparent paradox between the obvious accomplishments of biomedical research and the widespread disenchantment of the general public and its representatives in government is largely attributable to different points of view.

The nature and extent of these different conceptions can now be appreciated in the colder light of current reality. Thus, there are no "villains in this piece." Instead, there are honest differences in interpretation of the same situations from divergent vantage points.

The progress toward the original goals of improving the health of the American public has not lived up to inflated expectations. The medical community pointed to accelerated advances in provision of improved diagnostic and therapeutic technologies, but these technical triumphs did not conform to the elevated public expectations. The anticipated results were overly ambitious on the part of the public and overly optimistic on the part of the biomedical enterprise. The expectations were exorbitant in most areas of effort and unrealized for the most part. After all, the "killer diseases" had not succumbed to the massive attacks. The incidence of many major diseases is actually increasing.

Mounting disappointment with apparent progress and tangible advances has increasingly centered on congressional conviction that the biomedical community was too involved in efforts at understanding diseases with inadequate commitment to curing them. Congressional committee hearings have been increasingly concerned with shift in balance of programs from basic to applied research. Realistic distinctions between fundamental (pure), basic, and applied research and development are presented in Chapter 3. A natural response to the swelling waves of criticism of the NIH directorate was to develop programs designed to demonstrate the relevance of preceding research accomplishments and to expedite their entrance into common clinical practice.

Demonstrating and Enhancing Relevance. The underlying source of dissatisfaction among the critics was always the controversial issue of the magnitude of the return on the investment for research. The emphasis on basic research was repeatedly questioned and the demands for targeted research toward more specific and useful ends reached higher pitch. With increasing frequency, queries whether "too much energy was being spent on basic research and not enough on translating laboratory findings into tangible results for the American people," were audible even from supporters such as President Johnson. These questions persist to the present day.

Efforts to mend the rift between NIH and Congress were undertaken by instituting new programs designed to more clearly demonstrate the relevance of the research programs, including

- Clinical research centers in academic hospitals
- Regional medical programs throughout the country
- The Heart, Cancer, and Stroke Program
- Special centers of research (SCOR Programs)
- Categorical multidisciplinary centers in selected institutions
- Expanded applications of contract research and development programs

With the retarded growth rates in budgets and the diversion of increasing quantities of money toward large program projects and centers, the funds for individual research grants diminished. This process had the effect of gradually eliminating projects of questionable value and raising the overall standards of quality of projects supported by NIH.

In retrospect, it now becomes clear that the period from 1965 until 1973 was characterized by a fall from favor of the biomedical research community in the eyes of the governmental establishment. With the declining purchasing power of the budgets, new programs could be initiated only by curtailing existing ones. With changing administrative leadership in NIH and in the corridors of government, conscientious efforts to meet the growing demands for greater relevance and more tangible benefits were not enough to assuage widespread disappointment and disenchantment with the return on the massive federal investment over the preceding decades. The responses of NIH to the attacks from various quarters were initially defensive, then responsive, and, more recently, quite revolutionary; namely, long range planning of research (see Chapter 2).

Institutional Accountability: A Contemporary Challenge. The governmental granting agencies are all being caught up in a current of change which promises to have profound effects on their policies and priorities.

Widespread concern has surfaced regarding the escalation of size, scope, and complexity of governmental operations. New projects emerge and enlarge while old governmental programs persist, neither dying nor fading away. Agencies and activities initiated by statute persist with durability and permanence that generally defies efforts at turning them off or shutting them down. The bureaucracy appears to be in danger of losing control over the massive, diffuse, and enormously expensive programs. The net effect of such changes has been a deterioration in the accountability of the federal government and its component parts.

These important trends have stimulated a variety of legislative and administrative actions which are designed to improve the overall accountability of governmental programs. The nature, extent, intent, and potential significance of these trends are illustrated by a few specific examples:

- Sunset Laws
- Zero-based budgeting
- Reorganization Act of 1970
- Oversight Recommendations (House Committee on Science and Technology)

· The President's Biomedical Research Panel Report
· National Health Goals and Guidelines (National Health Planning and Resources Act, 1974 [11])
· Forward Plan for Health (FY 1978–82)

Each of these represents an intention to improve the policies and procedures by which governmental agencies perform their functions under conditions in which the responsibility and accountability are more clearly defined and more effectively maintained. The traditional approach to Congressional appropriations is to begin with the current level of support and debate the need for additional increments. Sunset Laws have been proposed to establish termination dates for governmental programs which could be renewed only after review. The intention is to provide a mechanism for discontinuing or reducing the size of efforts on a regularly recurring basis. More than 50 senators and more than 100 congressmen joined in sponsoring such legislation in the 94th Congress. The objectives of such legislation are clearly laudable but implementation would certainly be a monumental task in view of the number, magnitude, and complexity of programs requiring review. Zero-based budgeting is conceived as requiring comprehensive justification of the entire annual budget for each program, including the various components. The difficulties of instituting such a process are grave and no serious proposals have been advanced so far to apply the mechanism generally to the federal budget. Willis Shapely (12) studied these issues and concluded that this zero-based principle is being applied at present to the extent it appears practical and feasible.

Reorganization Act of 1970. The General Accounting Office has been assigned responsibility for actively pursuing specification and clarification of program goals with detail enough to allow informed judgements regarding the extent to which progress has been accomplished toward these stated ends. The approaches include requirements for the specification of goals, mile posts as indicators of progress, methods required to develop the data, and procedures by which this information will be collected, analyzed, and used to justify the funds authorized. A recent inventory of legislative acts disclosed requirements for such forms of evaluation included in 40 statutes, of which 15 were in the health and safety areas (13). There is a corresponding trend toward inclusion of increased requirements for program evaluation as specific elements in authorizing legislation.

Special Oversight Hearings. These hearings were conducted by the House Committee on Science and Technology to develop specific means of improving the annual reports of research and development (14). The proposal specifies the need for comprehensive overviews of the nation's various scientific and technological efforts as a whole rather than as a large number of unrelated projects and programs. These recommendations were clearly intended to encourage or require that the various agencies involved in support of research and development come up with explicit statements of goals, guidelines, policies, and priorities to an extent that had not been considered necessary until very recent times. Indeed, goals, policies, objectives, priorities, strategies, and performance criteria had never been developed by NIH for lack of both incentives and mechanisms. As long as the directions of research were established primarily by investigator-initiated projects and programs, the priorities of research were being established outside of that institution.

President's Biomedical Research Panel Report. A prestigious panel was established an an outgrowth of the controversy concerning the National Cancer Program in 1974 (15). The report was based on extensive public testimony (150 witnesses), written submissions, and staff analysis of specific issues. Certain of the key conclusions and recommendations are worth mentioning because many of the current trends in NIH appear consonant with these perceptions.

> *Missions of NIH:* In addition to vigorous programs of fundamental research, all Institutes should assume the same balanced roles in research planning with *comparable authority for program implementation.*
>
> *Application and Dissemination of Knowledge:* A formal structure for knowledge, *application*, and dissemination activities was recommended.
>
> *Formulation of the Research Budget:* Systems for developing budgets should be devised by which *research opportunities can be recognized* as well as assuring program balance.

The examples listed above are only a few of many evidences that NIH is being impelled by pressures toward long-range planning, more comprehensive oversight, greater fiscal responsibility, and more consistent justification for continuation of programs. The resulting changes in policies and operational modes will constitute an important transition for NIH from primarily a *bursar* of public funds toward a much more active role in the *initiation and management* of research programs in biology and medicine.

National Health Goals and Guidelines. The National Health Planning and Resources Act of 1974 (Public Law 93–641) called for issuance of national guidelines for health planning which set forth goals and standards with respect to supply, distribution, and organization of health resources. This Act stimulated a study directed toward the *first* statement of health goals which Congress has required (11).

This initial effort to develop concise statements of national health goals included definitions of relevant terms and a wide variety of goal statements from many sources in this country and abroad. Analysis of the various goal statements produced evidence of ambiguity and confusion regarding the distinctions among the goals, objectives, strategies, and other ingredients for a stable and consistent planning framework.

FORWARD PLAN FOR HEALTH
(FY 1978–82)

The Public Health Service published a forward plan for health in 1976 (16), the third in a series presenting a "frame of reference within which the PHS can examine major health issues." This plan incorporates the research and development proposals of the NIH and adds the broader concerns of improving the health status of the public and the delivery of medical care. Some of the salient features of this forward plan are summarized to illustrate the intent, magnitude, and scope of the effort along with elements of the tactical plan. The introductory statement by Dr. Theodore Cooper, Assistant Secretary for Health, Education, and Welfare, recognized the inevitable need for setting priorities when aspirations exceed resources. The essence of the tactical plan was:

- *Goal:* To help improve the health of the American people.
- *Objectives:*
  - To assure access to quality health care at reasonable cost.
  - To prevent illness, disease, and accidents.
- *Priorities:*
  - Strengthening the policy-making and priority-setting apparatus.
  - Containing health care costs.
  - Preventing disease and illness.
  - Increasing quality of health care.
  - Assuring that essential resources of the country are strengthened, including:
    - Modernization of health data system.
    - Strengthening the stability of the academic medical institutions.
    - Maintaining a stable and vigorous biomedical and behavioral research program.
    - Supporting a policy-oriented system of health services research.
    - Continually replenishing and targeting our manpower pool.
    - Assisting states and communities in the development of health services capacity in underserved areas.

The development of clearer goals and guidelines are specific responses to growing feeling of need for assuming more responsibility and leadership by the Institutes for initiating and implementing programs. The development of forward plans for health expressly covering five-year spans in the future are clearly a tangible step in this direction. The Health Policy Board representing the various component agencies of the Public Health Service (ADAMHA, CDC, FDA, HRA, HSA, NIH) meet regularly to advise the Assistant Secretary, DHEW, on key issues. Such meetings are intended to integrate and coordinate the efforts of these health-related agencies.

Knowledge development in the forward plan for health includes research priorities in three broad categories:

- Important cross-cutting areas of knowledge such as immunology, virology, basic genetics, nutrition, epidemiology, endocrinology, neurophysiology, neuropharmacology, and molecular biology of disease.

- New and expanded legislative mandates, specifically aging, diabetes, arthritis, occupational and environmental hazards, child health, sudden infant death syndrome, genetic diseases, alcoholism and drug abuse, and health services research.
- Sustained priorities for cancer and heart, lung, and blood diseases.

The document provides an overview of the major problems confronting the biomedical community at all levels from the most fundamental investigation requirements to the provision of quality health care at reasonable cost.

As a result of these and related factors, the last decade of consolidation or retrenchment under fire has been characterized by fundamental changes in the atmosphere surrounding biomedical research. The most significant consequences for NIH were summarized by Dr. Donald Fredrickson (17) as:

> The increasing competition for federal resources and self-imposed limits on Congressional appropriation limits.
>
> A marked restriction, for the present at least, in *growth* of purchasing power for science.
>
> A countervailing increase in expectation and demand that science tend to urgent practical problems.

The current trends toward increasing emphasis on accountability, forward planning, priority, and assessment of research and development efforts tend to run counter to a long-standing scientific stance and tradition. The "right" of a scientist to choose his own line of research and follow it wherever it may lead is widely defended as being desirable or even necessary for the fruitful development of scientific knowledge (18). The very process of setting national policies, goals, guidelines, objectives, priorities, and methods of assessment necessarily imply a narrowing of the freedom of choice by scientists. As large and growing proportions of the funds available for the research effort are channeled into programs for application or assessment of health services, the support of basic research enterprises is necessarily curtailed. The growing dependence of the biomedical research efforts, particularly in medical schools, on the government for support of their research and training programs, provides a powerful leverage that subtly or strongly diverts efforts of the individual investigator toward the objectives with high priorities expressed by the various granting agencies.

The scientific community recognizes and fears two major thrusts: (1) mounting pressures for applied research rather than fundamental investigations, and (2) over-regulation implied by increased accountability as it impacts the conduct of research.

TIMELINESS OF A COMPREHENSIVE REAPPRAISAL

The comprehensive review of the federal role in biomedical research contained within the Wooldridge report dealt primarily with equity of grant awards without consideration of the appropriateness of the targets, the priorities, or the relevance of the research to the scientific and national needs (10). The more recent report of the President's Biomedical Research Panel (15) focused mainly on the organizational and operational relationships and management of both biomedical and behavioral research as conducted by NIH and ADAMHA. The addition of "behavioral research" in the agenda is a subtle indication of a very broad expansion of the scope of health-related research. During the past two decades, the scope of medical and health care has been enormously expanded to encompass not only disease and disability, but also the impact of psychosocial and cultural stresses as they affect the ability of individuals to cope with their particular situations. This enlarged concept of "holistic" medicine that includes the whole person in its scope extends far beyond the traditional boundaries of biomedical research and practice. The setting of goals, objectives, priorities, and strategies for the future must take into account the complex interactions of many different disciplines which have never been considered in comprehensive overviews in previous years.

REQUIREMENTS FOR A COMPREHENSIVE, MULTIDISCIPLINARY REAPPRAISAL

Edward Burger (19) presented a strong case for a new review of the biomedical research enterprise which would necessarily reflect a breadth of points of view as opposed to a narrow spectrum of advocates of science. There is a clear need for appropriate analysis to support (or refute) arguments and conclusions that otherwise rest on judgment or advocacy. The current shift away from the dominant self-regulatory role of the biomedical research community is an adequate stimulus for such a broad-scale review. Forward plans should reflect the lessons learned from past experience with particular regard for the social impacts of technological triumphs. In our complex modern society, the changes wrought by biomedical research extend far beyond the bounds of medicine or health care. Consider just two examples. The high priorities that have been awarded the common causes of death have necessarily resulted in a progressively aging population. Such changes affect every thread in the fabric of our society: its cultural, economic, ethical, philosophic, legal elements at virtually all levels. More discretely, the technical successes represented by artificial kidneys, coronary bypass operations, or drug therapy of mental illness have broad impacts throughout our social structure. It is no longer sufficient that the members of the biomedical community establish research and development priorities in hopes that everything is going to turn out all right. Prime targets for the future should be based on constructive input by the most respected, accomplished, and competent representatives of the relevant disciplines. The traditional mode in the United States is to establish review groups comprised of experts, generally prominent figures with the greatest personal and professional interest in the outcome of the evaluation.

Reassessment of goals and guidelines by any group engaged in forward planning needs to be based on clear understanding of the current conditions, their origin, and significance. A major objective of this book is to explore some of these fundamental issues in hopes that this and similar efforts can provide added insight to the nature and scope of the present problems and factors for consideration in formulating forward plans for the future.

SUMMARY

1. Since World War II, the biomedical research enterprise of the United States has attained world leadership, a process that involved efforts at accomplishing in about 30 years scientific progress that required some 300 years for quantitative sciences of mathematics and physics.

2. The National Institutes of Health expanded explosively through generous Congressional appropriations substantially in excess of budgetary requests during the initial mobilization phase of growth.

3. The "golden years" of NIH expansion were arrested by unexpected criticism. In retrospect, the fall from favor of the biomedical research community was due in part to the development of a number of underlying misunderstandings based on the very different perceptions of the biomedical community as contrasted with the views of the general public and their representatives in government.

4. Pressures for long-range planning stem from leveling or declining budgets, increased requirements for accountability, fiscal responsibility in governmental agencies, and a growing conviction that the targets for programmatic development need to be developed in systematic fashion rather than purely in response to the academic interests.

5. Forward planning and fiscal accountability both require the identification and definition of missions (aims), goals, policies (guidelines), specific objectives, priorities, criteria of success and mechanisms of evaluation; features that have not previously entered into the arena of biomedical research support.

6. As a consequence of many trends, the relationships between the academic research community and the federal granting agencies are being dramatically altered. The roles of the various Institutes are being progressively expanded and the scope of biomedical research is extending into new areas such as behavioral and social sciences.

7. It is increasingly important for biomedical investigators to understand the organizational and operational mechanisms of federal granting agencies, their forward plans, and the ways by which investigators can adapt in order to maximize their contributions to knowledge, techniques, and technologies for the benefit of the nation's health.

REFERENCES

1. McKeown T, Lowe DR: *An Introduction to Social Medicine*, ed. 2. Oxford, London, Edinborough, Melbourne, Blackwell Scientific Publications, 1974.

2. McKeown T: *The Role of Medicine: Dream, Mirage, Or Nemesis.* London, The Nuffield Provincial Hospital Trust, 1976.

3. Flexner A: *Medical Education—A Comparative Study.* New York, Macmillan Co., 1925.

4. Strickland SP: *Politics, Science, and Dread Diseases: A Short History of United States Medical Research Policy.* Cambridge, Harvard University Press, 1972.

5. Strickland SP: Integration of medical research and health policies. *Science* 173: 1093-1103, 1971.

6. A chronology of major health legislation. In *Health in America, 1776–1976,* US Department of Health, Education, and Welfare, Health Resources Administration, DHEW Pub No (HRA) 76-616, 1976.

7. Henley C: Peer review of research grant applications at the National Institutes of Health. *Fed Proc* 36:2066-2068, 2186-2190, 2335-2338, 1977.

8. Cole S, Rubin L, and Cole JR: Peer review and the support of science. *Sci Amer* 237:34–41 (No 4), 1977.

9. Administration of Grants by NIH; Re-examination of Management Deficiencies. Report of the Fountain Committee, 87th Congress, 2nd Session, June 30, 1962.

10. Wooldridge D: Biomedical science and its administration; a study of the National Institutes of Health. Report to the President, The White House, Washington DC, 1965.

11. *Baselines for Setting Health Goals and Standards.* Papers of the National Health Guidelines: DHEW Publication No HRA 76-640, September 1976.

12. Shapley WH: Impact of Sunset Legislation and Zero-based budgeting on research and development. A report prepared for the Office of Technology Assessment. D77-4. January 31, 1977.

13. Krezo, G (Analyst, Congressional Research Service Library): Program Evaluation: Emerging issues of possible legislative concern relating to the conduct and use of evaluation in the Congress and Executive Branch. November 16, 1974.

14. Special Oversight Report #1. Review of the Annual Report of the Federal Research and Development Program—Fiscal Year 1976. Subcommittee on Domestic and International Scientific Analysis: Committee on Science and Technology. U.S. House of Representatives, 94th Congress, Second Session, Serial II.

15. Report of the President's Biomedical Research Panel. Submitted to the President and the Congress of the United States. DHEW Publication No. (S) 76-500, April 30, 1976.

16. Forward Plan for Health, FY 1978-82, Public Health Service DHEW, US Government Printing Office, Stock No 017-000-00172-8, August 1976.

17. Fredrickson DK: The government in biomedical research. *Fed Proc* 35:2538-2540, 1976.

18. Freedom in the Research System, in: *Science at the Bicentennial; a Report from the Research Community.* National Science Board, National Science Foundation, US Govt Printing Office 0-207-044, 1976.

19. Burger EJ: Science for medicine—time for another reappraisal. *Fed Proc* 34:2106-2114, 1975.

CHAPTER 2

Forward Planning of Health-Related Research

The biomedical research community is entering into a new phase of development with fundamental and profound significance to the future of academic faculties, practicing professionals, and ultimately the general public seeking health services. The preeminent position of science and technology at the end of World War II persisted in providing uninhibited and enthusiastic support of health-related research as described in the preceding chapter. The federal granting agencies supporting biomedical research were established on a relatively new and untried premise that most important issues for investigation could best be identified by the individual investigators through applications for grants awarded primarily on the basis of peer review of their scientific merit. The responsibility for problem identification, experimental specifications, data collection, fiscal accountability, analysis, reporting and dissemination of results was largely delegated to the individual investigator with superficial oversight by the institution in which the work was accomplished. The combination of rapidly escalating congressional appropriations for research coupled with grossly inadequate budgets for administration impelled agencies like the NIH to rely heavily on the scientific community who were riding on the crest of extremely great popularity.

New congressional initiatives, stimulated by a persuasive lay lobby, have launched some major changes in the organizational relationships and operational mechanisms of the main agencies supporting health-related research. Amendments in 1971 and 1974 to the enabling legislation that created the Cancer Institute initiated pervasive changes amounting to a major metamorphosis. The paramount importance of these is confirmed by Dr. Donald Fredrickson, Director of NIH, as follows:

A new state of transition now dominates the relationship between government and biomedical science. . . . It needs to be said. Having come into an inheritance of social responsibility it did not anticipate, *the old NIH is gone.* Its unparalleled growth, the relative privacy of its enterprise, and its solitary role in the federal support of the academic medical centers have become subjects for nostalgia. To the extent that this is true for the NIH, so is it true for biomedical science in general (1).

The implications of these statements are profound for the entire biomedical research enterprise. The underlying causes and consequences of the precipitous fall from public favor have stemmed from major misunderstandings and honest differences in perceptions between the public, representatives in government, and the biomedical community described in Chapter 1. The radical changes, which are currently manifest throughout the entire biomedical research effort, can be fully appreciated only by an awareness of the driving forces which impell them. It must be clear that the impetus toward forward planning, integration of research efforts, evaluation of research results, increased reliance on contracts as opposed to grants and many other signs are predictable responses to increasing clamor for greater control over science and technology in general.

CRISIS IN CREDIBILITY

The unbridled enthusiasm for science and technology as the wave of the future was dampened by a number of factors leading to growing demands for greater controls. The biomedical research community was caught up in a generalized "anti-science movement" that gathered force during the decade of the 1960s. There was a growing awareness both of the need for improved institutional control over funding and application of science and technology (1). The biomedical research enterprise was particularly sensitive to the mounting doubts and criticisms because of several related factors.

· Federal support of biomedical research had emerged suddenly without previous experience or tradition and had grown explosively without opportunity or provision for developing a sound administrative structure within the federal granting agencies.
· Lacking mechanisms or manpower to assume appropriate administrative accountability in disbursing public funds, a great deal of responsibility was delegated to the biomedical research community, including
    1. initiation of research projects,
    2. peer review of research grant applications,
    3. grant management and fiscal controls, and
    4. reporting results of research—mainly by publication in the scientific literature.
· Inevitable allegations were directed at loose management procedures, sup-

port of projects of questionable value, and inadequate monitoring of expenditures.

Notable progress in both research and health technologies failed to reach the exorbitant expectations which had been generated to develop and maintain widespread public support of this large national effort.

The vulnerability of the NIH was greatly increased with the loss of some of its strongest support on the death of Representative John Fogarty, the retirement of Senator Lister Hill, and the departure from Congress of Representative Melvin Laird to become Secretary of Defense. At the same time, Representative Fountain launched a new attack on NIH management. The undermining of congressional support was coincident with a series of changes in the administrative leadership in NIH and DHEW. Even the most sympathetic and powerful of proponents (such as President Lyndon Johnson) were heard to query whether too much energy was being spent on basic research and not enough on translating laboratory findings into tangible benefits for the American people. The same questions continue to plague the biomedical research community even into most recent times (see the Kennedy Hearings, ref. 2). At the heart of these doubts was the discrepancy between the high hopes of conquering cancer, curing heart disease, and controlling many other common diseases of the American people and visible progress toward these goals.

Undaunted by the growing skepticism regarding progress toward conquest of the great killers, the influential lay lobby became increasingly convinced that the firm foundation of basic knowledge had indeed been constructed and was now ready for launching massive attacks, particularly against cancer. The original Lasker lobby had been reinforced by medical scientists inside and outside of government. These advocates argued that conquest of the disease could be achieved by a bolder approach. A proposal by Mrs. Lasker led to the appointment of a special panel by the Senate Labor and Welfare Committee to advise the Senate on appropriate approaches to the cure of cancer. It was no accident that the panel was comprised of prominent and strong proponents of a greatly expanded attack on this dread disease. Obviously, cancer has no advocates and everyone is strongly opposed to it. However, the "lay lobby and some of its new friends decided that those in charge of NIH were not sufficiently against it and they said so" (3). Unfortunately, the underlying issues in this controversy have been seriously obscured by partisanship on all sides, and the final decision was a compromise that has had extremely significant repercussions in accelerating fundamental changes in policies and priorities at the NIH, which inevitably affect the entire biomedical research community.

PRESSURES FOR ACCELERATED PROGRESS

In the belief that the scientific conservatism of the NIH was retarding progress in cancer cures, the controversial proposal was made that the cancer program be organized as a separate agency reporting directly to the President.

The forces that molded and propelled the legislation were powerful. The discussions and presentations were highly polarized, emotional and biased (4). The proponents argued that the successes in cancer research had opened broad new vistas and promising opportunities for both understanding and controlling this dread disease. Honest differences of opinion concerning the validity of such assumptions were obscured by heightened controversy. The panel proposed legislation that would provide a separate and autonomous National Cancer Institute.

The leadership of both the NIH and the biomedical community were deeply concerned that splitting off the Cancer Institute from NIH might lead to progressive splintering of the Institutes of Health, endangering the future of the biomedical research enterprise.

The opposing views extended well beyond the political arena into the biomedical community, based on differences in perceptions of clinicians and basic medical scientists, along a historical pattern.

The controversy became so heated that the biomedical community came off the sidelines to a greater extent than ever before in applying pressures to retain the National Cancer Program within the NIH. The congressional representatives were confronted by a hotly contested issue involving strongly expressed divergence of views within the biomedical community regarding the wisdom of enlarging the attack on cancer and particularly with such preferential treatment as an autonomous Institute with direct channels of communication to the president.

The resolution of these divergent views took the form of a series of legislative acts that represent new and different approaches to the integration and planning of a National Cancer Program.

December 23, 1971. The National Cancer Act Amendments of 1971 enlarged the authorities of the National Cancer Institute and the National Institutes of Health in order to advance the national effort against cancer. The authority of the NCI Director was expanded, a National Cancer Advisory Board was established, and appropriations in excess of $400 million were authorized for 1972 with further increases in subsequent years.

July 23, 1974. The National Cancer Act Amendments authorized $2.565 billion over a three year period to extend and improve the National Cancer Program as well as $210 million over a three year period for cancer control programs. The Act also (1) established the President's Biomedical Research Panel to make a comprehensive investigation of federal biomedical and behavioral research, (2) extended the research contract authority, (3) provided that the Director of NIH be appointed by the President by and with the advice of the Senate, and (4) required peer review of ADAMHA grant applications and contract projects.

Major operational changes were introduced by these acts of Congress. To facilitate this process, the level of support for the National Cancer Program was increased four times between 1971 and 1976. The Director of the National Cancer Institute, with the advice of the National Cancer Advisory Board was instructed to "plan and develop an expanded, intensified, and coordinated cancer research program encompassing the programs of the National Cancer Institute, related programs of the other research institutes, and other federal and non-federal programs."

The mission of the National Cancer Program was extended beyond the relatively passive role of encouraging and responding to investigator-initiated projects. The new element was the need to engage in long range planning, identifying, defining, setting priorities, and integrating large-scale nationwide efforts directed at elucidating causes, exploring methods of management, and instituting demonstration centers for therapy on ambitious scales.

As a consequence, the National Cancer Program received a budget amounting to one third of the entire NIH research budget.

The lopsided distribution of the NIH budget among the various Institutes is indicated in Figure 2-1. The cancer budget towers over all other categories of human disease and disability as an indication of the extent to which it has attained topmost priority in this country. The NCI budget displays major shifts in the distribution of resources among the various components of the program.

The most significant change is the reduction in the spontaneous research grants as indicated by the black areas at the base of the NCI column in Figure 2-1. Less than 25% of the NCI budget is devoted to traditional grants of which less than half are competitive. This is a very much smaller proportion of the budget in support of investigator initiated proposals which loom relatively large in the budgets of all the other Institutes. The research grant proposals are increasingly channeled into areas of research designated by staff as having high priorities by a continuing distribution of announcements or requests for applications (RFAs) to laboratories indicating interest and competence. The combined effects of these policies and approaches has largely replaced the investigator initiatives by programmatic priorities originating with the National Cancer Program. Specifically, the budgetary provision for management, for construction, for cancer control, and for intramural research are largely under direct control of the NCI staff. The greatly expanded budgets for contracts provide a basis for a greatly increased number of projects with well-defined objectives, experimental methods, performance criteria, and overview. The special programs and centers also tend to represent the plans and perspectives of the NCI administration and its program plan. The scientific community is not excluded from the process of identifying important areas and arriving at priorities, but their role is substantially different than was true during the early days of the NIH.

The reliance on research grants remains quite prominent among the other Institutes of Health, as represented by the proportion of their budgets in Figure 2-1. Budget allocations for contracts are prominent in NCI and NHLBI. They are more prominent in all the Institutes than before 1970. The National Cancer Institute appears to represent a generously funded prototype engaged in exploring new mechanisms by which biomedical research

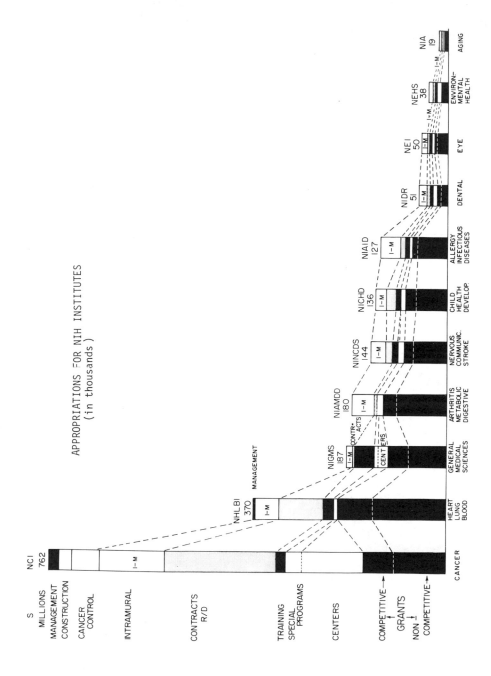

Figure 2-1. The size and distribution of the budgets of the Institutes of Health are illustrated for the year 1976. Reflecting the National Cancer Act Amendment (1974) the NCI budget is approximately one-third of the total NIH research budget and is largely Institute-initiated (data from FASEB Newsletter 9:2, 1976).

can be directed toward selected targets with improved integration of efforts and with greater accountability.

Congressional views of the importance of enhanced accountability are clearly reflected in many pronouncements. A representative example appeared in the Report on Appropriations (DHEW report #92–892, June 21, 1972) as follows:

> This Committee is equally concerned with the results that might be achieved from the investment of tax dollars at a time when greater accountability is somewhat overdue. . . . This Committee is convinced that the time has come when the health research resources of our nation must be better organized and address themselves to the problems at hand in a more systematic manner. . . . Greater accountability is possible in the field of health, and the Committee will expect all of the NIH to formulate 'blueprints' or health research strategies that will take into account the above factors.

THE NATIONAL CANCER PROGRAM: PROTOTYPE
FOR PLANNING

The National Cancer Act (Section 410b) has specifically called for annual reports of progress, as follows:

> The Director of the NCI shall, as soon as practicable after the end of each calendar year, prepare in consultation with the National Cancer Advisory Board and submit to the President for transmittal to the Congress, a report on the activities, progress, and accomplishments under the National Cancer Program during the preceding calendar year, and the plan for the Program during the next five years.

It was felt that this "rolling plan" mechanism would allow the National Cancer Institute, the president, and the Congress to take advantage of new opportunities as they arise. The National Cancer Program serves as a prototype for all the other Institutes for long-range planning of their programs. The rather generous budgets have made it possible for this challenging problem to be addressed with adequate resources. A staff of more than 20 people has been engaged in the development of plans and strategies for the National Cancer Institute on a continuing basis through annual updating.

FORWARD PLANNING AT THE NATIONAL CANCER
INSTITUTE: PROCESSES AND PROCEDURES

The National Cancer Institute, with participation by nonfederal scientists, has engaged in the development of a coordinated program in specified areas of cancer research (5). Current effort is based on previous experience with the special virus-cancer program and the chemotherapy program, which have been underway for many years. The aims of the plan can be paraphrased as follows:

- To represent to the public and Congress the relevance of various aspects of cancer research to practical objectives of prevention and treatment of cancer in man.
- To incorporate in a single framework *all* conceivable approaches to the attainment of these objectives in a way which is meaningful to laymen and acceptable to scientists.
- To respond to the mandates specified by Congress in cancer legislation.

The prime requirement was for a stable framework for cancer research that would be useful over extended periods despite the constantly changing progress and pressures affecting scientific biomedical disciplines. Seven major cancer objectives were defined (6a). They are summarized as follows:

1. Reduce the effects of external agents in producing cancers (i.e., carcinogens in the environment).
2. Modify individuals to decrease the likelihood of cancer development.
3. Prevent the conversion of normal cells into cells capable of forming cancers.
4. Prevent tumor establishment in cells already capable of forming cancers.
5. Assess accurately (*1*) the risk of developing cancer in groups and individuals and (*2*) the presence, extent, and probable course of existing cancers.
6. Cure as many patients as possible and maintain maximum control of the disease in patients not cured.
7. Restore patients with defects resulting from the disease and treatment to as nearly normal a functioning state as possible.

Objectives 1 through 4 are concerned principally with prevention, objective 5 with detection, diagnosis, and prognosis, objective 6 deals with treatment, and objective 7 deals with rehabilitation. This ambitious cyclical attack on the overall problem of cancer is graphically represented in Figure 2-2. The program is divided into two main sections, the research thrust in the hemicircle above and the control interventions in the hemicircle below. Seven major cancer objectives are listed for each of these two major thrusts under R1–R7 and C1–C8 (6c).

DEVELOPMENT OF THE NATIONAL CANCER PROGRAM PLANS

Since a national plan of such magnitude had never been developed previously a hierarchy of plans was devised to cover three major levels of program activities and is presented in three substantial volumes (6a, b, c).

The *strategic plan* took the form of recommendations for both research and control based on extensive advice and guidance from many different sources prepared biennially (6a).

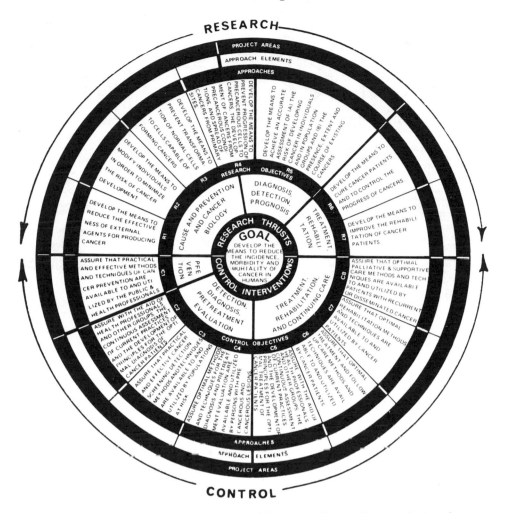

Figure 2-2. The strategy for planning the National Cancer Program is based on a hierarchy of components. Four research goals and seven research approaches are identified and specified in the compartments occupying the upper hemicircle. In accordance with recent planning efforts, the objectives oriented toward control of cancer have also developed and are displayed in the lower half of the figure. The hierarchies implied by this organizational concept are employed for refining objectives and pursuing strategies in an ongoing planning effort (6).

The *operational plan* (6b) contains descriptions of policies and procedures for initiating and managing the various components of the research and control components of the strategic plan, with five year projections for research, control, and support programs (updated annually).

Individual program plans consist of detailed proposals for the conduct of the many individual projects and programs (Fig. 2–3).

The national strategic plan includes both the program and implementation strategies in general terms. The Operational Plan includes the mechanisms for implementing the program and the management policies and procedures. The

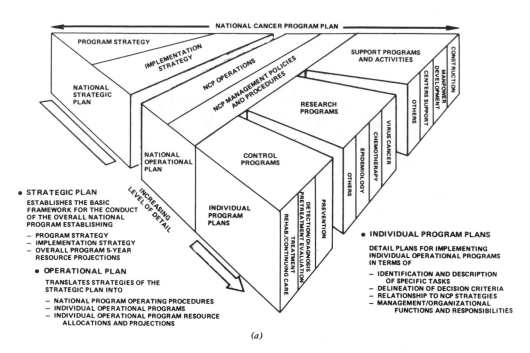

(a)

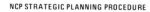

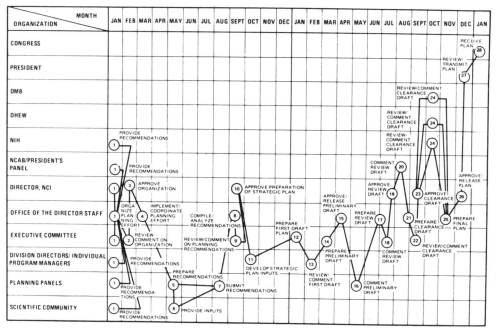

(b)

Figure 2-3. (a) Forward planning for the National Cancer Program involves a hierarchy of plans beginning with a large-scale strategic plan incorporating both programs and implementation strategies. With increasing levels of detail, the operational mechanisms and management procedures are elaborated. Finally, individual program plans for control, research, and support activities are developed. (b) The process of arriving at the various program plans is complex and comprehensive, involving input from a wide variety of sources, in government and in the scientific community. Recommendations and strategic plans are refined by iteration and then progress through channels. This process as illustrated occupies about two years (6).

Individual Program Plans are indicated under three headings, namely the support programs and activities, the research programs, and the control programs. The rather elaborate process by which the strategic plans are developed is indicated in Figure 2–3B. At the outset, input was sought from a wide spectrum of sources from within NIH, from advisory panels, and from the scientific community at large.

PARTICIPATION BY THE SCIENTIFIC COMMUNITY

The need for participation and endorsement by the nonfederal scientists was recognized from the beginning. At all stages, advice and guidance were sought from broad representation of the scientific community in the formulation of the national plan. Planning sessions were conducted in two phases. Phase one was concerned with the development of broad approaches to the attainment of each of the seven research objectives listed above. Phase two was concerned with the development of more detailed definitions of the various types of research needed for progress along each approach channel.

A broad and representative cross section of the scientific community was attained by developing a list of more than 1,000 names of prominent scientists and experts in the field. In addition, an extensive roster of expert consultants to NIH, the Director of NCI, and the National Advisory Cancer Council, plus 15 biomedical, professional, and volunteer societies were canvassed. Ultimately, 250 scientists and physician investigators participated in a national planning effort in a series of 40 planning sessions. The NCI "deliberately played a low-key role," so that the resulting plan would represent the work of the total scientific community and not just the NCI staff. More detailed planning was carried out by 39 members of the scientific community that developed the seven program objectives and 35 research approaches, with interrelationships between them. These reports served as the basic input to the planning sessions in phase two.

In addition to the development of specific research recommendations, the participants in phase two were asked to supply information regarding the present status of the research problems covered, the type of information required for future progress, the relative priority of the proposed research, estimates of probability of success, estimates of potential impact of research on the objectives, estimated duration of the proposed research, and estimates of the resource requirements. This information was compiled in 33 reports (one for each approach). Based upon this comprehensive initial effort, operational Forward Plans have been developed annually (6a,6c).

THE NCI PROGRAM STRUCTURE

The major research thrusts of the National Cancer Program are:

· Cause and prevention
· Detection and diagnosis

- Treatment and rehabilitation
- Cancer biology

Distribution of resources for research programs are indicated for the seven designated research objectives as illustrated in Figure 2-4.

External Causative Agents. Epidemiological studies have indicated the importance of environmental exposures to chemical agents in the development of cancer in various anatomical locations. (For additional details see Figures 4-3 and 4-4, Chapter 4.) The contribution of such carcinogens has been estimated variously up to 80% by some investigators (7). This area of endeavor has been most attractive because of a common belief that most carcinogens are man-made and therefore may be subject to control or elimination by regulations. It has proved to be much easier to collect data on carcinogenic properties of chemicals than to decide what to do next. The exploration of chemical carcinogens remains an extremely prominent component of the overall search for elucidation of the causes of cancer.

INDIVIDUAL PROGRAM DISTRIBUTION SUMMARY

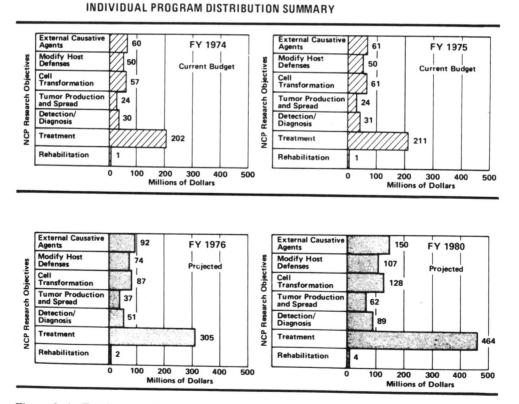

Figure 2-4. Fundamental investigations into carcinogenesis and mechanisms of spread are encompassed in the top four categories. The distribution of resources for FY 1974–1980 is heavily oriented toward treatment as the largest single item. The large appropriations for diagnostic, therapeutic, and rehabilitation programs are responsive to public demands for relevance (6b).

Modify Host Defenses. The likelihood of developing cancer is believed to be influenced by individual genetic inheritance and also the effectiveness with which the body's defense reactions can contain or control cellular proliferation. The nature and extent of immune reactions as protective mechanisms against developing cancer and containing its spread has created a great deal of interest in cancer circles.

Cell Transformation. The factors which lead to uncontrolled cell division are of undoubted importance in carcinogenesis. Many different cells in the body divide under normal circumstances and never give evidence of entering into excessive proliferation. The factors which precipitate abnormal cell division or interfere with maturation and specialization of cells are of fundamental biological importance in this context (see also Fig. 4-4).

Tumor Production and Spread. The factors which influence the growth of tumors and their tendency to spread and metastasize involve many diverse considerations such as the size, location, and complications produced by mechanical impingement. Growing tumors must be able to stimulate the elaboration of expanded blood supply to nourish the rapidly growing cells. The tendency to invade surrounding tissues may be dependent on the ability of the growing tumor to overcome its resistance to spread (Fig. 4–4c).

Detection/Diagnosis. The early recognition of cancer is regarded as an essential requirement to effective treatment, particularly in those types which are prone to rapid growth and spread.

Treatment. During the past three decades, available therapeutic procedures have greatly expanded in several directions. The traditional approaches of surgery and radiation have been supplemented by various forms of chemotherapy. Obviously, definitive therapy of high effectiveness has evolved for only a small fraction of cancer patients (such as leukemia and Hodgkin's disease), and concern has recently surfaced regarding recurrence of these many years later. There is also justified concern that radiation therapy may be carcinogenic. The very large and rapidly growing portion of the budget which is devoted or proposed for treatment is impressive in view of the relatively unsatisfactory state of current therapeutic modalities. There are some who believe that cancer therapy not only prolongs living but also prolongs dying. The allocation for rehabilitation appears to be extremely conservative from that point of view.

Potential Complication: The Rich Get Richer. The preeminent position of cancer as the prime target for NIH research is inherently strengthened by a generous budget, which can accommodate a very large planning effort. The resources expended for planning take the form of extensive documentation in several volumes containing masses of data and new and intriguing avenues of research. This kind of material is obviously more impressive to the decision makers in executive and legislative branches of government than the relatively limited efforts that can be generated by the other, less affluent

Institutes. This is inherently a process by which the "rich get richer and the poor get poorer."

RATIONALIZING RESEARCH SUPPORT: THE NEW DIMENSIONS

The conduct of research is essentially an exploration of the unknown or at least the examination of uncertainties. Such activities do not lend themselves to planning or logical sequencing of the sort commonly employed in the solution of technical problems. Charting courses toward unknown destinations is fraught with uncertainty. Even more challenging is the development of a reasonable and responsible program of research and development directed at mechanisms for curing or controlling disease or disability. The National Cancer Program summarized above is clearly responsive to the intent of Congress as implied by the relevant cancer legislation. It has the effect of assigning the responsibility for programmatic development to the National Cancer Institute. Reliance on input from the scientific community is retained but the accountability is clearly shifted from investigators and their support institutions to the federal agency. The process of long range planning necessarily involves much more detailed specification of the targets and the mechanisms for approaching them. It is possible to identify a series of steps progressing from general to specific which can be anticipated in the process of developing and pursuing research. For purposes of present discussion, some important levels in this hierarchy are briefly defined in Table 2-1. These terms do not conform to any official document or definition and are presented here merely to indicate the sense in which the terms will be employed in the remainder of this publication.

KEY COMPONENTS OF PROGRAMMATIC PLANNING OF RESEARCH

The enabling legislation that authorizes the formation of an agency or arm of government contains statements of *aims* which are generalized indicators of the "intent of Congress" regarding the *mission* of the organization. The statements of aims are frequently vague enough to encourage the development of a consensus in the legislative arena. For example, the enabling legislation establishes their missions as supporting research and training for the purpose of elucidating, recognizing, curing, and controlling the category of disease(s) specified in the name. (The programs developed by the various Institutes were initially oriented toward strong programs of basic research, which was not strictly in accordance with the "intent of Congress.")

The *objectives* are represented by targets that are much more specific than the stated goals. These shorter range *objectives* are attacked in accordance with *priorities*, preferably assigned in accordance with clearly established criteria.

TABLE 2-1. Essential Ingredients for Rationalizing Research Support (brief definitions for present purposes)

AIMS
Stated reasons for developing the various governmental agencies in very broad terms.

MISSION
The designated role or function of agencies based upon the interpretation of the wording of the enabling legislation.

GOALS
The general aspirations of groups or agencies are developed to indicate the long range results toward which the efforts will be directed.

POLICIES
The operational guidelines to be employed in efforts to attain the goals, expressed as policies.

OBJECTIVES
Specific targets which are believed to be attainable within the constraints or time available, selected in accordance with priorities.

PRIORITIES
The rank ordering of targets in accordance with stated or operational criteria for the distribution of resources, effort, and time.

STRATEGIES
The mechanisms by which agencies or investigators approach or attack the specific targets or objectives.

PROPOSALS
The plans, programs, or research designs which specify the means by which objectives are to be attained.

EVALUATION MECHANISM
Processes by which the effectiveness and relevance of research accomplishments can be judged.

ASSESSMENT
Appraisal of the outcome(s) of research efforts and of the consequences of success (preferably quantitatively).

The methods and procedures employed in the attack on research problems are commonly regarded as *strategies* that lead to the development of specific *proposals* containing plans, research designs, and supporting data.

Evaluation mechanisms have received increased emphasis as an essential component of research and development, particularly for projects that are supported by research grants. The traditional approach to evaluation of the outcome of research supported by grants has been generally permissive.

The extent to which the research enterprises of the NIH were progressing toward the goals of the Institutes could not be accurately assessed from the records maintained in the Bethesda headquarters. As a result, the annual testimony by the administrative scientific leaders before Congressional committees was characteristically vague when they were asked to demonstrate progress or to distinguish between the basic and applied research efforts. This problem is considered in more detail in Chapter 3.

The impacts of the forward-planning programs on the various Institutes and other governmental agencies are having profound effects on the biomedical research enterprise of this country. The individual Institutes are adapting to this new era of Institute initiatives by circulating requests for applications

(RFAs) to appropriate laboratories, by increasing their commitment of funds to contracts and by developing special centers for specific research, development, and diffusion of techniques and technologies. These alterations in both philosophy and operational mechanisms are natural consequences of growing pressures for greater governmental accountability.

ORGANIZATIONAL OBSTACLES TO RATIONAL FORWARD PLANNING

Long-range planning was not a recognized need during the period of rapid growth when the research targets were plentiful and each experiment elicited more questions than were answered. Priorities were not an issue while appropriations regularly exceeded the budget request from the various agencies (see Fig. 1-6). Slowing of growth rates and leveling of budget allocations has imposed more stringent requirements for evaluating current status, developing priorities, and looking farther into the future.

Forward planning of research and development is extremely difficult at best. Without definitive data and understanding of the current status of the enterprise, the process is replete with frustrating obstacles. Implementation is difficult when programs must be inserted into inconsistent or cumbersome organizational relationships. In retrospect, there were many things that might have been done better to avoid some immediate problems. The participants in this drama were all dedicated and conscientiously attempting to create a whole new enterprise by attempting to divert a growing flood of project proposals into an incongruous organizational framework developed by incremental additions of Institutes in response to political and public pressures.

During the postwar expansion of NIH, the successive addition of Institutes was a natural response to the popular and political concerns regarding the most prevalent of the dread diseases. The orchestrated public fears of cancer and heart disease placed them at the top of the national priority list. Subsequently, interest in other forms of disease and disability emerged and were incorporated into these or additional Institutes. The incremental addition of components in the NIH reflected continuously shifting pressures converging on different targets from different directions. Unfortunately, these additions were adopted in rather rapid succession with great enthusiasm and without a clearly defined organizational framework into which the new additions could be inserted to provide internal consistency. The current organizational format of the NIH has significant deficiencies to be considered below. They stem from the three stages of progression summarized in Chapter 1. The mobilization phase was a period of extremely rapid and unbridled growth with Institutes being added both individually and in groups (see Table 1-2). These incremental additions made it possible to accommodate a wide variety of new opportunities but inevitably led to overlapping efforts due to poorly defined areas of responsibility.

CATEGORIES OF INSTITUTES IN NIH

No specific organizational framework had been conceived when the first two categorical Institutes were established to focus on cancer (a disease) and the heart (an organ), respectively.

Each of these Institutes set about developing programs directed at their designated targets. The subsequent additions were Institutes oriented toward the organs such as teeth, nervous system, and eye, or to other diseases such as arthritis, metabolic disease, infectious disease, etc. Even more general categories were represented by child health and human development or general medical sciences.

The nature of the problem is amply illustrated by a few examples. A research project directed at the "role of streptococci in the development of rheumatic heart disease in children" could be logically encompassed under infectious disease (NIAID), heart disease (NHI) or childhood disease (NICHD). Similarly, any program oriented toward the elucidation of the relationships between diseases, organ systems, environmental influences affecting different age groups could be reasonably incorporated into the programs of several of the Institutes. Since each of the Institutes undertook to develop expansive programs broadly representing the categorical designations, their different "territories" exhibit an extremely high degree of overlap. For such reasons, the Division of Research Grants was established to receive all the grant applications from investigators and to distribute them for study section review and Institute support on rather arbitrary grounds. This complicating feature could have been avoided to some degree by the development of an organizational framework specifically designed to accommodate projects in terms of anatomical components, disease entities, age, or environmental considerations, but not all simultaneously. The Institutes of Health can be classified for convenience into three different categories (Table 2-2).

Dr. James Shannon (8) rationalized the categorical support structure of NIH on the basis of two rather simple propositions:

· No simple discipline-oriented structure could be identified around which the full spectrum of biomedical research could be organized. A unique and universal classification of research along the lines of traditional academic disciplines was regarded as unattainable.
· Diseases could be grouped around medical and surgical specialties. Each group could serve as the focus for a research strategy, with common sharing of relevant fundamental research. Applied and developmental programs could emerge as opportunities arose. "This could have the added advantage of being socially understandable and still amenable to balancing scientific opportunity with perceived societal needs" (8).

It was obviously expedient to take appropriate advantage of demonstrated public interest. Incremental additions provided an enormous flexibility during exuberant growth in the mobilization phase when there was little need to justify the research efforts to either the public or their representatives in government.

TABLE 2-2. Three Categories of Institutes

Disease or Cause-Oriented Institutes:
  Cancer (NCI)
  Arthritis, Metabolic and Digestive Diseases (NIAMDD)
  Allergy and Infectious Diseases

Organ-Oriented Institutes:
  Heart, Lung, and Blood (NHLBI)
  Dental (NIDR)
  Neurology, Communicative Disorders, and Stroke (NINCDS)
  Eye (NEI)

Combined Categories:
  General Medical Sciences (NIGMS)
  Child Health and Human Development (NICHHD)
  Aging (NIA)
  Environmental Health Sciences (NIEHS)

Disease-oriented Institutes of Health deal with identifiable pathological processes, notably cancer (NCI), arthritis, and metabolic and digestive disease, (NIAMDD), allergies and infectious disease (NAIAID). The mandate of each Institute encompasses most or all organs of the body. Organ-system orientation is exemplified by the Heart, Lung, and Blood Institute (NHLBI), Dental Research (NIDR), Eye (NEI), and Neurology, Communicative Disorders, and Stroke (NINCDS). Conglomerate or combined categories encompass a diversity of broad areas. For example, the Institute of General Medical Sciences was originally intended to cover basic research efforts that were common to several Institutes or not readily identified with any one. Child Health and Human Development (NICHHD), and the newly developed Institute on Aging (NIA) are age-dependent designations. The Institute of Environmental Health Sciences deals with noninfectious hazards to health through factors or chemical substances in air, water, food, and other contacts at home, at work, or during other activities. Alcohol, drug abuse, and mental health are self-explanatory, broad in concept, and extend beyond traditional medical concerns into psychosocial and even socioeconomic considerations.

Three-Dimensional View of NIH. The eleven Institutes currently comprising the NIH can be illustrated by means of a three-dimensional model (Fig. 2-5). For this purpose, organ-oriented Institutes (NHLB, NINCCDS, NEI, and NIDR) are displayed on a vertical axis. The disease-oriented Institutes, listed on a horizontal axis, are concerned with the causes and manifestations of pathological processes. NIAMDD contains a mixture. The combined categories are assembled along the third dimension representing the age-oriented (NICHHD, NIA) and nonspecific categories (NIGMS, NIEH). Other related agencies are omitted ADAMHA, Center for Health Services Research, and so on. For present purposes, consider only the problem of a three dimensional organization in NIH illustrated in Figure 2-6.

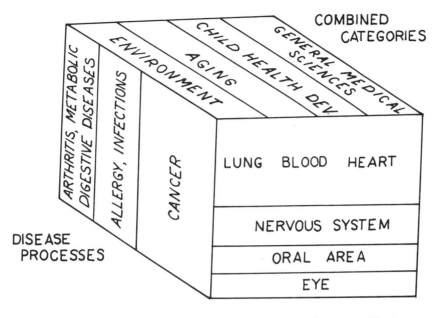

Figure 2-5. Disease-oriented, organ system-oriented, and composite Institutes of Health are presented schematically on the faces of a cube to illustrate the fact that their areas of responsibility are broadly overlapping and not clearly defined. As a consequence, the various Institutes tend to incorporate many common elements in their programs and investigator-initiated projects could be channeled to more than one and often to several different Institutes for review and funding. These uncertainties represent organizational obstacles to forward planning.

The operational significance of this odd organizational format is indicated by the problem repeatedly faced in allocation of resources. Each of the Institutes derives a budget from the Congressional appropriation and proceeds to allocate the total among the several components under its jurisdiction. A substantial majority of research objectives can and are being addressed by several Institutes in both intramural programs and extramural grants and contracts. Specifically, disease entities, such as cancer, infections, metabolic diseases, and environmental exposures have an impact on most organ systems and age groups. Similarly, the various organ systems are susceptible to the various disease processes at all ages to varying degrees. The basic science endeavors—immunology, virology, microbiology, genetics, physiology, pathology,—are relevant to all diseases, all organ systems, and all ages. As a consequence, consistent and rational approaches to priorities and resource allocation are beset by organizational obstacles of extreme complexity.

The categorical organization of NIH has not been spared criticism. A "mixed bag of arguments" against the present categorical structure of NIH was acknowledged by Dr. James Shannon, who remained convinced that

DEPARTMENT OF HEALTH, EDUCATION, AND WELFARE
Public Health Service

| National Institutes of Health | Health Services Admin. | Health Resources Admin. | Center for Disease Control | Food and Drug Admin. | Alcohol, Drug Abuse Mental Health Administration (ADAMHA) |

3 NIH BUREAUS: National Cancer Institute | National Heart, Lung, Blood Institute | National Library of Medicine

9 OTHER INSTITUTES: NIDR (Dental) | NIGMS Gen. Med. Science | NINCDS Neurol. Commun. | NICHHD Child Health | NIAID Infect. Dis. | NEI Eye | NIEH Environ. Health | NIA Aging

APPROPRIATIONS (FY 1976, expected 1977)

NATIONAL INSTITUTES OF HEALTH			ALCOHOL, DRUG ABUSE, MENTAL HEALTH ADMINISTRATION		
Activity	FY 1976	Coalition 77		FY 1976	Coalition 77
Cancer	762.6	793.9	NIMH (Mental Health)		
Heart, Lung, Blood	370.3	403.0	Research	92.9	105.0
Dental	51.4	55.5	Training	85.1	112.0
Arthritis, Digestive	179.8	212.6	Rape Prevention	3.0	5.0
Neurological, Communicative	144.7	159.0	Community Mental Health Centers		
Allergy	127.2	147.7	Initial Operations	24.0	36.0
General Medical Sciences	187.4	210.0	Planning	1.5	1.5
Child Health	136.6	147.5	Consultation & Education	4.0	14.0
Aging	19.4	27.4	Continuation (old law)	162.2	150.0
Eye	50.3	54.4	Continuation (new law)	--	--
Environmental Health Sciences	37.8	52.7	Conversion	20.0	20.0
Research Resources	130.3	137.0	Facilities	0	5.0
Fogarty Center	5.7	8.0	Financial distress	4.0	15.0
Library	29.2	35.5	NIDA (Drug Abuse)		
Buildings and Facilities	54.0	65.0	Research	34.0	37.4
Director's Office	15.3	16.5	Training	10.0	11.0
			Community Programs	174.1	205.0
TOTAL, NIH	2,302.1	2,525.7	NIAAA (Alcoholism)		
			Research	11.8	20.0
			Training	7.5	11.0
			Community Programs	12.9	175.0
			TOTAL, ADAMHA	702.4	989.3

Figure 2-6. the components of the Department of Health, Education and Welfare with major responsibilities for health-related research are illustrated in an organizational framework. The National Institutes of Health encompass three bureaus, nine Institutes, and several support functions. The budgetary allocations for these components are indicated bottom left. The Alcohol, Drug Abuse, Mental Health Administration is being endowed with increased responsibility for research and the budget for this component is presented (lower right).

little would be accomplished now by efforts at simplifying the internal structure (8). The broadly overlapping areas of responsibility among the Institutes made widespread duplication of effort almost a certainty and greatly complicated the ability of the Institutes to respond in satisfactory manner to demands for detailed justification leveled at them by unsympathetic critics. The ambiguity of the organizational relationships undoubtedly contributed to the difficulties of responding convincingly to charges of loose management practices by the Fountain Committee. The long-range planning required during the present stage of transition is most certainly complicated by gross uncertainties regarding the territory covered by each of the Institutes of NIH.

ORGANIZATIONAL FRAMEWORK OF THE NATIONAL INSTITUTES OF HEALTH

The current organizational framework of NIH is indicated in relation to other components of the Department of Health, Education and Welfare in Figure 2-6. The Assistant Secretary for Health in DHEW has responsibility for six health-related components—specifically, the NIH, Health Services, and Health Resources Administrations, the Center for Disease Control, Food and Drug Administration, and the Alcohol, Drug Abuse, and Mental Health Administration (ADAMHA). The NIH and ADAMHA are positioned at opposite ends of the chart for conveniently presenting the relative magnitude of the budgetary allocations for years 1976 and 1977, respectively. The National Cancer Institute and the National Heart, Lung, and Blood Institute have been designated as bureaus, reflecting their great size and scope. The National Library of Medicine is also classified as a bureau, presumably because of its unique responsibility for accumulation, storage, and retrieval of masses of information from all sources.

The nine other Institutes of Health are substantially smaller than NCI and NHLBI and represent a diverse mixture of problem areas. In addition, the NIH encompasses six research and service divisions concerned with processing research grants, provision of research resources, computer applications, vital statistics, and many other essential elements. The Alcohol, Drug Abuse, Mental Health Administration is also an assembly of categorical Institutes dealing with the three main elements in a broad program of psychosocial concerns, mental health, drug abuse, and alcoholism.

The budget for ADAMHA is expanding as suggested by the proposed jump from $700 million to nearly $1 billion as the bottom line in Figure 2-7. The original programs were directed toward the management of problems of alcohol, drug abuse, and mental health. More recently, the importance of engaging in research in these areas has been recognized and emphasized. The past few years have witnessed a growing commitment to research in behavioral and social sciences, not only in ADAMHA but in virtually all of the Institutes of Health.

The organization of NIH and related agencies is being complicated by current trends toward the inclusion of "soft sciences" as integral parts of health-related research. The modern definition of health and health care has extended beyond considerations of sickness of physical disability to include the ability of each person to function as effectively as possible within the social and cultural environs in which he lives. There is general recognition that a wide variety of external factors can produce signs and symptoms similar to those from organic disease. The stresses of modern living are suspected of being centrally involved in many of the most prevalent health problems. Environmental, cultural, and social stresses are now believed to contribute to poor health, disease, and disability.

FORWARD PLANNING PROCESS:
NIH DIRECTORATE

Dr. Donald Fredrickson, Director, National Institutes of Health, has instituted "forward-planning" sessions with the personnel of each Institute as a part of the budgetary process (9). These sessions are designed to contribute to the development and justification of the next year's budget. The assembled staff of each Institute is invited to specify projects and

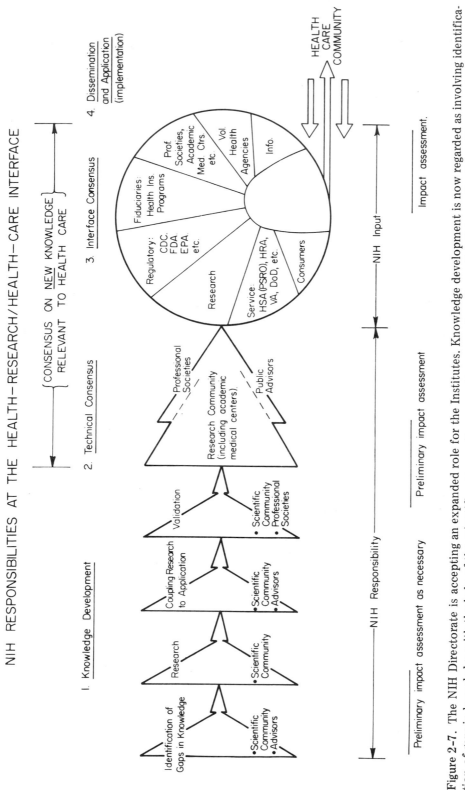

Figure 2-7. The NIH Directorate is accepting an expanded role for the Institutes. Knowledge development is now regarded as involving identification of gaps in knowledge with the help of the scientific community, supporting research and coupling it to applications. Consensus in the research community is now regarded as a step of importance in determining the relevance of *new* knowledge to health care (10).

programs they identify as having highest priorities, with justification for their choices. The bases for their priorities are explored by considering the relationships between opportunities and need. By the end of these discussions, the Director of NIH and his staff have achieved better personal understanding of the objectives of each Institute and are therefore much better prepared to present and defend them.

With this information in hand, the budgets of each Institute can be carefully considered in relation to the overall NIH budget. The individual Institutes have the immediate responsibility of developing consensus and appropriate mechanisms for identifying gaps in knowledge, scientific opportunities, outcome, and diffusion of the information to the biomedical community. The new look at NIH involves much greater institutional initiative in encouraging increased research activity in directions deemed crucial for future progress on the basis of forward planning processes.

EXPEDITING APPLICATIONS OF NEW KNOWLEDGE

The administration of NIH has responded to the requirements for increased responsibility for the effects of research on the quality and cost of health care. Specific proposals were advanced in a working document issued by the Office of the Director, NIH, February 28, 1977 on the Responsibilities of NIH at the Health Research/Health Care Interface (10). The NIH leadership has accepted the responsibility for improved processing of information so that "clinically applicable" information is:

· Systematically identified
· Validated for efficacy and safety
· Assessed (where appropriate) for cost
· Distributed to the health care community in useful and accessable form

Specific approaches to the problem included the identification of opportunities, gaps, and lags in research applicable to health and disease problems. Developing stronger information base in response to these needs, relating the new knowledge to existing concepts, coupling research to application, and validating research results in terms of safety, usefulness, and relative effectiveness (see Fig. 2-7).

Technical consensus is proposed as a process for evaluating the suitability of a given intervention for introduction into practice. Increased involvement in clinical trials to accomplish these ends is specifically implied. Improved mechanisms for diffusion of information in the community of practicing physicians are also proposed. Thus, the process of accelerating the transformation of basic knowledge and concepts into tangible health benefits is exemplified by the establishment of a new Office of Medical Applications of Research in the Office of the Director of National Institute of Health.

Office of Medical Applications of Research, National Institute of Health. Dr. Seymour Perry assumed direction of this new office as a response to mounting pressures from the public, expressed by their representatives in Congress. The growing need for such a function was expressed by the NIH Director as follows:

> It seems clear that in the future, the NIH and the rest of the scientific community must assume greater responsibility for the effect of research on the quality and cost of health care. The need for assuring effective transfer of useful new knowledge across the "interface" between biomedical research and the health care community and systems is a major issue (Testimony before the Health Subcommittee, Senate Labor and Public Welfare, June 17, 1976).

A process was described in a directive of February 1977 for systematic identification and evaluation of clinically relevant research information and its effective transfer to the health care community (Fig. 2-7). The identification and validation of appropriate knowledge for clinical applications to disease prevention, detection, diagnosis, treatment, and rehabilitation can be attained by the development of "technical consensus." Each Institute director is charged with responsibility to design credible identification/validation/consensus-seeking processes to meet the needs of the particular research areas with appropriate expert advice. The numerous and obvious sources of advisory competence would be used in various combinations to address the individual topical areas. They would be supplemented by lay-professional groups, general and specialized organizations such as American Cancer Society, American Heart Association, or Cystic Fibrosis Foundation.

The implications of this effort are extremely broad. It provides a visible mechanism by which relevant new knowledge can be more swiftly brought to bear on the practice of medicine. In the past, the accumulating mass of medical research output has been dispersed to the scientific community through scientific journals and meetings mainly from the initiative of the scientific invetigators. New technologies need to be evaluated at early stages of application to avoid premature adoption of inadequately tested techniques by an excessively enthusiastic clinical community. The Office of Medical Applications of Technologies coordinates and facilitates orderly transfer of innovations to practice when they are adequately developed and assessed.

Forward planning implies a need for clearly defined goals, objectives, and priorities to arrive at rational distribution of resources. By what criteria should priorities be established for programs that could be added or expanded equally well in two, several, or even all the various Institutes? Equitable and scientifically sound distribution of research resources among such tightly interwoven areas of responsibility would require both clear policies and guidelines and extremely effective internal integration within and among the individual Institutes involved. With each Institute naturally inclined to protect its turf and expand its areas of responsibility, such dilemmas are vulnerable to resolution on the basis of political considerations or arbitrary decisions.

FORWARD-PLANNING PROGRAMS IN THE
INDIVIDUAL INSTITUTES OF HEALTH

Program Planning and Evaluation offices have been established in each of the 11 Institutes of Health and the National Library of Medicine, the Division of Research Resources, the Division of Research Grants and other components of the institution. Representatives are responsible for the development of forward looking plans, either as a full-time responsibility or as a portion of an overall administrative responsibility. The magnitude of the planning effort is clearly dependent upon the size of the Institute as it affects the resources available for the planning effort. None of the other Institutes is able to mount a program as well endowed as that of the Cancer Institute.

The forward-planning efforts being conducted by the individual Institutes elicit from a wide variety of advisory sources timely topics for research each year. In order to respond to the options and priorities that are presented in this manner, increasing proportions of the budgets of the various Institutes are being devoted to Institute-initiated research projects.

A variety of different mechanisms are employed. For example, specific requests for grant applications are now being distributed to appropriate laboratories as a means of indicating to the scientific community the areas that are being particularly emphasized by the individual Institutes. For this purpose, the laboratories having particular expertise in these areas are being identified and invited to submit to the Institute their research capabilities. The biomedical investigators who are specifically involved in research having particular interest to the various Institutes are now being alerted to the availability of funding for identified topical areas. By this means, the ongoing evaluation of the unmet needs for research are being satisfied through mechanisms which are developed by the staff of each Institute. These may take the form of individual research projects. On the other hand, some Institutes are sponsoring the development of major centers for research and development strategically located within prestigious academic institutions across the country.

FORWARD-PLANNING PRIORITIES IN
"DISEASE-ORIENTED" INSTITUTES

Biomedical research programs have become highly dependent on continuing grant and contract support in order to sustain scientific progress and the integrity of their laboratories. Successful competition for grants and contracts implies a need for investigators to be aware continuously of the current policies and future trends in priorities of the various granting agencies. The best indications of future priorities are to be found in the forward plans being generated and updated by each Institute. To provide some specific examples, key elements have been selected from recent forward plans and other releases from the individual Institutes. The following summary will not do justice to the overall programs of these organizations, but will bring into sharper focus the major mechanisms by which investigators could gain insight into areas of involvement and responsibilities sponsored by the different institutions.

NATIONAL CANCER PROGRAM

The magnitude, forward-planning program, and major directions of the National Cancer Program were discussed in the preceding paragraphs. This is by far the largest and most comprehensive research effort being supported within DHEW. The size and scope of the program are so great that virtually all other health related research efforts are affected by the existence of this ambitious program. By virtue of the inherent overlap in areas of responsibilities, many of the programmatic areas in the cancer program are shared to varying degrees by other Institutes. The magnitude of the available funding from NCI undoubtedly serves as an attraction to individual investigators seeking funding for their research programs. Many of the problems at issue in cancer are very fundamental (i.e., genetics, hereditary cell proliferation, cell metabolism, virology, immunology). Furthermore, cancer can affect many different organs and tissues of the body, either directly or through complications. Diagnostic methods used to detect cancers can be used for diagnosis of other ailments as well. The epidemiology of cancer implicates conditions in the environment that can affect other functioning organ systems (such as smoking in cancer and heart disease). For these reasons, a very large proportion of the total health related research effort is being accommodated under the general umbrella of the cancer program.

The availability of generous quantities of research support is sufficient to attract many scientists, causing them to divert or tailor research interests toward cancer to gain such support. This process is encouraged by the widespread distribution of requests for applications (grants) and requests for proposals (contracts) issued from Washington in large volume. When investigator-initiated research grants are sent to NIH, the Division of Research Grants often has several different Institutes to which a particular project could be justified. There is a natural tendency to channel promising grants toward the Institutes with the largest available resources. The net effect of such trends is to divert a very large proportion of the total biomedical research competence in certain key areas into the cancer program. The entire biomedical research effort may well benefit greatly from the generalized application of fundamental research conducted under the cancer program. For example, new insights into the basic principles of mutogenesis, virology, immunology, or cell metabolism may be equally applicable to cancer or to other kinds of diseases. On the other hand, the concentration of resources on cancer could be conceived as depriving or depleting efforts in other important areas such as arthritis, diabetes, or more common illnesses. The mechanisms of forward planning for cancer can be expected to serve as an example to the corresponding long-range planning in other Institutes. In this broad context, the entire biomedical research effort is being significantly affected by the National Cancer Program.

The National Cancer Program has had an enormous impact extending far beyond the biomedical research community to encompass the entire population, confronted on all sides with warnings regarding the potential hazards of cancer-producing chemicals in the environment. The complex problems involved in assessing the possible causative role of chemicals in producing various cancers is shared with many other agencies such as the National Institute of Environmental Health Sciences, the Food and Drug Administration, the Environmental Protection Agency, the Department of Agriculture, and many other agencies of government. The magnitude of the problem is indicated by the fact that some 550 chemical agents are currently under study, but some 33,000 are believed to be in common use from among the 4,039,907 chemical entities reported (11) to be listed in the Chemical Abstracts service of the American Chemical Society. The complications of this massive effort are unpredictable but great caution must be used to avoid severe, unwarranted economic dislocations and cancerphobia in epidemic proportions among some segments of society. The gaps in our knowledge regarding causes of uncontrolled cell proliferation and epidemiological evidence for chemical carcinogens are considered in more detail in subsequent sections (see also Fig. 4-4).

The Cancer Biology Program is oriented toward understanding molecular and biological processes, involving diverse disciplines such as cell biology, molecular biology, ultrastructure analysis, genetics, physiology, pathology, genetics, morphogenesis, developmental biology, immunology, pathology, and "other related disciplines." Such fundamental areas are of common interest and involvement of various Institutes

The areas of responsibility of the various Institutes of Health have very blurred borders, resulting in enormous overlap of interest, particularly with respect to the more fundamental issues. The nature and extent of such overlap is difficult to assess for lack of firm data. A rare example was a review by the Division of Research Grants (12) of the levels of support for immunology (and virology) in the various Institutes. Immunology would superficially appear to be a special province of the Institute dealing with allergy and infection. However, this review indicated major investments by seven institutes. By far the largest number of projects in both immunology and virology was found to be included in the Cancer Program (see also Table 3-5 in Chapter 3). The appropriate distribution of support between the NCI and the NIAID remains unclear.

ALLERGY AND INFECTIOUS DISEASES

The National Institute of Allergy and Infectious Diseases (13) reported that "sure foundations" have been developed for the conquest of the two categories of diseases for which it has prime responsibility. Infectious disease research is directed toward a wide variety of pathogens, particularly viruses, common bacteria (cocci), and "non-conformist" microbes (Rickettsia, actinomycetes, mycoplasms). The enormous progress in prevention and control of infection is currently threatened by the development of the long-feared resistance to antibiotics. The clinical applications of microbiology are many and mostly obvious. However, the conquest of infectious disease is far from complete. Some of the most common ailments of mankind are due to infectious agents that have effectively resisted all previous efforts, notably colds, "flu," certain diarrheas, hepatitis, and many others.

Research in microbiology is concentrated on characterizing the cell membranes and exploring the toxic products of microorganisms. Virology is not only a concern of NIAID but extends to most of the other Institutes to varying degrees. The most familiar bacterium (*E. coli*) has assumed a stellar role in a drama that has captured the imagination of the scientific community and the general public, namely genetic manipulation by means of recombinant DNA.

Research on the immune systems is an area of critical significance to NIAID and to a majority of the other Institutes of Health. Attention has been focused increasingly on using human leucocyte antigen (HLA) sera of potential importance for recognizing individual disease states—ankylosing spondilitis and certain cancers. Clinical implications of immunology include "immune complex diseases" in the form of injurious antigen-antibody complexes, which can be filtered or trapped in small blood vessels such as kidney glomeruli. Antigen-antibody complexes are used as irritants to produce experimental "atherosclerosis." Asthma is an extremely common and debilitating allergic disease being approached by both basic research and treatment centers. Individuals, especially infants, with immune deficiences are extremely susceptible to infections.

At first sight, allergies and infectious diseases would appear to be rather explicit and well-defined categories, yet the implications of immunology, virology, genetics, and infections permeate many components of biomedical research.

ARTHRITIS, METABOLISM, AND DIGESTIVE DISEASES

The forward plan (FY 1979–1983) for the National Institute of Arthritis, Metabolism, and Digestive Diseases (14) necessarily covers a very broad mandate as indicated by its name. The inclusion of digestive diseases in the title (1972 P.L. 92–305) brought renewed emphasis to this important area. The areas of responsibility include arthritis and connective tissues diseases, diabetes, and other metabolic disorders, disturbances of endocrine glands, digestive system and nutrition, diseases of the kidney and urinary tract, and orthopedic problems involving blood, bone, and skin. The health problems encompassed by these manifold problems are not generally included among the "killer diseases," but they represent an extremely important spectrum of diseases and disabilities. For example, arthritis affects at least 22 million Americans with untold suffering. Some 10 million people suffer from diabetes. Estimates indicate that 48,000 Americans die each year of irreversible kidney failure despite an end-stage renal program (dialysis) costing about

$650 million (1976). Ample justification can be advanced for increased emphasis on these and the other disease-oriented conditions embraced by the NIAMDD.

Fundamental research efforts include investigation of connective tissues and causes of inflammation as occur in arthritis and other related conditions. Human leukocyte antigens have been associated with certain arthritic diseases and are of interest to several other Institutes. The basic science issues encountered in mebabolic diseases are widely disseminated among the various Institutes.

The management of metabolic diseases and disabilities tends to be relatively restricted to NIAMDD. However, complex relationships can be demonstrated between metabolic and nutritional diseases, kidney ailments, cardiovascular disease, pregnancy, developmental malformations, obesity, and other clinical areas. Overlapping areas of involvement abound among conglomerate Institutes, including child health, human development, aging, mental health, and many others. The orthopedic program is focused on bone growth, congenital abnormalities, tendon and hand research, biomechanics of skeletal system, artifical joints, biomaterials and orthotics, trauma, shock, and fracture healing. These are readily rationalized in clincial perspective, but the permutations on the more basic levels are less obvious.

The Institute also encompasses organ-oriented categories of diseases, including bones and joints (orthopedics), kidney disease, digestive diseases, and hematology. A Congressional initiative has given impetus to work on cystic fibrosis. The current mandate of the Institute has been complicated and obscured by its multidimensional scope.

ORGAN-SYSTEM ORIENTED INSTITUTES

Institutes with specific organ orientation appear to have fairly definite boundaries and disease processes that are readily identified with their structure and functions. Thus, pneumonia, hyperthyroidism, and cirrhosis are each associated with a specific organ. Each organ system is also affected by generalized systemic disturbances or by complications of pathological processes in other organs. The nature and scope of the research and development programs of the organ-oriented Institutes can best be appreciated in terms of programmatic areas being emphasized in their long-range plans.

HEART, LUNG, AND BLOOD INSTITUTE

The largest of the organ-oriented Institutes encompasses three functionally related components, the heart and vascular system, lungs, and blood. Twenty program elements are currently included in the (NHLBI) plan focused on diseases or disfunctions specific to the anatomical components (Fig. 2-8). The intent of the Institute is to engage in a continuous process of analysis

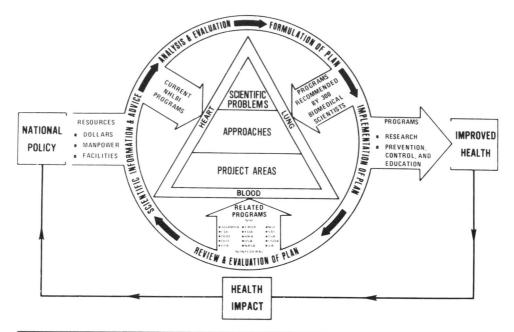

HEART AND BLOOD VESSEL DISEASE	LUNG DISEASE	BLOOD DISEASE AND BLOOD RESOURCES
Arteriosclerosis	Structure and Function of the Lung	Bleeding and Clotting Disorders
Hypertension	Emphysema and Chronic Bronchitis	Disorders of the Red Blood Cell
Cerebrovascular Disease		
Coronary Heart Disease	Pediatric Pulmonary Diseases	Sickle Cell Disease
Peripheral Vascular Diseases		Blood Resources
Arryhthmias	Fibrotic and Immunologic Lung Diseases	
Heart Failure and Shock	Respiratory Failure	
Congenital and Rheumatic Heart Diseases	Pulmonary Vascular Diseases	
Cardiomyopathies and Infections of the Heart		
Circulatory Assistance		

Figure 2-8. Under the 1976 legislation, the primary missions of the NHLBI are to conduct and support research to increase fundamental and clinical knowledge about cardiovascular, pulmonary, and blood systems. The schematic representation of these efforts illustrate the concept of continuing input, output, and feedback as part of a commitment to forward planning by the Institute. Twenty key targets of high priority are presented (15).

and assessment of current programs, formulation of new plans, and evaluation of their results, as indicated schematically in Figure 2-8. In the current context, attention is directed to the list of fiteeen related federal programs listed within the lower arrow (specifically ADAMHA, CDC, DOD, DOT, EPA, ERDA, FDA, HRA, HSA, NASA, NSF, SAS, SSA, USDA, VA), as well as other nonfederal activities. The program strategy developed by the Institute (15) for any individual condition includes an ordered sequence of:

· Acquisition of new knowledge (basic and clinical research)
· Testing and evaluation of promising hypotheses (clinical trials)
· Application of existing knowledge (education, demonstration, and control)

A prime example of this continuum is represented by the approach to hypertension (15). The underlying cause(s) of elevated blood pressure are unclear or unknown. However, effective mechanisms for lowering the blood pressure have been developed and put into widespread clinical use. To this end, a major campaign of public education and mass screening was initiated by the Institute, a most unusual role for a research institution (16). However, the relatively modest investment was greatly expanded through the Bureau of Community Health Services involving participation by state and local organizations. A statistically significant reduction in mortality has been reported to result from a massive high blood pressure detection and follow-up program. The apparent risks of stroke, heart failure, and kidney failure have been reduced, particularly in older people.

The Division of Lung Diseases became a recognized component of the National Heart and Lung Institute in 1969. Further reorganization took place in 1972 when the Institute was elevated to bureau status with six division level components, including Blood Diseases and Resources. The Division of Lung Diseases has been recently reorganized into four branches, including Structure and Function; Airways Diseases; Interstitial Lung Diseases and Prevention, Education, and Manpower (17). Fundamental investigations predominate in the structure and function branch (including growth and development). The airways disease branch deals with asthma (in concert with NIAID), chronic obstructive lung disease, bronchiolitis, and cystic fibrosis. Hypersensitivity pneumonitis (immune lung disease) is a key target in the Interstitial Lung Diseases and Prevention, Education, and Manpower Branches. The pediatric program has been dispersed among the other branches rather than appearing as a separate component.

Thus, the NHLBI encompasses a group of anatomically related components; the various programs parallel or overlap corresponding programs in many of the other Institutes of Health. The strong clinical orientation of the NHLBI program is quite clearly consistent with the persistent public and political pressures for relevance. Furthermore, a large proportion of "flexible funds" are allocated for a series of large and costly clinical trial programs (16).

Clinical Trials. The effectiveness of therapeutic approaches is explored through cooperative efforts by selected investigators in several institutions following common protocols and working within clearly defined guidelines.

The major clinical trials currently being supported by the Institute include the following (18):

- Aspirin Myocardial Infarction Study
- Coronary Artery Surgery (bypass operations)
- Hypertension Detection and Follow-up
- Coronary Primary Prevention Trial (cholesterol reduction)
- Multiple Risk Factor Intervention Trial (risk reduction)
- Neonatal Respiratory Distress Syndrome
- Inhibitors in Hemophilia
- Extracorporeal Membrane Oxygenator Study
- Clinical Trial on Mild Hypertension (VA study)
- Nocturnal Oxygen Therapy Trial

There is urgent need for more definitive information on effectiveness of therapeutic measures, but other regulatory agencies of government might be more appropriate mechanisms for such assessment. (For additional discussion, see Chapter 6.)

A glance at the list of programs of the NHLBI (Fig. 2–8) and the list of clinical trials above discloses that a relatively few organ-specific ailments account for a very large proportion of the Institute's activities. Thus, atherosclerosis, hypertension, arrhythmias, heart failure, acquired and congenital malformations of the heart, respiratory distress syndrome, hemophilia are conditions that are unequivocally within the preview of the Institute and are only remotely represented by the relatively nonspecific disease-oriented or compositive Institutes.

NATIONAL EYE INSTITUTE

The National Eye Institute was created by separating this entity from an earlier association of blindness with neurological diseases. The eye institute is the most explicit and highly focused of all, and its boundaries are correspondingly well defined. The research program of the National Eye Institute provides investigator-initiated research project grants to the extent of 77% of extramural funds in the forward plan for FY 1980 (19). Opportunities and unmet needs for research have been identified and used to guide individual investigators in the formulation of project grant applications. Center grants and contracts are used to a lesser extent (9% and 7% of the 1980 extramural budget, respectively). Center grants to institutions already actively involved in quality research projects are preferred to "outreach" programs. Research contracts are used in support of clinical trials, involving fixed protocols, or for development of specialized research resources (instruments and animal models). Contracts are used when the following conditions apply: (1) the topic is of national importance, (2) the concept and design of the study is developed by NEI staff with advisors, (3) collaboration is required among a number of institutions, (4) the NEI has the staff resources to assume responsibility for management as well as the sponsorship of the study.

Most of the contracts have been awarded for clinical trials of new therapies for diabetic retinopathy. The NEI "is most comfortable" with multiprotocol projects whose parts can be separately reviewed and funded on their own merits. Future program plans are expected to retain the present balance between basic (45%) and applied (55%) research.

Forward planning for the Eye Institute is more extensive than most "smaller" Institutes. The process was initiated in 1975 with the establishment of six panels of experts in the areas of (1) retinal and choroidal diseases (principally diabetic retinopathy), (2) corneal diseases, (3) cataract, (4) glaucoma, (5) sensory and motor disorders of vision, and (6) vision research training. Special attention was accorded 24 different research topics included under these main headings (20).

The enigmatic etiology of retinal changes associated with diabetes requires extensive basic research. More than one third of blindness in the United States is due to vascular diseases of the retina and choroid. Diabetic retinopathy is one of the prime areas of involvement. In addition, senile macular degeneration and sickle cell retinopathy have vascular components of prime interest. These three vascular manifestations have obvious relations to the Institutes dealing with metabolism, aging, and cardiovascular system.

Another key problem is glaucoma, which is now suspected of having a metabolic (corticosteroid) as well as a "mechanical" component in the elevation of the intraocular pressure (21). A major clinical trial has been undertaken to determine if photocoagulation of these lesions by means of lasers can retard or impede the extension of lesions. The lesions are related to the vascular system as affected by a metabolic disease. This particular element in the program is inherently interdisciplinary in its scope. In contrast, the other main categories of corneal diseases, cataract, glaucoma, and sensory motor disorders are peculiar to the eye. Obviously, there are peripheral concerns with infections, immune reactions, neuromuscular controls, and other elements represented in other Institutes. However, most of the concerns of the NEI are specific to the eye.

NATIONAL INSTITUTE OF DENTAL RESEARCH

The National Institute of Dental Research was one of the early additions to the National Institutes of Health (immediately following the National Heart Institute). Effective collaborative relationships were established early with the National Bureau of Standards, through which a number of invaluable contributions have emerged. Of particular importance was the development of specialized dental materials. Very high speed dental drills were also a product of this important interaction.

Dental diseases extend beyond the care of teeth and include periodontal diseases, craniofacial anomalies, and other oral and pharyngeal disturbances. The forward plan FY 1980–84 (22) lays particular stress on caries and on periodontal disease, with programs on facial deformities (malocclusion, cleft lip, maxillofacial injuries) and soft tissue diseases such as infections and cancer. The anatomic focus on the oral cavity provides the basis for integration of the research and development programs. Initiatives on pain control and behavioral studies broaden the scope of endeavors substantially. Continuing collaboration with the National Bureau of Standards in developing dental materials and instruments has been encouraged by a Senate appropriations directive. The research efforts of the program have been strengthened by provision of additional funds specifically for collaborative research (contracts) by which the Institute initiatives can be pursued more directly and effectively.

NEUROLOGICAL, COMMUNICATIVE DISORDERS AND STROKE

The nervous system is the primary anatomical focus of this Institute. Blindness was removed from its area of responsibility with the creation of the National Eye Institute discussed above. Both basic and applied research are represented in the Institute's intramural and investigator-initiated extramural grants program. The areas of interest encompass the full spectrum of both function and diseases affecting this vital system. Important examples are epilepsy and convulsive disorders, encephalitis, and other infectious invasions, particularly those related to early life. An ambitious collaborative program using contracts calls for analysis of data from 50,000 pregnancies to explore neurological and mental development of the offspring.

Communication disorders have been added to the Institute's area of responsibility. Hearing deficiencies are of particular importance, not only in the aging population, but also in the very young. If auditory deficiences are undetected during the first year(s) of life while the speech centers should be developing, serious speech defects are generally encountered that require literally years of intensive remedial correction at enormous expense. Improved hearing aids and other sensory aids for the hearing impaired are being developed using contract mechanisms. The effects of noise on auditory sensitivity is also within the scope of the research enterprise.

The National Research Strategy for Neurological and Communicative Disorders (22) has been organized in accordance with certain common themes. For this purpose the major neurological disorders were grouped according to the growth and development of the nervous system. Developmental disorders and neuromuscular conditions common in childhood are specified, along with the degenerative diseases of older age groups. A second part deals with assaults to the nervous system in the form of infections, neoplasms, stroke and trauma (including toxic elements in the environment). Thirdly, the human nervous system is viewed as a "master coordinator and orchestrator of behavior" that can be affected by failures of communication, both internally and in relation to the external world. Deafness and communicative disorders are striking examples of conditions that block interpersonal relations and isolate victims from society. The emotional disorders and behavioral problems receive increased attention in common with many of the other Institutes of Health.

Brain damage due to tumors, hemorrhages, or cerebral occlusion is an important element in the program. These areas have mutual interest with other Institutes such as NCI and NHLBI. The applications of biomedical engineering are involved in the provision of substitutes or supplements for the neurologically handicapped and diagnostic technologies. Engineering applications are a prime responsibility of one of the Composite Institutes (NIGMS).

COMPOSITE OR AGE-ORIENTED INSTITUTES

NATIONAL INSTITUTE OF GENERAL MEDICAL SCIENCES

The original mandate called for an Institute for "the conduct and support of research and training in the general or basic medical sciences and related natural and behavioral sciences which have significance for two or more Institutes or are outside the general area of responsibility of any other Institute." (From PL 87-838 Sec. 442.) According to the forward plan FY 79-83 (23), a major thrust of the Institute is directed toward research on the body's responses to acute trauma and burns.

Genetic diseases also have high priority in addition to the more basic research on cellular and molecular basis of disease. Attention has been focused on properties of cell membranes including physicochemical and molecular aspects of the problems of cell metabolism, hormone action, immune reactions, and cell division. Clearly these are concerns of fundamental interest to many other Institute programs.

Biomedical engineering is devoted to applied research and development of materials, instruments, and methods involving engineering science, physics, mathematics, and analytical chemistry. Automated clinical laboratory equipment has been a major thrust of the program.

Genetics is being investigated through gene mapping in humans and mutations in lower forms, such as insects and bacteria.

The *pharmacology-toxicology program* is intended to improve medical therapy by increased understanding of drug actions. Included is an active program on agents that stimulate production of interferon, an antiveral protein that has been long under study by NIAID as a promising mechanism for controlling virus diseases for which neither immunization nor definitive therapy are available. These include such common conditions of colds and flu (see also Fig. 4-6). In addition, the metabolism of drugs as well as their deactivation are under exploration.

Clinical Physiology Program supports special areas of clinical medicine such as anesthesiology, trauma, burns, and behavioral and psychological aspects of chronic pain.

NATIONAL INSTITUTE FOR CHILD HEALTH AND HUMAN DEVELOPMENT

A multidisciplinary approach is used by NICHD to address the problems that occur during perinatal periods and development processes of children (24). Reproductive biology is devoted to studying the full range of phenomena associated with reproduction from ovulation and spermatogenesis to intrauterine development and the birth process. *Developmental biology* is the term used to cover the changes from egg fertilization through infancy, maturity, to old age.

The Institute's support of basic studies on hormonal receptors focuses primarily on contraceptive development and cures for infertility. Recent research at the Institute has shown that genetic makeup affects the response of the fetus to both hormones and foreign chemicals entering by way of the placenta; responses that affect its protection against toxic materials and the occurrence of congenital defects.

The Institute is committed to a major investment in fetal and perinatal medicine, as well as major initiatives in the areas of reproduction, pregnancy, and infancy.

Additional funds in the president's budget for FY 1979 provide opportunities to develop initiatives of which a substantial portion will be directed toward adolescent health and the prevention of unwanted children. The Institute is continuously confronted by the apparently conflicting aims—mechanisms for increasing fertility and also means of controlling population growth, and providing positive alternatives to abortion.

An increasing emphasis is evident in the areas of behavioral, social, and cultural influences in childhood that contribute to unhealthy habits or interfere with proper nutrition.

The Institute gives high priority to 10 specific program areas as follows:

- High risk pregnancy
- Fertility-Infertility
- Congenital defects
- Sudden infant death syndrome (SIDS)
- Child development
- Nutrition
- Mental Retardation
- Contraception development
- Contraceptive safety
- Population and family dynamics

In addition, the Human Learning and Behavior Branch supports studies in human communication, learning disabilities, and personality development (25). The intramural research program is divided into basic research covering developmental neurobiology, biomedical sciences, molecular genetics, and social and behavioral sciences. Clinical research is carried out by Developmental Pharmacology Branch, Neonatal and Pediatric Medicine Branch, Pregnancy Research Branch, and Endocrinology and Reproduction Research Branch.

The increasing concern and concentration in the areas of social and behavioral sciences, epidemiology, and biometry are represented in this Institute and in the closely related Institute on Aging.

INSTITUTE ON AGING

Before 1974, the older age groups were encompassed by NICHHD. The Institute on Aging is the most recent addition to the Institutes of Health. Senior citizens are a large and growing segment of society, prone to develop many and varied problems affecting their health, psychological, and socio-economic status. The congressional mandate was to further the study of the aging process, "the one biological problem common to us all." Senior citizens are often excluded from full life by physical infirmities resulting from advancing age, and complicated by economic, social, and psychological factors associated with aging. A prime objective of NIA is the extension of the healthy middle years of life (26).

A Division of Research Priorities has been established to consider biological and social factors in three categories (27):

- Biomedical sciences
- The behavioral and social sciences
- Human services and their delivery

The biomedical research effort is oriented toward elucidation of the aging process at the cellular level (structure, biochemistry, genetics, and physiology), the normal physiological changes with age, and immunological changes. Diagnostic criteria of aging and factors affecting susceptibility to disease and brain disorders are specified as topics of concern. Changes in metabolism and nutritional requirements are also included (28).

Behavioral and social science research is generally oriented toward reduction of dependency, mechanisms for maintaining income, the retirement process, individual interactions, social competence, and integration. Clinical psychology and psychiatry are of particular importance to the aging population (29). Human services and delivery systems involve the exploration of mechanisms for providing the special needs of the aged such as medical care, home care, mental health, nutrition, and housing, transportation, institutional care, and comprehensive approaches to provide a "full range of services."

The Institute on Aging inherently contains areas of concern and responsibility that overlap virtually all the other Institutes and extend far beyond the traditional boundaries of health care into social, economic, and legal spheres.

ENVIRONMENTAL HEALTH SCIENCES

Noninfectious substances and factors in the environment that can cause human disability, disease, and premature death exemplify the mandate of the National Institute of Environmental Health Sciences (30, 31). In the present era of cancer concern, the potential hazards of carcinogenic substances among the enormous number of chemicals introduced into modern societies was mentioned in relation to the Cancer Cause and Prevention Program of NCI. The Toxic Substances Control Act of 1976 mandates that substances must be tested for safety *before* introduction into commerce if a "reasonable risk to human health may occur." Each year 700 to 1,000 new compounds are introduced in commercial quantities that represent hazards to human health for reasons that are poorly understood at present.

The forward plan of the NIEHS is based on the realistic assumption that most agents are not toxic enough or present in sufficient quantities to threaten human health if their potential risks are recognized and control is instituted on the basis of an adequate data base. The Institute is located in the research triangle in North Carolina, geographically separated from the main NIH campus in Bethesda, Maryland. As the necessary environmental data base is established for specific disease entities, the information will be supplied to the categorical Institute(s) charged with responsibility for the disease.

The present research programs in environmental health sciences are based on two comprehensive and broad-based task forces exploring research needs in relation to human health and environment (32, 33). A provision of both general and detailed recommendations were developd by groups of experts. The scope of the efforts is suggested by the following main headings:

· General atmospheric pollution
· Occupational health and safety
· Food, water, and multiple sources
· Selected problems of special environments (neighborhood, home, hospital, etc.)
· Physical environmental factors (i.e., various types of radiation)
· Transport and alteration of pollutants, waste disposal, and natural sources of toxicants.
· Environmental measurements of chemicals for assessment of human exposures
· Biologic mechanisms and determinants of toxicity
· Carcinogenesis
· Mutagenesis
· Reproduction, teratology, and human development
· Behavioral toxicology (i.e., CNS toxicants)
· Organ systems; environment and disease
· Methods and resources for estimating disease risk in humans.

Environmental Health Science Centers. Seven centers have been established to cover the broad areas of:

· Heavy metal intoxication (especially behavioral, neurological, and renal effects)
· Aerosol toxicology and respiratory disease and epidemiology
· Occupational diseases
· Carcinogenesis and mutagenesis
· Pharmacology and metabolism of toxic substances
· Biometry, biostatistics, and experimental modeling of pollutants through time and space

Intramural programs of the NIEHS supplement the activities of these centers.

This brief summary of environmental factors indicates the widespread hazards to the health and well-being of individuals and groups of citizens of all ages. The environmental health sciences have significant impact on all the various organ systems of the body to various degrees. Since the other disease-oriented Institutes have areas of responsibility widely dispersed among the various organ systems, they necessarily supplement, overlap, or duplicate research and development efforts.

OVERVIEW OF RESEARCH PLANS: NATIONAL INSTITUTES OF HEALTH

The average biomedical scientist is confronted with a pressing need to keep up to date with the changing policies and priorities in the various granting agencies from which he derives research support. The annual updating of the forward plans of the various institutes often involves major shifts in emphasis that could have significant impact on decisions regarding the most appropriate thrust of research grant applications. Gaining access to the current versions of forward plans is not simple, particularly since many investigators are not informed regarding their existence or imminent release. A very useful summary of the research plans of the National Institutes of Health has been developed under the title "Research Plan FY 1981-83" (34). It includes tabulation of some of the major thrusts and changes in program orientation of the NIH along with summaries of the programs of the individual institutes including major changes which are being effected. This document can serve as a directory to the research programs encompassed by the individual Institutes, a kind of guidebook to help investigators thread their way through the complex meshwork of overlapping areas of responsibility.

TERRITORIAL BOUNDARIES: THE NEED FOR CLARIFICATION

The process of forward planning by the various Institutes is inevitably complicated by ambiguity regarding their areas of responsibility. The natural tendency of any organization to compete for territorial turf is a strong incentive to encompass accessible and relevant areas of research. Appropriate allocation of spheres of involvement and avoidance of undesirable overlap requires internally consistent organizational relationships. The fact that the various Institutes of Health fall into at least three distinctly different categories oriented toward organ systems, pathological process and age-oriented or composite target areas inevitably induces extensive overlap in the areas of responsibility (see Fig. 2-5). Each of the institutes tends to embrace relevant fundamental and functional issues, pathophysiology and clinical management of the conditions within its orbit. The current efforts toward rationalizing programs through comprehensive forward planning have little chance of avoiding repetition and redundancy without clearer differentiation of the organizational relationships. At the risk of appearing presumptuous, one possible approach to clarifying the area of responsibility of the various Institutes of Health is presented schematically in a tiered organizational framework (Fig. 2-9).

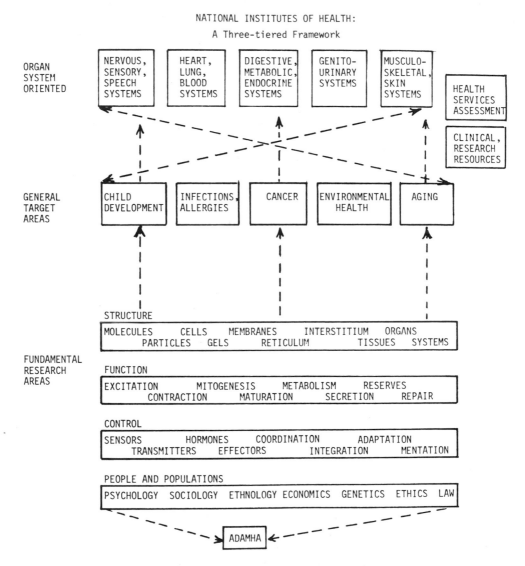

Figure 2-9. The operational boundaries between biomedical research agencies might be more concisely demarcated by means of a three-tiered framework. Each organ system is subject to a specific set of diseases and disturbances, and is represented by various clinical specialties. Hazards to life and health represented by each of the General Target Areas can affect any or all of the organ systems. Fundamental research on a variety of topics in different levels is an essential ingredient of each of the organ systems and general target areas, creating an essential requirement of communication and cooperation among all of the components (including ADAMHA).

AREAS OF INSTITUTE RESPONSIBILITY

The essential components of the national biomedical research effort can be arranged in an internally consistent format based on three tiers. The health care delivery system is largely based on organ system orientation. The nervous system is the sphere of interest of neurologists and neurosurgeons. Ophthamologists and otolaryngolosists care for disturbances of vision, hearing and speech. Cardiologists and cardiac surgeons take care of heart diseases. Blood is the province of hematologists. Gastroenterologists, proctologists, and endocrinologists focus on diseases of the digestive tract and hormonal control mechanisms. Obstetricians, gynecologists, nephrologists and urologists deal with the genito-urinary system. Rheumatologists, orthopaedic surgions and dermatologists are responsible for supporting structures (bones, joints, muscles, and skin). Central to each of the specialty areas are diseases or disabilities that are specific to the organ system. Thus epilepsy, multiple sclerosis, Parkinson's disease, otosclerosis and glaucoma obviously are restricted or relevant only to the nervous and sensory organs. Atherosclerosis, hypertension, asthma and anemia are equally organ-specific. These few examples are representative of the large and diverse array of specific kinds of malfunctions that can be identified for each tissue, organ or system.

In addition, all tissues or organs are affected to varying degrees and ways by many different factors in the middle tier of Figure 2-9 and labeled General Target Areas. Congenital malformation can occur in any tissue of the body. Developmental defects in infants and children can be manifest in many different ways, including physiological, psychological and pathological malfunctions. Allergies and infections can produce disturbances in virtually any tissue or organ. Cancer cells can emerge or metastasize in various tissues and organs. Environmental hazards can contribute to the production of cancer and many other diseases or malfunctions. The aging process also can induce functional or degenerative changes in a wide variety of locations. The major research efforts carried out in the general target areas are clearly applicable to many or all of the organ systems in the top tier.

Fundamental research can be considered in terms of the many different structural elements in cells, tissues and organ systems. The function of living organisms and their control are also subject to fundamental investigation. Expanded scope of the biomedical research enterprise now extends beyond the ailments of individual patients to include the problems of groups or populations. The contribution of stresses of modern living to holistic health requires research in such areas as ethnology, psychology, economics, and many other disciplines previously neglected. As mentioned above, the behavioral and social sciences have been widely adopted into the areas of responsibilities of the various Institutes of Health.

In retrospect, the areas of responsibility of the different Institutes of Health might have been more clearly defined using an organizational framework like that illustrated in Figure 2-9 during the exuberant expansion phase of NIH development. Now that many of the Institutes have embraced approaches that are widely overlapping, the process of sorting out the boundaries is fraught with great difficulty. The forward planning process may not succeed in attaining its ultimate usefulness unless mechanisms can be developed for clarifying the borders between the areas of responsibility among the various institutes.

SUMMARY

1. The National Cancer Act of 1971 and the subsequent amendments (1974) specified the need for undertaking large scale programmatic planning of the National Cancer Program and provided the budgets for staff to engage in this effort. The forward-planning program of the NCI is very comprehensive and appears to serve as a prototype for increasing the planning effort of all the other Institutes of Health.

2. The categorical organization of NIH evolved through incremental addition of three different categories of Institutes, specifically disease-oriented, organ system-oriented, and composite Institutes. The lack of consistency in assigning missions has resulted in ambiguity and uncertainty about the scope of mission of each Institute. Any of the Institutes can easily justify incorporating into its programs areas of interest that are equally well situated in several other Institutes. Conversely, virtually any research proposal could be accepted by more than one, and often many, of the Institutes.

3. The lack of clearly defined areas of responsibility greatly complicates the process of forward planning in the Institutes of Health and contributes to the uncertainty faced by individual investigators attempting to interpret the unmet needs for research. The fluctuating waves of emphasis as new plans emerge can only confuse the scientific community attempting to adapt to the changing scene in Washington.

4. A brief survey of the forward plans of the various Institutes of Health discloses both substantial uncertainty and ambiguity regarding the most appropriate sources of support, particularly for the more fundamental and cross-cutting issues (such as virology, immunology, genetics, molecular biology, biomedical engineering, etc.) The picture is further complicated by the greatly increased emphasis on "soft sciences" such as behavioral sciences, sociology, and even socioeconomic and legal aspects of health. These added areas of responsibility are finding increasing expression not only in the Alcoholism, Drug Abuse, and Mental Health Administration (ADAMHA), but also in the various Institutes comprising NIH.

5. The growing demands for forward planning, fiscal responsibility, and accountability on the part of governmental agencies are difficult to meet with organizational components having ambiguous and overlapping areas of responsibility and insufficient budgetary provisions for staff required for forward planning and for internal communication, integration, and monitoring of this huge and dispersed research enterprise.

6. One significant change in the NIH has been a pronounced shift from the role of bursar of public funds into a manager of research programs

through increasing reliance on Institute-initiated programs and greater reliance on requests for applications (grants) and requests for proposals (contracts).

REFERENCES

1. Frederickson, Donald S: The government in biomedical research. *Fed. Proc.* 35: 2538-2540, 1976.
2. Culliton B: Kennedy Hearings; year long probe of biomedical research begins. *Science* 193:32-35, 1976.
3. Strickland SP: Medical research; public policy and power politics, in Cater D and Lee PR (ed): *Politics of Health*, New York, Medcom Press, 1972.
4. Rettig RA: *Cancer Crusade: the Story of the National Cancer Act of 1971.* Princeton, NJ, Princeton University Press, 1977.
5. Carrese LM: The national planning effort; the need for a comprehensive national plan, its organization and implementation. *Natl Cancer Inst Monogr* 40:21-24, 1974.
6a. The Strategic Plan, National Cancer Program, January 1973, DHEW Pub No. NIH 74-569.
6b. Operational Plan FY 1976-1980, National Cancer Program, August 1974.
6c. 1976 Annual Plan for FY 1978-1982. National Cancer Program, December, 1976.
7. Higginson J: The role of geographical pathology in environmental carcinogenesis, in: *Environment and Cancer*, 24th Annual Symposium on Fundamental Cancer Research, Baltimore, The Williams and Wilkins Company, 1972.
8. Shannon JA: The American experience with biomedical science. In *Health in America 1776-1976*, U.S. Public Health Service, DHEW Pub No (HRA) 76-616, 1976.
9. Personal interviews with Dr. Donald K. Fredrickson, Director, NIH; Dr. Dewitt Stettin, Deputy Director for Research, NIH; Dr. Seymour Perry, Office of Medical Applications of Research, NIH; Dr. Louis M. Carrese, Deputy Director, National Cancer Institute; Dr. Claude Lenfant, Director, Pulmonary Disease Division, NHLBI; Dr. Robert Ringler, Deputy Director, National Heart, Lung, Blood Institute.
10. Responsibilities of NIH at the Health Research/Health Care Interface. Memorandum from the Director, National Institutes of Health, Washington DC, February 28, 1977.
11. Maugh TH: Chemicals; how many are there? *Science* 199:162, 1978.
12. Jones JA: NIH support for immunology research FY 1975. Research and Evaluation Branch, Division of Research Grants, NIH, DHEW, April 7, 1977.
13. Krause RM: *Sure Foundations:* A report of the Director, National Institute of Allergy and Infectious Diseases, DHEW Pub No. (NIH) 77-1220, 1976.
14. Forward Plan FY 1979-83, National Institute of Arthritis, Metabolism, and Digestive Diseases.
15. Fourth Report of the Director, National Heart, Blood Vessel, Lung, and Blood Program, DHEW Pub No (NIH) 77-1170, 1977.
16. Levy RI (Director NHLBI): Statement Before the Subcommittee on Health and Long Term Care. Select Committee on Aging, House of Representatives, Thursday, July 21, 1977.
17. Division of Lung Diseases. Report to Advisory Council of the National Heart, Lung, Blood Institute. December 2-3, 1976.

18. Fact Book for Fiscal Year 1976, National Heart, Lung, and Blood Institute, DHEW Pub No. (NIH) 77-1172.
19. Forward Plan, FY 1980-84, National Eye Institute, Director's Overview Statement.
20. Vision Research: A National Plan, 1978-1982. The 1977 Report of the National Advisory Eye Council, DHEW Pub No (NIH) 78-1258.
21. Forward Plan, FY 1980-84, National Institute of Dental Research, January 30, 1978.
22. National Research Strategy for Neurological and Communicative Disorders National Institutes of Health DHEW (Draft) February 26, 1979.
23. Forward Plan Submission, FY 79-83, National Institute of General Medical Sciences.
24. Forward Plan FY 1980-84, National Institute of Child Health and Human Development, April 10, 1978.
25. Research Program of the NICHD. Office of Research Reporting, National Institute of Child Health and Human Development, DHEW Pub No (NIH) 77-83, August 1977.
26. Epidemiology of Aging. National Institute of Child Health and Human Development, DHEW Pub No. (NIH) 77-711.
27. Butler RN: Mission of the National Institute on Aging. *J Am Geriatrics Soc* 25: 97-102, 1977.
28. Announcements of National Institute on Aging Programs. NIH Guide for Grants and Contracts, Vol 7, No 12, pp 1-28, September 1, 1978.
29. Our Future Selves: A Research Plan Toward Understanding Aging, DHEW Pub No 77-1096.
30. Forward Plan 1980-84, National Institute of Environmental Health Sciences, Director's Overview Statement.
31. James EY, Kingman GM: The National Institute of Environmental Health Sciences, a perspective, 1977.
32. Man's Health and Environment—Some Research Needs. Report of the First Task Force for Research Planning in Environmental Health Sciences, US Govt Printing Office, March 10, 1970.
33. Human Health and the Environment—Some Research Needs. Report of the Second Task Force for Research Planning in Environmental Health Science, DHEW Pub No (NIH) 77-1277, 1977.
34. Research Plan. (FY 1981-1983) National Institutes of Health DHEW, Draft April 1979.

Part Two

Research Requirements

The urgent need for a major basic research effort became increasingly recognized as essential for elucidation of normal function and responses to stresses and to pathological processes. Paradoxically, most granting agencies have consistently disclaimed ability to distinguish between basic and applied research. The biomedical leadership is increasingly required to account more specifically for the proportion of research support allocated to basic as opposed to applied research, a question which has often been answered quite evasively. To facilitate presentations in this book, some operational definitions of various categories of research are presented and discussed in Chapter 3. Operational definitions of research categories are proposed including fundamental, functional, targeted, clinical investigation, and clinical evaluation to facilitate efforts at achieving balance in future research planning.

Recent evidence has disclosed that the lag times from successful feasibility to practical utilization of important contributions to health care have varied from a few months to more than 50 years. In contrast, some technologies have been developed and disseminated throughout the medical community so rapidly that they became widely used before their usefulness had been established. The factors that affect the rates at which innovations are converted into practical and useful additions to clinical practice are essentially unknown and unexplored.

The mechanisms for monitoring the current output from more than 10,000 research projects are insufficient to recognize and to avoid repetitive or redundant research or to recognize significant gaps in the overall research efforts. Some mechanisms are suggested to indicate theoretical possibility of monitoring and assessing the outcome from current research efforts as well as accounting for the financial input.

Progress toward the identifying ultimate etiology for the major causes of death and disability has been much slower than the monumental successes in control and eradication of many infectious diseases. There appears to be ample justification for more concentrated effort toward "targeted" research, referring to intensified exploration of causes and cures of disease and disability (Chapter 4).

CHAPTER 3

Priorities and Strategies for Forward Planning

The rapid evolution of the biomedical research enterprise in this country bore greater resemblance to a spontaneous popular crusade than to a deliberately planned approach to intricate scientific problems. For example, the addition of a succession of categorical Institutes in the NIH without an overall organizational framework was a response to political opportunities. These were opened up by the bold and insistent strategies of the lay lobby on the one hand, and the conservatism of the scientific community on the other, modulated by Congress to produce an unparalleled rate of growth. The participants in this process were all fully dedicated and conscientious in their intentions and desires to control or cure various important diseases. The gross differences in their perceptions inevitably led to numerous misunderstandings as detailed in the preceding chapters. The lack of mutual understanding and the divergent viewpoints were largely ignored during the rapid expansion of the mobilization phase, when soaring appropriations easily accommodated expanding projects, new programs and created whole new enterprises as new opportunities surfaced. This enthusiastic and free-wheeling approach was interrupted by a growing criticism based primarily on obvious differences between results anticipated by the public and accomplishments of the scientific community. The most persistent and strident differences in perception resulted from three fundamental sources of misunderstanding:

· A common misconception that the acquisition of new knowledge is converted into tangible benefits to mankind through a sequence beginning with "basic" research and progressing through applied research to the development of new processes, procedures, or technologies.

- A failure to distinguish between technical and theoretical obstacles to progress in research and development.
- Semantic confusion regarding the distinctions between "basic" and "applied" research and development.

STRATEGIC MISCONCEPTIONS

The American approach to health problems, environmental hazards, the conquest of space, or the development of an atomic bomb typically involves the mobilization of massive resources focused on major problems with great energy. This process is designed to produce rapid progress but necessarily involves a sacrifice of efficiency through duplication of effort or encounters with unexpected complications or contingencies. A typical American innovation is the bulldozer that rides over obstacles with a massive concentration of power. The organizational ability and American ingenuity has startled the world during two world wars, the Manhattan project, and the manned space program. Massive mobilization of resources for an assault on social or political problems has proved to be highly successful when the targets are clearly defined and well understood. This approach disclosed deficiencies when applied to conquest of disease.

CONCEPT OF A CONTINUUM OF HEALTH-RELATED RESEARCH

New information, gleaned from fundamental research, is commonly believed to be converted into tangible benefits for mankind by a sequential process (Figure 3-1a). According to this perception, progress flows along a linear path. Basic research efforts produce new knowledge, which is disseminated rapidly and widely by scientific publications. The accumulated information is then used by people engaged in "applied" research and development to produce new processes, procedures, or devices. When new innovations are proved to be practical, effective, and safe by animal and clinical investigations and trials, they are introduced into medical practice through demonstration programs. This progression from basic research to health practices in a sequential or linear fashion has been presented consistently as the rationale for support of basic research (i.e., in the Forward Plans for Health, ref. 1). The schematic diagram in Figure 3-1a illustrates the NIH strategy. The growing political pressures for payoff for the huge investment in basic research have tended to divert increasingly large portions of the available resources into applied research, clinical investigation, clinical trials, and demonstration programs, often before adequate understanding has been achieved by basic research.

The common concept that research and development processes follow a sequential progression from basic investigations to human benefits is an attractive illusion, which can be both useful and misleading. There is an unstated assumption that the channeling of resources into basic research will

CONCEPTS OF BIOMEDICAL PROGRESS

A. SEQUENTIAL STEPS

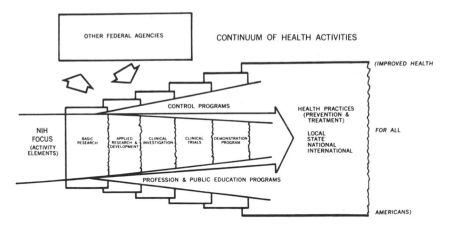

B. FRONTAL ASSAULT ON DISEASE OR DISABILITY

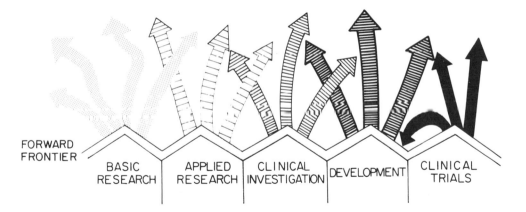

Figure 3-1. Concepts of Biomedical Progress. (*a*) The forward plans at NIH (and other agencies) are based on a concept of a "continuum" representing the conversion of new knowledge from basic research to health practices through a sequential progression as indicated by the arrow (1). This chain of events can sometimes be identified in retrospect but not in terms of either current activities or projections into the future. (*b*) Since the care of sick people cannot await the deliberate sequential process displayed above, health-related research and development can be more accurately portrayed as a frontal attack occurring simultaneously at all levels from basic research to clinical evaluation.

inevitably lead to innovations and to benefits to mankind along a sort of innovation chain. Widespread belief in this process has been engendered in the minds of the public, their representatives in Congress, and even in the scientific community. However, this linear progression rarely occurs in the development of any innovation along a single pathway, because large amounts of diverse information and experience must be accumulated, consolidated, integrated, and focused on a problem in order to arrive at a solution (see Fig. 3-2). For this reason, logical, sequential steps from initial observation to finished product can be recognized only retrospectively and rarely, if ever, in a prospective, or forward-looking manner. An additional implied assumption is that the necessary theoretical obstacles have been clarified by basic research before a strategic sequence can be planned and implemented. The principal tragedy of the last 30 years has been the apparent necessity to embark on major clinical trials and demonstration programs in response to public and political pressures, before the necessary fundamental research has provided the solid basis for such an attack. The inevitable result has been a wide-scale frontal attack (Fig. 3-1b), instead of a spear-headed invasion (Fig. 3-1a).

The health professions have always been required to engage in diagnosis and therapy of diseases and disabilities with mysterious causes and ineffective therapies. Suffering humanity cannot wait for the slow and deliberate progress required for the scientific attack on the diseases which trouble mankind. Clinical practice has always been dependent on whatever diagnostic and therapeutic resources are available, while the biomedical research effort engages in both basic and applied research and development simultaneously and somewhat independently. As a consequence, all the segments of the medical community are struggling to attain a known objective, which is hidden by the fog of ignorance beyond uncharted terrain. Basic or fundamental research is inherently the process of following obscure and tortuous pathways, many of which have no clear and direct relevance to the ultimate objective. In those circumstances where the basic research has cleared away the theoretical obstacles to progress, a massive attack can be mounted in a logical progression like that employed by NASA (Fig. 3-2). Notable examples include the rapid progress toward a successful vaccine against poliomyelitis once the specific viruses had been identified and grown on embryonic tissues. The repair of congenital heart defects demonstrated rapid progress when the diagnosis could be established by cardiac catheterization and heart-lung machines became available. When the underlying and theoretical foundations are grossly inadequate, the broad, frontal attack illustrated in Figure 3-1b may appear attractive, but it has far less prospect of providing the desired return on investment within any predictable time frame. The efficiency or the scientific logic, deeply desired by all concerned, is often deficient and disappointing. For these reasons, it becomes imperative that a clear distinction be drawn between technical and theoretical obstacles to progress in research and development.

DIFFERENTIATING TECHNICAL AND THEORETICAL OBSTACLES

The most convenient way to illustrate the nature and significance of the distinctions between technical and theoretical obstacles is to describe some examples. The scientific community is frequently challenged by the query, "If we can land a man on the moon, why can't we cure cancer?" This has been a compelling argument in support of a massive attack on dreaded killers such as cancer, heart disease, stroke, and other common, chronic diseases. A closer look will reveal the weakness of this apparent logic. When President Kennedy responded to the challenge of Sputnik with a declared intention to put a man on the moon within a decade, he was establishing the space policy for the subsequent 10 years. The fundamental knowledge required to place a man on the moon was very solid and at hand. The position of the moon in relation to the earth could be predicted with extreme accuracy through centuries of studies by astronomers. World War II had greatly stimulated production of technologies for the maintenance of normal human function under extremely unfriendly environmental conditions, extending from the deserts to the tropics. Physiological requirements for maintaining human function were well established, and mechanisms for maintaining a viable environment within an enclosed compartment in the rarefied atmosphere of space had been well established. Long-standing experience with communications over long distance was clearly adequate for the task. Two major obstacles remained, both of a technical nature. There was a need to develop sufficient power to propel rockets beyond the earth's gravitational field. Extremely precise guidance and control was promised by the emergence of sophisticated computer technologies. Thus, the major obstacles to placing the man on the moon were technical rather than theoretical (Fig. 3-2).

Gravity is a universal experience for all living creatures on earth; its properties, manifestations, and characteristics are known in great detail. The influence of gravity can be lessened by going into outer space, but progress toward directly overcoming the effects of gravity on earth has been essentially ineffectual over an extremely long period of time. Valid arguments could be advanced in favor of a national policy committed to developing mechanisms for overcoming the force of gravity. Benefits would be enormous. Consider the enhanced ability to transport materials with little energy expenditure from one place to another. If the public support could be generated and maintained at sufficiently high levels, Congress might appropriate budgets for a massive attack on the problem through a planned process like that of NASA. It can be predicted with considerable confidence that an expenditure ten times that employed for NASA would probably have revealed little or no progress toward the objective. Levitation would continue to be an illusion that could be provided only by professional magicians. (Fig. 3-2).

These two extreme examples clearly distinguish the differences between theoretical and technical obstacles and their significance in determining the direction and approaches of a research enterprise. Solid, scientific foundation for the NASA program was based on a long and productive history of mathematics, astronomy, physics, chemistry, and engineering (see Chapter 1).

The rapid progress toward the production of an atomic bomb by the Manhattan Project is another favorite example of a major enterprise that appeared to overcome all obstacles and produce dramatic results through the mobilization of massive resources. At the beginning of World War II, atomic theory had been advanced to the point that the composition and structure of nuclei could be pursued through quantitative analysis. An accidental observa-

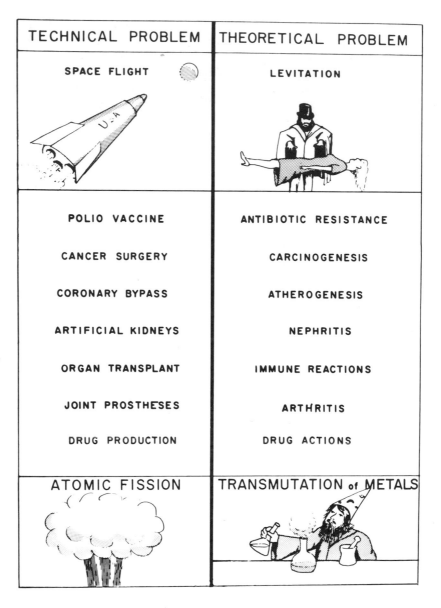

TECHNICAL PROBLEM	THEORETICAL PROBLEM
SPACE FLIGHT	LEVITATION
POLIO VACCINE	ANTIBIOTIC RESISTANCE
CANCER SURGERY	CARCINOGENESIS
CORONARY BYPASS	ATHEROGENESIS
ARTIFICIAL KIDNEYS	NEPHRITIS
ORGAN TRANSPLANT	IMMUNE REACTIONS
JOINT PROSTHESES	ARTHRITIS
DRUG PRODUCTION	DRUG ACTIONS
ATOMIC FISSION	TRANSMUTATION of METALS

Figure 3-2. The distinctions between technical and theoretical obstacles to progress are illustrated by the "conquest of space" in contrast with "overcoming gravity." Technical biomedical problems can be overcome by mobilizing and integrating efforts. Theoretical problems defy massive attacks pending elucidation of fundamental concepts by basic research or serendipity.

92

tion by Otto Hahn in Berlin indicated that a controlled reaction was attainable, a prospect initially unrecognized by him. Neils Bohr learned of the accident and relayed the destructive implications to a number of refugee scientists, including Szilard, Fermi, and Teller. Thus, theoretical obstacles were cleared to the release of enormous amounts of energy by a process of transmuting metals, an objective with long history.

The Manhattan Project brings to mind another extreme example—the theoretical problems faced by the alchemists. Modern chemistry can be traced back to the trial and error gropings of alchemists dedicated to finding ways to transmute base metals into gold. This was a long-range, precisely defined, and highly desirable research goal. However, the fundamental knowledge was totally inadequate. The entire wealth of the medieval world could have been channeled into a greatly expanded effort in alchemy, without affecting progress toward the transmutation of metals. This process is somewhat reminiscent of the problems confronted by the research community engaged for many years in the cancer chemotherapy program, devoted to identification of chemicals that have the effect of killing the rapidly-developing cancer cells and sparing normal tissues. Such an attractive objective has limited prospects of success without some accidental discovery that would clarify basic or fundamental issues. The search for an effective chemical could have been approached on a much more rational basis if the essential differences between cancer cells and normal cells had been well established through fundamental research. Even better, a knowledge of the mechanisms responsible for uncontrolled multiplication of cancer cells would have served far better as a launching pad for an exploration of cancer chemotherapeutic agents. This complex issue is discussed in greater detail in the next chapter (Chapter 4).

INDISTINCT DEFINITIONS OF BASIC VS APPLIED
RESEARCH AND DEVELOPMENT

The persistent demands that the health-related research enterprise shift its emphasis strongly from basic research toward applications has become progressively more strident. Biomedical investigators have consistently replied that *all* biological research, basic *and* applied, is intended for ultimate application and benefit to patients. The scientific leadership has professed inability to draw distinctions between basic and applied research. This stance has effectively preserved flexibility in the pursuit of individual research efforts as well as the distribution of grant and contract resources on a national scale. The key phrases "basic research" and "fundamental knowledge" have been converted into stimuli for conditioned reflexes by the reluctance of the biomedical community to apply more concise criteria for distinguishing between the stages of progress from fundamental, or pure science, toward applications. Senator Edward Kennedy, announcing impending hearings on health research, stated, "At root, medical research is dedicated to uncovering new knowledge—for science's sake—not for the conquest of specific diseases or development of new technologies" (2). During their initial stages, the Kennedy Committee hearings were oriented toward attempting to determine the proportion of resources that were being disbursed for basic research by the organizational components of NIH and ADAMHA. The vague answers provided by the leadership of NIH and other agencies clearly failed to satisfy the Congressional committee. There has been a progressive tendency for basic research to be identified in the minds of critics as intellectual pursuits of somewhat self-serving scientists. Applied research has become synonymous with tangible benefits to the public and the political constituency. This semantic problem is not confined to biomedical areas, but clearer definitions were employed in a National Science Foundation report for the Senate Budget Committee (3, 4).

> Research is systematic, intensively directed toward fuller scientific knowledge or understanding of the subject studies. Research may be classified as either basic or applied.

> In basic research, the investigator is concerned primarily with gaining a fuller knowledge or understanding of the subject under study.

> In applied research, the investigator is primarily interested in a practical use of the knowledge or understanding for the purpose of meeting a recognized need.

> Development is systematic use of the knowledge and understanding gained from research, directed toward the production of useful materials, devices, systems, or methods, including design and development of prototypes and processes. It excludes quality control, routine product testing, and production.

These definitions appear to draw clear distinctions between the three different investigative categories of activities: basic research, applied research, and development. Despite general agreement on these terms, the various agencies of government consistently express difficulty in distinguishing basic research (see Table 3-1.) These definitions seem vague and evasive. It seems timely to consider more specific and detailed distinctions between the identifiable stages in the pursuit of progress toward methods of managing disease and disability as it affects the American public.

RATIONALIZING BASIC AND APPLIED RESEARCH REQUIREMENTS

As a general principle, basic research is directed at enhancing understanding of *theoretical problems* while applied research and development is oriented toward overcoming the technical obstacles to the development of tangible benefits to mankind. The characteristics of technical and theoretical obstacles are fairly easily distinguished at the extremes. In the middle ground, these differences become less distinct.

Operational definitions are employed at NIH to designate categories of

TABLE 3-1. Distinguishing Between Basic and Applied Research*

Agriculture Department: Basic research is generally inseparable from other research in both planning and conduct.

Environmental Protection Agency: There is no official differentiation between basic and applied research in EPA . . . which research falls into which category is open to debate.

Smithsonian Institution: For basic research, the end product is commonly the advancement of scientific knowledge in general. The goal of applied research is usually described as discovery of new scientific knowledge with a specific objective in mind.

Energy Research and Development Administration: The concept poses difficulties whenever the utility of the expected results is a criterion for choosing research tasks. (Different definitions of basic research are used in different contexts within ERDA.)

National Institutes of Health: "Although these conceptual distinctions can be made, it must be noted that basic and applied research form a continuum, and a specific research project may be basic from one point of view and applied from another. This fact makes it difficult and in some cases meaningless to speak of research as either basic or applied; it is usually more meaningful to speak of research as having basic and applied aspects."

National Science Board: Most agencies indicated that the same research project could be considered basic by the performer of the research and applied by the provider of funds; a difference in viewpoint that leads to serious anomalies in statistical data on support of basic research.

*From Basic Research in the Mission Agencies. Agency perspectives on the conduct and support of basic research, National Science Board, 1978.

research as part of this differentiation. Clinical trials and developmental contracts have been placed in the A (for "applied") category (5). Activities related to technology transfer have been designated under T (for "transfer"). The area of research training is also designated with a T. Finally, that which is left has been called S (for "science base"), representing activities which are primarily investigator-initiated intended to add to the fund of knowledge. These four categories have been designated as the SATT system, for the purpose of categorizing new initiatives. The development of operational categories to facilitate allocation of resources is clearly an important and necessary step. This process will vividly illuminate the need for more specific and understandable operational distinctions between the various kinds of research and development.

OPERATIONAL DEFINITIONS FOR RESEARCH AND DEVELOPMENT (A TENTATIVE PROPOSAL)

The differences between highly complex issues can rarely be clearly designated by simple statements as evident in the obfuscations between basic and applied research mentioned above. The multitude of activities which are embraced by the term biomedical research is far too complicated to readily fit into two large and inclusive categories. Definitions which are based upon operational aspects of the various activities can draw clearer distinctions between phases of research and development. For this purpose, a tentative proposal is advanced to illustrate the possibility of attaining these objectives (Table 3-2).

Fundamental ("pure") Research. The term *basic research* has come to embrace so many different kinds of activities, that its use commonly produces semantic confusion. Several subdivisions of basic research can be identified and defined. The most fundamental research is often designated "pure" research, signifying that the objective of the exploration is to gain knowledge and understanding without concern or responsibility for the ultimate relevance or application of the derived data. There is a clearly recognized place in our society for "pure" research. Many of society's greatest benefits have been derived from observations and insights by highly talented persons whose activities were not concerned at all with the practical applications of their activities. However, the number of creative persons capable of making substantial contributions to "pure" science is exceedingly restricted (see also Chapter 7).

The United States is well endowed with large numbers of people who have superior technical competence. In contrast, only exceptional people have that special scientific creativity that provides insight into complicated theoretical problems. Relatively few people are endowed with the spark of creativity that permits them to overleap the current limitations on human concepts and arrive at wholly new insights or discoveries. Such unique individuals most commonly function alone or as leaders of small, select teams. In the British tradition, such talent needs to be carefully and selectively identified, provided with adequate support with long-term funding, and encouraged to engage in free-ranging explorations with the utmost scientific freedom (see Chapter 7). This should not necessarily excuse the investigators engaged in fundamental research from periodic reports or reviews of progress, but it should place little or no limitations on the scope or content of their enterprise, so long as it remains demonstrably productive. The category of fundamental research should be reserved for investigators with well established reputations as being productive, innovative, and creative by critical judgement of their peers. Examples of fundamental or pure research which are cross-cutting and of significance to virtually all areas of biomedical science would include molecular biology, genetics, immunology, and neurochemistry as typical examples (6). Generous and long-range support of the most innovative intellects in the country engaged in pure research on such subjects can easily be defended as an investment of great value, regardless of the ultimate practical applications of their output.

Thus, fundamental research is characterized by exploration and analysis of underlying principles. Strategies may be based on a "hunch" or involve quantitative studies and analyses that are not targeted toward any particular application. The experimental objects of study are usually envisioned as small and discrete units, such as cellular and subcellular structure and function. On the contrary, a very wide choice of levels, extending from molecules to mammals and even to populations, can be encompassed by this term. Such research is normally conducted in academic or Institute laborator-

TABLE 3-2. Distinguishable Categories of Research and Development

	Research					Development		
Characteristics	Fundamental Research	Functional Research	Targeted Research	Clinical Investigation	Clinical Evaluation	Technology Transfer	Diffusion Production	Marketing
Goals	Adding to Stores of Knowledge in the Form of Data, Relationships, Concepts					Development and Distribution of Useful, Effective, Reliable, Safe Procedures, Techniques, and Technologies		
Objectives	Elemental analysis, underlying concepts	Structure, function, control of organs	Pathophysiological cause and cure of diseases	Diagnosis, therapy, course of disease, and disabilities	Safety, utility, benefits of technology	Development of new drugs, devices, and procedures	Providing access to innovations	Distribution, maintenance of medical materials
Strategies	Quantitative analytical studies of elemental functions	Exploration elucidation of organ functions	Quest for intimate causes and cures of diseases	Clinical signs symptoms, data, course, therapy, rehabilitation, complications	Assessing effectiveness, safety, reliability, validity	Experimental prototype production, testing	Design, produce reliable drugs, devices	Develop sales and maintenance capability
Experimental Objects	Wide choice molecules to mammals, cells to populations	Potentially extrapolated to mammals	Potentially extrapolated to human patients	Human subjects or patients	Human subjects or patients	Drugs, devices, procedures	Health care personnel and medical institutions	
Institutional settings	Academic or institute laboratories	Principally academic and institute laboratories	Academic, institute governmental industrial laboratories	Hospitals, clinics, laboratories	Hospitals, clinics, laboratories, F.D.A.	Biomedical engineering, industrial laboratories	Industrial, sales, facilities	
Time frames	Unpredictable extended commitments	3–7 yrs.	3–7 yrs.	3–5 yrs.	2–4 yrs.	uncertain 3–10 yrs.	2–3 years.	Indefinite

ies, and the time frame is unpredictable because the objectives cannot be clearly defined (Table 3-2).

Functional Research. The basic medical sciences of biochemistry, anatomy, and physiology are oriented in general toward the study of the normal function. A knowledge of normality is clearly necessary for the detection and understanding of malfunction. During the past 30 years, a substantial proportion of the research commonly called "basic" would be included within this category. The information gained from such studies is clearly relevant to an understanding of disease, but it does not appear to the average citizen as relevant to the care of patients.

The exploration of the structure, function, and control of tissues and organs of various species can be either descriptive, quantitative, or analytical explorations of features which potentially can be extrapolated to mammalian organs. Such research is also conducted primarily in academic or Institute laboratories, and the appropriate time frames extend from five to seven years for a major project (Table 3-2).

Targeted Research. The study of malfunction or pathophysiology of organs and systems has distinct relevance to disease processes, and yet may fall between fundamental research and clinical applications. Implicit in these studies are the responses of organisms and organs to stress. The initial focus may center on the time-course of malfunction or disease, on the reserves which are depleted by disease processes or the potential mechanisms for alleviating the consequences of these malfunctions. Searches for *causes* and *cures* can be used as an oversimplified catch phrase to identify the ultimate objective of such investigations (see Chapter 4).

The basic medical sciences of pathology, microbiology, and pharmacology are nominally oriented more closely toward elucidation of the nature and causes of pathological processes or therapeutic approaches by means of drugs and related agents. The fact that the prime targets of these disciplines are inherently oriented toward either malfunction or perturbation of function makes their output appear more relevant to attacks on disease. Many foreign schools have departments of *pathophysiology*. Such departments are oriented toward the study of the causes and mechanisms that are central to malfunction, diseases, and disabilities. This is a role that has not been adequately covered by the traditional American basic medical sciences and deserves consideration as a possible addition to the research enterprise of this country (see also Chapter 7). A common strategy is the simulation and/or analysis of abnormal function or responses to stresses. The experimental objects are usually selected in the hope that results can be extrapolated to human subjects or patients.

Functional and "targeted" research have distinguishing features which are indicated more extensively in Table 3-2. Research in these categories merits relatively long-term support but more concisely defined objectives and more consistent and effective monitoring of progress than is appropriate for fundamental research. Some adverse reactions of critics may stem from a sense that the past emphasis has been excessive on normal physiology and insufficient on pathophysiology.

Clinical Investigation. The patterns of signs and symptoms, the characteristics of syndromes, and the courses of illness are the primary areas of study of clinical investigation. Elaboration of clinical signs, symptoms, and laboratory data required for diagnosis is a key feature of this category. In addition, the mechanisms for effective treatment or management, along with complications that may occur, and the process of rehabilitation are all encompassed in this area. In general, the experimental objects are human subjects or patients, although mammalian prototypes may be employed in such studies as well. These explorations tend to be carried out in clinics and in clinical laboratories. The time span is of varying duration—typically three to five years.

There are at least two recognizable roles for clinical research. The traditional responsibility has been to define and describe as objectively as possible a wide variety of malfunctions, diseases, and disabilities and plot the course of these ailments or illnesses. This process includes the need to specify the kinds of diagnostic tools which are required for recognition and monitoring of diseases, and also the development of new and therapeutic approaches. Until relatively recently, medically trained clinicians were the principal source of innovations in terms of both diagnostic and therapeutic technologies. The last 15 years have witnessed the evolution of a powerful combination between clinicians and biomedical engineers in the joint specification of requirements for new techniques and technologies, the design of prototypes, evaluation for effectiveness, and finally production on the industrial level. The success of this process is manifest in the large and evergrowing array of sophisticated technologies, which are now commonplace in standard medical facilities (see Chapter 5).

Clinical Evaluation. By virtue of the rapid progress that has occurred in the development of new diagnostic and therapeutic techniques, there is a large and growing need for more formal mechanisms to evaluate the effectiveness, safety, and cost/benefit of newly developed processes, procedures, and techniques. In the past, clinical evaluation has been largely included as part of the process of development. Such assessments are an extension of the standard engineering type of evaluation required to establish safety and efficacy of new devices or procedures. In the past, there has been a widespread tendency among the medical professions to enthusiastically adopt new diagnostic and therapeutic technologies before they have been properly evaluated for effectiveness and cost/benefit (see the section on technology assessment in Chapter 5).

Outcome analysis as a means of evaluating the effectiveness of the interventions by medical facilities and services is an obligation of clinicians that has not been very well developed thus far (see Chapter 6). In view of the enormous progress made in developing objective and quantitative diagnostic tools, their use in monitoring the course of illness and the evaluation of effectiveness of therapy has been seriously neglected. The program of clinical trials recently mounted by the Heart, Lung, and Blood Institute is a specific example of an embryonic effort in this extremely important category of clinical investigation. Lacking this crucial information, the priorities for expenditure for facilities and services in hospitals all over the country cannot be established on rational grounds. Mechanisms for collecting the essential information are poorly developed and exorbitantly expensive at present. This issue will be discussed in more detail in relation to health services research in Chapter 6.

DEVELOPMENTAL PROCESSES: ULTIMATE OUTPUT OF RESEARCH AND DEVELOPMENT

The growth of medical electronics and sophisticated medical technologies has proceeded at such a rapid rate during the last 10 years that there seems to be little need for any encouragement in this area if the preceding steps had been adequately managed. However, it is important to distinguish the production and diffusion of technologies clearly from other forms of research to be certain that the mechanisms for stimulation and control are appropriate to the needs (Table 3–2).

TRANSFER OF TECHNOLOGIES

Clinical investigators function at an invisible interface between their patients, basic medical scientists, and biomedical engineers. The typical lack of knowledge and experience of physicians with technical problems is in part responsible for an intolerance to devices that do not perform consistently and well. However, the process of refining experimental prototypes into reliable, consistently operative devices is enormously expensive (see also Fig. 3–3b). Medical markets should be established before they are released for wide-spread public use. Unfortunately, the current mechanisms for establishing these characteristics are seriously impeding progress of the transfer of technology into clinical practice.

CONVERSION OF KNOWLEDGE INTO USEFUL TECHNOLOGIES

The common perception that basic research leads to new technologies has been discussed and illustrated in Figure 3–1A. Such an idealized version has been called the "innovation chain" by Haeffner (7). He proposed an alternative model composed of two parallel pathways, one leading toward knowledge as the output of research, while a separate pathway was involved in the creation of new and innovative devices or technologies. All previous research efforts have contributed to vast stores of knowledge and experience. The persons who are engaged in a search for new masses of knowledge rarely undertake the process of exploiting the available information. Haeffner's concept, adapted to the present discussion, incorporates the contributions and mutual interactions of fundamental, functional, targeted, clinical research and development. From these various sources are accumulated the knowledge, concepts, and experience of previous and current investigative activities. The vast store of information is a reservoir, which can be called on by innovative scientists as the source of vital information regarding unmet needs, conceptual approaches, successful experimental designs, and experimental prototypes (Fig. 3-3b).

The process of developing new research, diagnostic, or therapeutic devices is initiated most commonly as a recognition of unmet need. Envisioning a new technology is a creative process that can occur to a select few people, but even fewer are in positions to respond appropriately. Indeed, the identification of need is relatively useless without an idea or practical approach by which it can be met. A basic medical scientist or a clinician in academic life has relatively few incentives and even less opportunity to pursue such goals, even if this is viewed as desirable. The rapidly emerging field of biomedical engineering has been the principal pathway by which such a process can proceed most effectively. Alternatively, collaborative efforts can be established between basic medical scientists, clinicians, engineers, and/or industrial corporations. In any case, the concept leads to feasibility studies and the development of experimental prototypes. A fairly large number of such activities proceed to this level. However, there is a critical stage of development that requires the construction of a number of prototypes that are sufficiently reliable and dependable that they can be subjected to evaluation or clinical trial. The process of developing refined experimental prototypes is exceedingly expensive and is beyond the financial capabilities of most research laboratories. Most industrial corporations are wary of investing the large sums required without some assurance that there is a market. However, the availability of the market depends in turn upon successful clinical evaluations. For these reasons production of reliable prototypes for evaluation represents a large *missing link* in the process in many instances. In contrast, there are disturbing examples of intuitively useful new instruments emerging upon the scene and being accepted with exorbitant enthusiasm without appropriate evaluation (see also Chapter 5).

The process of converting fundamental information and experience into goods and services is extremely complex and therefore unpredictable. It is frequently difficult to understand how the process can be so very rapid in some instances and so frustratingly slow in others. In the case of biomedical techniques and technologies, we are simultaneously confronted with vivid examples of both precipitous and tardy transfer of technology into widespread clinical applications.

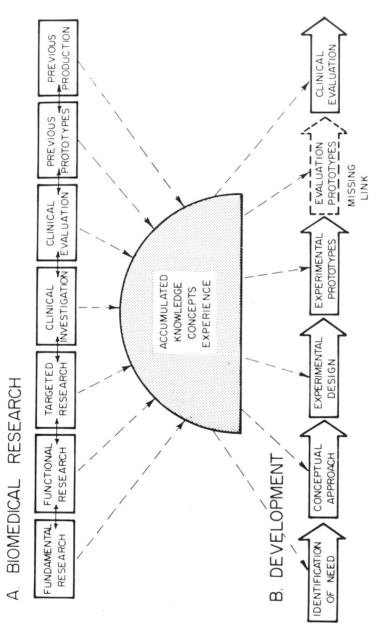

Figure 3-3. The development of new techniques and technologies for health care can be portrayed as two parallel pathways: (*a*) The accumulation of knowledge and experience through a wide variety of research activities. (*b*) The identification of an unmet need, coupled with ideas or concepts for new or improved approaches. The production of effective and reliable evaluation prototypes is often a "missing link" because it involves large financial risks (see text).

DIFFUSION OF DEVELOPMENTS:
TOO FAST OR TOO SLOW?

The development, production, and diffusion of new devices poses a strange paradox. On the one hand, there are many examples of sophisticated and expensive technologies that have emerged and been rapidly expanded at enormous expense and so rapidly that there was inadequate time for a critical evaluation of their effectiveness, safety, and contribution to the health of the nation. Notable examples include the rapid expansion of facilities for open heart surgery, intensive care of coronary patients, computerized axial tomography (CAT scanners), and coronary bypass operations. These familiar examples stem from a very much longer list containing a mixture of both diagnostic and therapeutic technologies, which are contributing greatly to the overall costs of health care delivery. Their contribution to the health of the recipients remains unsettled. These techniques and technologies undoubtedly have obvious potential for contributing to the health of the nation, particularly if they are appropriately utilized. The resolution of this paradox will ultimately require extensive study of the research and development process itself: an enterprise which has only just begun in recent years.

Comroe and Dripps (8) accepted the challenge of attempting to demonstrate that objective and scientific techniques could be used to justify the national biomedical research priorities. They were stimulated by Project Hindsight, a study by the Department of Defense indicating that 20 important military weapons were developed with little contribution by university research. Furthermore, scientists were stated to contribute most effectively when their effort was mission-oriented. The lag times between initial discovery and final application were believed to be shortened when the work was in areas "targeted" by the sponsor. To test such views, the "top ten clinical advances" in cardiovascular and pulmonary medicine and surgery of the last 30 years were selected for study, and a extensive literature review was undertaken on the following:

· Open heart surgery
· Cardiac resuscitation, defibrillation, pacing
· Intensive cardiovascular and respiratory care
· Chemotherapy and antibiotics
· Vascular surgery
· Medical treatment of coronary insufficiency
· Oral diuretics
· New diagnostic methods
· Drug treatment of hypertension
· Prevention of poliomyelitis

Some 6,000 published articles were examined, of which 3,400 specific reports were regarded as important in the development of 137 essential bodies of knowledge. The report of this study is summarized in Figure 3–4 with some specific examples of the various lag times between initial discoveries and the clinical applications of a variety of important methods and devices (9). For purposes of clarification, these various developments have been organized under diagnostic methods and therapeutic techniques and have been placed in appropriate positions on a time scale extending from 1895 to the present (Fig. 3-4).

Clinical applications of x-rays demonstrated a very rapid conversion from initial discovery to practical application. Roentgen rays were discovered in 1895 and within one year had been used to make x-ray photographs of human bones. Before the turn of the century, Thomas Edison had designed and developed a functioning fluoroscope for clinical applications. Angiography became a clinical reality within a year after the synthesis of organic iodides in 1929. An image intensifier was readied for clinical use six year after image intensification had been demonstrated by Chamberlain in 1942. The development of clinically useful ultrasonic flow sensing devices proceeded within seven years from the original design of an ultrasonic flow sensor. Echocardiography using ultrasound required approximately 13 years to be developed. Twenty-four years passed between the first electrocardiogram on a frog and the design and development of an electrocardiograph for use on humans. Electrocardiographic signs of arrythmias and infarction were established after elapsed times of seven and eight years, respectively. The ability to transmit electrocardiographic information by telephone was delayed 51 years after the necessary technology was available. Applications of radioisotopes as tracers varied in lag times from 4 years for their use in the study of circulation time to 27 years for their use in detecting blood volume. The development of laboratory instruments varied in duration from 5 years for gas analyzers to 71 years for the development of strain gauge pressure sensors. Some of these extensive lag times would give credence to the concept that there exist in the modern research laboratories large numbers of potentially useful devices that have not yet been exploited. The reverse argument could be used for those examples in which the developments proceeded with extreme rapidity as in the case of x-ray visualization. A contrasting trend is obvious in the case of the computerized axial tomography (CAT scanner), which has spread widely through the United States with unbridled enthusiasm before its ultimate utility has been established. The discrepancy between the lag times observed for x-ray, electrocardiography, ultrasound, and radioisotopes is difficult to interpret since they are all important diagnostic methodologies (Fig. 3-4).

Therapeutic techniques have also exhibited extremely and unexpectedly long time-lags. Most notable is penicillin, which was delayed 64 years from the observation by Tyndall (1877) of antagonism between bacteria and penicillin. Fleming's observation that penicillin lyses strep colonies was made in 1929, and penicillin emerged in the early 1940s.

Some of the time delay ascribed to surgical procedures may be unrealistic. For example, the development of coronary artery bypass by Favaloro (1968) followed by 27 years the observation that most occlusions of the coronary arteries are in the proximal 4 centimeters of the coronary branches. Such an observation might have indicated possibilities rather than actual applications. Similarly, the development of artificial organs as functional and anatomic substitutes generally took relatively long periods, with the exception of the use of plastic prosthetics for heart valve replacements.

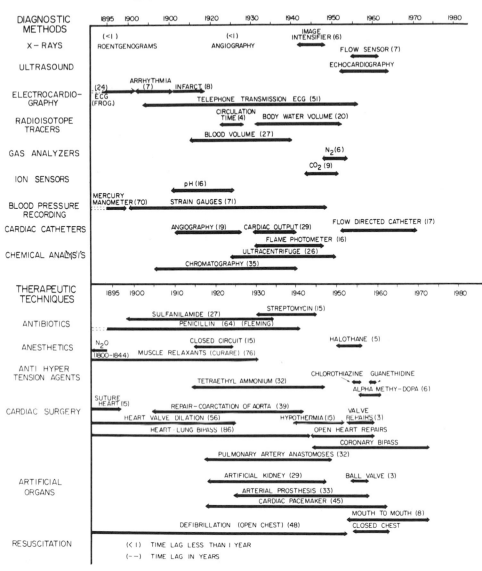

LAG TIMES FROM INITIAL DISCOVERY TO CLINICAL APPLICATION

Figure 3-4. The time elapsing between initial discovery and clinical application of a variety of diagnostic and therapeutic innovations varies from less than one year (i.e., roentgen rays for x-ray imaging) to more than 50 years (i.e., antibiotics). Obviously, these developments have not proceeded along a linear pathway (see Fig. 3-1). The factors responsible for the long time lags are not obvious and have rarely been explored (8–10).

Analysis of the processes and outcomes of research is relatively new and untried. There is pressing need for mechanisms to illuminate the process; namely, a more critical evaluation of the outcome of investment in research and development. For example, Alexis Carroll performed virtually every necessary technique used in vascular surgery today between 1902 and 1910, with the exception of the use of the dissecting microscope and of plastic tubes, neither of which had been discovered at that time. However, his work was not pursued by others and was virtually neglected until 1940 (10).

In view of the potential importance that could be derived from knowledge regarding the productivity and outcome of research activities, deficiencies in information in this area are astonishing.

CRITERIA FOR CATEGORICAL BALANCE

Death rates and life expectancies have been regarded as the crucial criteria of health status ever since death certificates became required in the early nineteenth century. There can be little question that the dreaded killer diseases have preempted the attention of the nation and the major emphasis of our biomedical research effort. In view of history, it is not surprising that cancer and heart disease have occupied such dominant positions in the mounting of the biomedical research enterprise. Death as an unequivocal end point seemed an appropriate index in the years before more accurate diagnoses were generally available. However, there are now many reliable sources of information on the prevalence and incidence of serious chronic and acute illnesses that also could subserve the role of indicators of the national health status. Continued reliance on death rates as the prime indicator of national health status seems somewhat inappropriate when the population explosion is one of the major societal concerns of modern times. For this reason, it seems appropriate to examine some other potential criteria as the basis for attaining better balance in the distribution of resources in support of biomedical research efforts (see also Chapter 6).

CAUSES OF DISABILITY

Disability from disease is much more common and has a distribution that is very different from the leading causes of death. Despite enormous progress in preventing, curing, and controlling communicable diseases, the incidence of disability from infections remains more than 10 times greater than from cardiovascular disease and several hundred times more common than death from any heart disease or cancer (Table 3-3).

Obviously, the most common infections (such as colds, influenza, and pneumonia) appear relatively innocuous when compared to mortality from any disease, particularly cancer. The incidence of disability from infections is some 300 times greater than mortality from cardiovascular heart attacks. There seems to be justification for some revision in our national biomedical research priorities. We have no yardsticks that permit comparison of the relative importance of one death from heart disease and 300 patients suffering from infections of mild or serious degree. However, it seems quite probable that our present priorities would be very different if the traditional and current goals of medicine were to *avoid or to alleviate suffering* rather

TABLE 3-3.

Major Causes of Death 1975		Prevalence of Disabilities[a]	
Cardiovascular diseases	979,180	Infections	224,000,000
Acute heart attack	328,670	Common cold	100,000,000
Subacute and chronic heart		Influenza	80,000,000
disease	319,740	Pneumonia	3,000,000
Cerebrovascular diseases (e.g.,		Gonorrhea	840,000
strokes)	195,630	Streptococcal sore throat,	
Arteriosclerosis and other		scarlet fever	430,000
arterial and capillary diseases	54,610	Cardiovascular	28,410,000
Hypertensive diseases	17,570	High blood pressure, hyper-	
Cancer	371,740	tensive heart disease	22,950,000
Digestive organs and peri-		Coronary heart disease (heart	
toneum	101,880	attack, angina pectoris)	3,940,000
Respiratory system	88,460	Cerebrovascular disease (stroke)	1,730,000
Genital organs	43,160	Gastrointestinal	21,900,000
Breast	32,570	Stomach and duodenal ulcers[b]	—
Lymphatic and hematopoletic		Ileitis and colitis	1,000,000
tissues	20,480	Respiratory	—
Infective and parasitic diseases	72,760	Chronic sinusitis	20,600,000
Pneumonia		Hay fever	10,800,000
Influenza		Mental and emotional	20,000,000
Diabetes mellitus	35,890	Arthritic	20,250,000
Respiratory diseases	26,120		
Emphysema	18,410		
Acute and chronic bronchitis			
and bronchiolitis	5,670		
Birth injury, difficult labor, etc.	15,200		
Congenital anomalies	14,380		

[a]Figures are rounded estimates for annual cases and have been compiled by the Department of Health, Education and Welfare and also by charitable foundations devoted to assisting in alleviating or curing the major illnesses.

[b]About 10% of the population is estimated to suffer from stomach and duodenal ulcers at some point during their lifetimes.

Carney, Thomas P., *Chemistry in Medicine, Chemical and Engineering News*, 55:28-36, December 1977.

than to *prolong life at any cost*. This statement does not represent an argument for curtailing research into cancer and heart disease but rather a plea to place our priorities in somewhat more rational and scientific perspective.

The priorities used for distribution of research resources should not be derived from a single criterion such as mortality, limitation of activity, hospitalization, days in bed, and so on. Criteria that would take into account these and other considerations would appear to have a valuable place in assessing the relative importance of various illnesses as a basis for appropriating resources for both research and health services. For such purposes,

Black and Pole (11) evaluated 54 different types and categories of disease in terms of five indices chosen to represent types of burdens on the health services. Indices used were as follows: inpatient days, outpatient referrals by general practitioners, general practitioner consultations, morbidity, and mortality. The first three of these indices were related to the use of resources, and the remaining two were related to severity of illness. This approach toward a more comprehensive basis for priority listings has been extended further by the National Center for Health Statistics.

The National Center for Health Statistics has undertaken a program to evaluate the magnitude of the burden of illness in terms of a variety of categories (12). The impact on health services by common chronic conditions has been explored in terms of the extent to which activity is limited, the requirement for medical attention, the number of bed-days per year, and the extent to which the affected patients requested health services (Table 3-4). Cardiovascular conditions, arthritis, and back problems obviously ranked very high in all categories. These were chronic conditions reported in interviews of civilian, noninstitutionalized populations. Heart diseases cause long-term limitation of activity for a large number of people, and more bed days than any other condition. Hypertension impelled the largest number of people to seek advice from a physician during the year.

BURDEN OF ILLNESS IN THE UNITED STATES

The dimensions of the burden of illness can be extended by including a more comprehensive set of criteria including the potential years of life lost, inpatient days, physician office visits, work-loss days, disability in accordance with social security administration records, limitation of major activity, and bed days. The ranking of 16 diagnostic categories in accordance with these dimensions are presented in Figure 3-5. It is interesting to note that diseases of the circulatory system ranked highest in three of the eight indices of burden; respiratory illness ranked highest in three indices as well. The burden due to cancer is less clear, ranking second in only one index of burden and fourth in two indices. Malignancies either cause death rather promptly or are considered cured within a relatively short period of time, resulting in a relatively low prevalence of cancer. At any particular time, there are large numbers of people classified as suffering from hypertension, heart disease, diabetes, arthritis, and other conditions that are controlled rather than cured, but have a far more favorable survival rate than most cancers. Obviously, no single approach is adequate for assessing the relative importance of these widely varied health problems. There is very little prospect of a consensus regarding which methods are preferable. However, there is also little doubt that a multiplicity of considerations should be included in any mechanism employed to develop priorities on which to base the relative distribution of resources for both health services and biomedical research activities.

TABLE 3-4. Impact of Selected Chronic Conditions—United States

Condition	Prevalence	Causing Limitation of Activity	Medical Attention in Past Year	Number of Bed Days per Year	Bothered a Great Deal or Some	Now Under Treatment or Medication Recommended by Doctor
All heart conditions	10,291	4,281	7,729	129,667	4,847	6,031
Coronary heart	3,370	1,988	2,880	52,912	1,915	2,613
Arthritis	18,339	3,228	7,629	66,020	13,864	6,675
Back Problems	8,018	1,964	2,646	32,072	5,573	N/A
Diabetes	4,191	1,245	3,462	24,308	1,425	3,085
Hypertension w/o heart	12,271	1,092	9,890	24,542	3,792	7,301
Asthma	6,031	1,031	3,637	34,980	4,746	3,100
Stroke	1,534	782	1,118	38,503	845	973
Emphysema	1,313	590	785	19,038	847	566
Hernia	3,191	511	1,781	15,636	1,420	594
Ulcer	3,360	366	1,979	21,163	2,369	2,053
Bronchitis	6,526	261	4,666	23,494	4,953	1,299
Hay fever	10,826	162	3,800	6,496	8,314	3,692
Sinusitis	20,582	144	6,710	14,407	15,169	4,507
Hemorrhoids	9,744	68	2,777	6,821	5,661	1,871

National Center for Health Statistics, Health Interview Survey. Selected years 1968–1972.

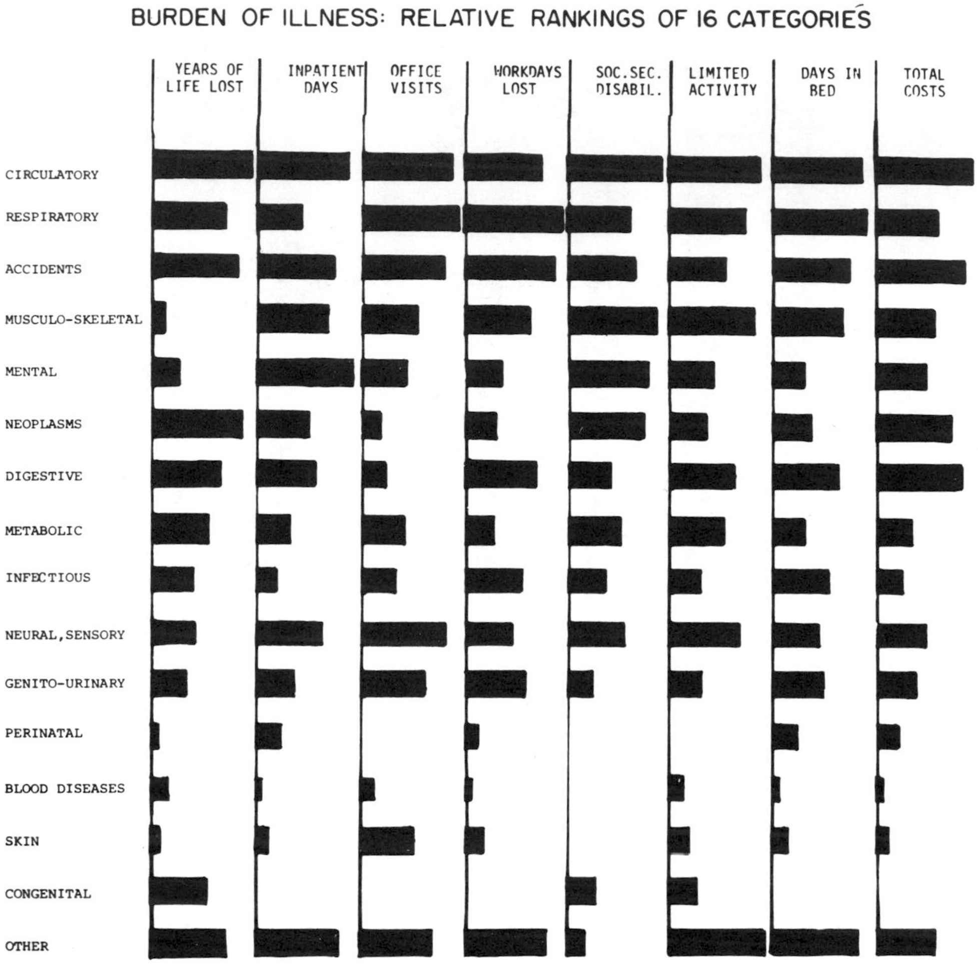

BURDEN OF ILLNESS: RELATIVE RANKINGS OF 16 CATEGORIES

Figure 3-5. The burden of illness on the American people involves many factors in addition to mortality rates or prevalence. The relative rankings of the 16 categories of ailments are represented by horizontal bars. cardiovascular disease ranks first or second in all factors but one. The ranking of the various factors in the vertical columns indicates the nature and relative magnitude of the load imposed by each category (12).

ASSESSING RESEARCH PROGRESS AND STATUS: REDUCING REDUNDANCY

The forward-planning process extends far beyond the requirement to identify current gaps in knowledge, targets of opportunity, or health problems that deserve additional research attention. There is an implicit requirement to make priority judgments regarding which of the unlimited opportunities for research deserve the most resources. Such judgments depend on both ability to forecast future needs and—equally important—to be aware of the current status of knowledge and research efforts. In other words, it is necessary to identify what is known and what issues currently are under study. The outcome of the previous and current research efforts needs documentation to avoid unnecessary and wasteful duplication and redundancy.

At an earlier time, the biomedical community was so small and so intimate that an experienced investigator could assess rather accurately the status of research in his own area. This situation is no longer the case. The magnitude of the research effort in this country and in other countries has grown enormously. The volume of biomedical publications has become so great that assessing the current status of research is most often judged by the quantity of money being expended on research or by the number of publications in various categories while neglecting the assessment of content within these publications. The magnitude of the problem of current research assessment is indicated by the total number of publications being produced continuously by this huge enterprise. For example, publications in *Med-Line* from January 1972 to July 1974 amounted to 573,248 publications. A similar tally of articles in 1973 in the *Science Citation Index* disclosed that about 70% were in clinical medicine, and the remainder were in more basic biomedical research (13). It is necessary to include the publications from other countries as well as our own. The *Science Citation Index* in 1973 disclosed that scientists in the United States were the authors of 42% of all biomedical papers, whereas the British output was approximately 10% of the total—with a budgetary allocation only 5% of that of the United States. West Germany and France accounted for 7% and 6%, respectively, a major change from the situation earlier in this century when these countries clearly dominated the field of medical research. The overall quality of research in theUnited States and the United Kingdom is indicated by the fact that the publications from these countries tend to be cited more commonly than those from any other country, both in absolute numbers and in relation to their contribution to the total.

REPETITIVE AND REDUNDANT RESEARCH

It is generally acknowledged that experimental observations should be confirmed by other investigators to establish their validity. There is little consensus on how many repetitions are required for this purpose. However, a critical examination of the categorized indices of the medical literature discloses a very large number of papers dealing with the same topics, suggesting very extensive repetition of identical or similar experiments. The same impression is gained by attending annual sessions in scientific meetings in which the papers in successive years sound extremely familiar. For example, electrocardiography has been used intensively for the detection of arrhythmias or infarction of the heart for longer than 50 years (see Figure 3-4). The number of observations, experiments, and reports on this subject must number in the tens of thousands, so one might expect the subject to have been thoroughly drained of substance. Yet the torrent of proposals, projects, and papers in this area persists without much decrement. Similar observations can be made with reference to a vast number of "favored topics" in medical research enjoying popularity over the past few decades. A few examples of a long list would include observations using cardiac catheterization, radiography, isotope tracer techniques, ultrasonic methods, and countless others. Similarly, the medical literature is still replete with articles dealing with the therapeutic effects of antibiotics, vascular surgery, defibrillation, and a multitude of traditional drugs. Aspirin has been widely used for more than a century and yet is the subject of a mammoth clinical evaluation (see the section on the clinical trials of the NHLBI in Chapter 2).

The ultimate impact of experimental results obtained in any given year is extremely difficult to estimate. Of the 573,248 publications between 1972 and 1974, relatively few can reasonably be expected to be adjudged as representing tangible advances 5 or 10 years later. The sparse data available on the outcome of past and present research efforts provide few answers to these vital questions. It is the very nature of research, particularly at the fundamental or theoretical level, that very large investments in exploratory efforts are required for each forward step. While no one could reasonably expect most research projects to provide tangible addition to our fund of knowledge, the current trends toward forward planning of research demands more complete information about the current state of knowledge and present projects to arrive at rational priorities and strategies in pursuit of the aims of the various agencies and Institutes.

The National Institutes of Health alone support approximately 13,000 projects. Eight of the Institutes at NIH have acknowledgments for more than a thousand publications a year (14), and four of the Institutes receive more than 2,000 annual acknowledgments of support in biomedical publications (1973). The publications from Institutes tend to be divided rather evenly between journals representing the fields of clinical medicine and journals representing more basic biomedical research (14). The citation of the basic research papers by other authors is far greater than among clinical reports or publications of applications. Basic science research has greater impact than clinical investigations judging by much more frequent citation by other authors. There is increasing interest in the utilization of the frequency of citation of articles as a measure of the impact of the research on the scientific community. If an article is never cited, it has made little impact and only slight contribution to the useful scientific knowledge. On the other hand, articles which are frequently cited clearly have a greater significance in affecting the course of scientific pursuits (15).

MECHANISMS FOR MONITORING RESEARCH PROGRESS

There is decreasing likelihood of significant information remaining unpublished these days, since the incentives for publication are very strong by investigators aspiring to professional advancement and the maintenance of research support. However, none of these mechanisms really deals with the problem of the overall content of the research efforts in terms of the nature of the major research thrust and the progress which has been made toward their stated objectives. Mechanisms for improving the process of assessing progress of science have value for both grantors and grantees.

The monitoring of research results is much more thorough and stringent in intramural than in most extramural programs. The intramural research programs in NIH and elsewhere generally have thorough updating of the progress and contributions of these laboratories on an annual basis. The objectives of the intramural laboratories can be clearly specified, and the staff can be selected on the basis of interest that conforms to these priorities. The annual requirement for justification of the budgets for these laboratories also provides ample motivation for the review of their performance and progress. The collaborative programs carried on by the means of contracts, renewable on an annual basis, are generally monitored relatively closely in terms of both the magnitude of the expenditures and the outcome of the effort. In contrast, very little reporting is requested or required of investigator-initiated projects.

INSTITUTE INITIATED PROGRAMS

The Institute initiatives, which are mounted by means of requests for proposals (RFPs) are implemented by means of contracts. Requests for grant applications (RFAs) also modulate or orchestrate investigator responses. In both instances, the Institutes have an opportunity to guide the directions of a portion of its extramural research effort to a degree considerably greater than is true of the spontaneous investigator-initiated grants. The bulk of research carried out on the basis of research grants (RO1) generally represents commitments of from three to five years, with a requirement for a brief annual report and a final report to be submitted by the investigator. In the past there has been little effort to extract the information from these reports, which tend to lie dormant in the files at NIH. Instead, there is an implied assumption that the scientific community will appropriately recognize the content of this mass of information through publications and through scientific meetings, and use it appropriately. Lacking means by which the outcome of this research is evaluated deprives the reviewing bodies of the information required to assess the effectiveness, the current thrusts of research effort, and the extent to which there is repetition, duplication, and redundancy among the many different research channels. This problem is further complicated by the fact that health-related research is actively pursued in many other agencies of government (see Chapter 2).

EXTRAMURAL GRANTS

The available mechanisms for assessing the current status of research and the progress toward the objectives of the various programs are seriously deficient. The magnitude and directions of the research activities in the overlapping areas of interests of the various Institutes and agencies are not clarified by the current mechanisms in use. In general, the methods used for the purpose depend on assembling information about easily countable characteristics, such as the number of projects, the quantity of money being dispersed, and the number of publications that result.

The Number of Projects. The number of projects funded by the various Institutes is the most readily available information on research thrusts. The assignment of individual projects to the various Institutes is accomplished by the Division of Research Grants (DRG), in accordance with their interpretation of the contents of the proposals. By virtue of the large overlap in areas of interest and research in the various Institutes, it is often difficult to get an overview of the total effort in any particular area. The number of projects supported by the NIH are assembled in two different reference lists. One is devoted to the individual projects and is organized on the basis of the supporting Institute, the name of the investigator, the site of the research, and the title of the project. In addition, there is a cross-reference listing, which represents the various projects under various categories of research objectives. Clearly, the use of a project title composed of 52 letters or less is a totally inadequate basis for judging the content of research projects, program projects, or centers.

Distribution of Resources. In order to meet its financial responsibilities, the NIH maintains an extensive inventory of information regarding the budgets which are supporting the thousands of research projects sponsored by the various categorical Institutes and their subdivisions. For lack of more comprehensive information, every reliance is placed upon financial features of the research programs in the review of current activities and in the formation of forward plans. Even this information has serious deficiencies when used to assess the magnitude of the efforts in research areas that encompass several of the Institutes. The Division of Research Grants can respond to requests from Institutes for the production of an overview of the financial expenditures by the various Institutes in specific research or topical areas. The magnitude and distribution of the research efforts supported by various Institutes and other agencies is largely obscure for lack of definitive data. One of the few examples was a report by the Division of Research Grants on the distribution of research support for immunology in various institutes studied at the request of the NIAID (Table 3-5). Support of immunology was found to be widely distributed through ten of the eleven Institutes. The National Cancer Institute dominated the field with almost twice as much investment as the Institute on Allergy and Infectious Diseases. A similar situation was found to occur in the case of virology as well. These distributions of research effort might be appropriate or even optimal but there is currently no basis for judgment. The nebulous boundaries between the various Institutes of Health virtually assure a broad scale overlap of programs without obvious mechanisms for assessing the utility or validity of the current or planned allocations in terms of overall impact or effectiveness.

Content Coverage. None of the mechanisms described above provides very much insight into the nature and content of research activities. Each project

TABLE 3-5. Distribution of Resources for Research on Immunology (Totals of Projects, Program Projects and R/D Contracts—in thousands)

	NCI (000)	NIAID (000)	NIAMDD (000)	NHLBI (000)	NIGMS (000)
Immune chemistry	$367	$4325	$348	$425	$80
Immunogenetics	2664	3590	286	14	1238
Immune response	7071	11071	2489	1530	399
Immune pathology	2748	3118	672	2130	465
Autoimmune reactions	81	2111	1843	2539	25
Neoplasm immunology	31177	181	138	141	49
Infectious diseases	608	3251	214	101	–
Organ transplants	1184	1218	1763	1735	83
Immunotherapy	16548	6160	22	607	62
Adverse drugs	524	307	–	570	109
Hypersensitivity	17	1633	42	162	128
TOTALS (000)	$62,989	$36,965	$7,817	$9,954	$7,638

*Additional projects included NICHD (63), NINCDS (54), NIDR (36), NEI (32), and NIEHS (14).

From Jones, JA: NIH Support of Immunology FY 1975 Research and Evaluation Branch, Division of Research Grants, NIH, DHEW, April 7, 1976.

is necessarily accompanied by a summary or an abstract which is prepared by the investigator and sent to the Smithsonian Institution for storage and retrieval. This information can be accessed by virtue of key words underlined by the investigator to indicate his evaluation of the principle issues involved in the research project. This valuable store of information has not been fully exploited for the purpose of getting insight into the total research activities in the various channels of biomedical research activity. It represents an example of a means by which the investigators could and should be given additional responsibility for conveying, in easily retrievable form, the nature and intent of their research efforts. (13)

Investigator Intentions: Proposed Review Process. There appears to be a need for an improved mechanism by which the scientific community can have access to extensive and consistent data regarding current status of research in various topical areas. The best sources of such information are the investigators. The mechanism should be simple, widely applicable, consistent, and readily interpreted. In view of the masses of data involved, the recording format should be computer compatible. An example of a format that might be used in addition to or in lieu of the current abstract of the grant or contract proposals is illustrated in Table 3-6.

The General Research Category indicates the level of the research effort as envisioned by the investigator in planning the proposal. The reviewing bodies would be in position to assess the extent to which the proposal conforms to the stated intent and evaluate it accordingly. The scale of the research target from molecules to groups of people could be indicated by inserting the appropriate letter in the square near the right hand margin. If

TABLE 3-6 Indicators of Investigator Intent (Tentative Proposal)

To aid in the assessment of the current health-related research effort and the development of appropriate priorities by the Federal Granting agencies, each investigator is requested to carefully check those items listed below that best describe the purpose and approach of the investigation proposed in the accompanying application for research grant or contract. INSERT MOST APPROPRIATE NUMBERS OR LETTERS IN THE SQUARES ☐ ON THE RIGHT HAND MARGIN.

GENERAL RESEARCH CATEGORY

1	2	3	4	5	6	Insert Appropriate Letter or Number ☐
FUNDAMENTAL	FUNCTIONAL	TARGETED	CLINICAL INVESTIGATION	CLINICAL EVALUATION	TECHNICAL DEVELOPMENT	

SCALE OF RESEARCH TARGET

A.	B.	C.	D.	E.	F.	G.	H.	
Molecular	Subcellular	Cells or Tissues	Organs	Organ Systems	Whole Person	Groups	Other ____	☐

SPECIFIC RESEARCH INTEREST

1. FUNDAMENTAL

A MOLECULAR	B VIROLOGY	C MICROBIOLOGY	D IMMUNOLOGY	E GENETICS	F METABOLISM	
G SECRETION	H EXCRETION	I DIFFUSION	J TRANSPORT	K MOTILITY	L EXCITATION	
M DIFFUSION	N MEMBRANES	O RECEPTORS	P MITOSIS	Q REPLICATION	R AGING	☐
S BEHAVIOR	T OTHER ____					

2. FUNCTIONAL (Organ system oriented)

A	B	C	D	E	F
NERVOUS	SENSES	CARDIOVASCULAR	RESPIRATORY	GASTROINTESTINAL	URINARY

G	H	I	J	K	
REPRODUCTIVE	MUSCULAR	SKELETAL	RETICULOENDOTHELIAL	ENDOCRINE	

L OTHER _____ ☐

1	2	3	4	5	6
METABOLISM	EXCITATION	CONTRACTION	EXCRETION	SECRETION	DIGESTION

7	8	9	10	11	12
CIRCULATION	TRANSPORT	REPRODUCTION	SENSATION	ADAPTATION	COGNITION

13	14	15	16	17
CONTROL: Neural	Chemical	Hormonal	Integration	Coordination

18 Other _____ ☐

3, 4, or 5—TARGETED, CLINICAL INVESTIGATION, OR CLINICAL EVALUATION

A	B	C	D	E
NERVOUS	SENSES	CARDIOVASCULAR	RESPIRATORY	GASTROINTESTINAL

F	G	H	I	J	K
URINARY	REPRODUCTIVE	MUSCULAR	SKELETAL	RETICULOENDOTHELIAL	ENDOCRINE

L OTHER _____ ☐

TABLE 3-6 (Continued)

ORGAN SPECIFIC* (Disease or disability peculiar to specific organs such as multiple sclerosis (CNS), atherosclerosis (CV) emphysema (Resp.), Peptic ulcer (GI), Nephrosis (GU), etc.) ☐

Please insert name of organ specific ailment _____

NON SPECIFIC DISTURBANCES ☐

2 CONGENITAL	3 INFECTIONS	4 INFLAMMATIONS	5 ALLERGIES	6 HYPERACTIVITY
7 PROLIFERATION	8 DEGENERATION	9 AGING	10 UNCOORDINATION	

11 OTHER _____

TARGETS OF INVESTIGATION (Please specify under Principal Aims) ☐

20 Dx Symptoms	21 Signs	22 Chemical tests	23	24 Clinical Lab	25 Imaging
26 Monitoring course of illness	27 Rx Symptomatic	28 Pharmaceutic	29 Physical		
30 Remedial	31 Curative	32 Outcome	33 Preventive	34 Immunization	
35 Health maintenance	36 Risk avoidance	37 Healthy habits			

118

the investigator indicated that his specific research interest lay in the General Research Category number 1 (Fundamental Research), he could identify more concisely the nature of his approach by inserting a letter corresponding to one of the list ranging from molecular to behavior or insert his own if none obviously applies. Incidentally, the tabulation of content of blanks labeled "other" could provide valuable insight into what additional types need to be added to the form. They would also indicate something about the nonconventional areas that might deserve additional attention. A similar approach would be available to the person planning to conduct functional research by identifying the organ system and the function of the organ system under study. For this tentative example, details of interest among researchers investigating disease processes under the categories of targeted, clinical investigation and clinical evaluation might be able to indicate their topic of research interest by identifying the organ system and the nature of the disease process as a second step. Two categories of disease s are listed, namely organ specific (named) or nonspecific pathological processes which affect the organ under study. Finally, the targets of the investigation can be specified in terms of the clinical signs, symptoms, data sources, diagnostic efforts or therapeutic approaches.

The combination of the eight letters and numbers appearing along the right hand margin of the table would provide a wealth of information on the nature and distribution of the national research effort if it could be routinely compiled, analyzed, and distributed. Such information could serve a useful purpose for investigators wishing to avoid unnecessary duplication of effort in his selection of research areas. It would also indicate areas which are not very actively pursued and might warrant additional programs. The status of the research effort would be more accurately known to the scientific leadership, the granting agencies, and ultimately the elected representatives of the people. The form presented in Table 3–5 is not intended to be a specific proposal but rather an example to illustrate that such an approach is feasible and possibly worth further consideration.

Division of Research Grants: An Extended Role. Since the Division of Research Grants serves all the Institutes by selecting reviewers and distributing applications for study section and council review, it serves as a logical clearing-house for continuous inventory of the magnitude and nature of the total extramural research effort. The increasing requirements for comprehensive information covering the research and development efforts of all the Institutes of Health clearly suggest an expanded role for the Division of Research Grants as the most appropriate organization for providing an updated inventory of such activities. In addition to the current role of summarizing the resource distribution, the Division of Research Grants could be awarded additional funding and staff to provide a greatly extended effort at monitoring the input of investigator initiated research proposals. Information about the ongoing contract and intramural programs within the various Institutes might be included in this repository for completeness. The Division of Research Grants could be an appropriate organizational component for such independent overviews of current research projects to avoid the inherent bias which inevitably results from selfassessment. There would be advantages in providing incentives and resources for this organization to develop new and innovative mechanisms for collecting information of the general sort suggested by Table 3-5.

The National Library of Medicine: Expanded Roles. The National Library of Medicine is a unique institution, having a potential that extends far beyond serving as a repository of medical publications and periodicals. Whereas the Division of Research Grants can monitor the incoming and current research emphasis, the National Library of Medicine could be delegated the responsibility for reviewing the content and the status of research from previous years. The National Library of Medicine responds to requests for searches of the medical literature originating with individual physicians, scientists, and professionals, as well as appropriate organizations. Perusing the list of literature searches discloses no systematic or organized basis for the selection of the topics to be explored. Despite the rather arbitrary selection of topics and the relatively limited number of different topics that have been explored, these lists prove extremely useful when their content matches the current needs of an investigator. This process could be enormously expanded using the computer facilities to which the National Library of Medicine has access. Of particular importance would be the development of new methods for identifying the content of grant and contract programs in a meaningful and reliable fashion. For example, the Library of Medicine might undertake a much more comprehensive review of the content of research embodied in the abstracts available through the Smithsonian Institute. The problem is too huge to undertake arbitrarily and requires a systematic format by which it would be possible to identify the topics of particular interest, significance, and timeliness in terms of the current decision-making process within the National Institutes of Health and other organizations. For this purpose, it would be desireable to have a mechanism by which an independent organization such as the National Library of Medicine could undertake unbiased reviews of the medical literature in key topic areas in accordance with a standard format and selected on the basis of priorities which have been carefully elaborated. More specifically, the various Institutes of Health are currently engaged in trying to develop consensus among the scientific community involved in various areas of research regarding the important next steps which deserve high priority in research funding. As these efforts for developing consensus emerge, the National Library of Medicine could undertake systematic literature reviews of the prescribed areas and provide the important background required for a more scholarly approach to the development of consensus. The Library could use the *Science Citation Index* as a means of eliciting information about which are the key articles in the medical literature on certain principal topics.

Additional information could be rather painlessly obtained by a simple form added to the research grant application form. At the present time, the number of bibliographic citations in the research grant proposals is arbitrarily limited. This was intended, no doubt, to reduce the stress on the reviewing bodies in terms of limiting the number of articles they might be inclined to peruse in arriving at their priorities. However, the investigators who are applying for research grants are likely to be most knowledgeable regarding the most important and significant contributions to research areas from the past. On this basis, it might be possible to require the investigators to provide more extended lists of bibliographic citations of the literature with an asterisk indicating each article regarded as being particularly important and critical. This process would provide an extended source of bibliographic citation stemming from individuals who are most actively engaged in research in various fields. The Division of Research Grants could provide copies of these bibliographic citations to the Library of Medicine where the results could be quite readily assembled and analyzed for future use. This would be a relatively small imposition on the scientific community and ultimately yield rather rich rewards in terms of a more comprehensive approach to an evaluation of the key contributions to research in many different areas. It would also provide an indication of the current status of knowledge in these areas of value in arriving at priorities for long-range planning.

Improved Medical Coding Mechanisms. The mounting problems of acquiring, storing, and retrieving medical information is becoming so serious that modern medicine is threatened with drowning in its own prolific excretions in spite of high speed computers. The categorization of topics in the biomedical literature is extremely subjective and complicated to a significant degree by the fact that many terms have several meanings, and several meanings may be conveyed by the same term. Efforts at standardizing medical terminology have helped resolve such issues to a limited extent, but there is really no prospect of rendering medical nomenclature clear, concise, and computer compatible. The task of restructuring the medical nomenclature would be momentous—like the transition into metric units. However, it is possible to demonstrate that such an effort might be successful by suggesting a specific approach and format.

Communication by means of traditional terms does not fully utilize our ability to transmit information. A new type of terminology is needed based on consistent and logical principles that pack information much more concisely and unambiguously than present systems do using specific requirements such as the following:

· Each letter, syllable, and sequence should have maximum intelligible content.
· The system should combine flexibility with consistency.
· Computer compatibility should be assured (i.e., by an alphanumeric system).
· Additional data and new knowledge should be readily accommodated with minimal reorganization of terms.
· Definitive diagnosis should be conveyed by specification of the nature, site, and extent and functional disturbance of the disease or disability.

A cumulative, compact, and computer compatible nomenclature could be devised on the basis of the following general principles (16). First, individual letters could be employed to stand for words and phrases. "NASA" adequately conveys the meaning of the words National Aeronautics and Space Administration, and is not often confused with NATO or with any other government agency. Although words synthesized from initials sound at first like nonsense syllables, familiarity and common usage enable them to become adapted as meaningful units of speech. The quantity of information packed into a single word could be greatly increased by utilizing each successive letter to denote a particular category of meanings. In the decimal system, position of a number to the right or left of the decimal point indicates uniquely the multiples of 10 which it represents. If letters are substituted for numbers, it becomes possible to assign a categorical meaning to each successive letter. For example, the first letter of a word could be a consonant selected to identify one of the major organ systems: n for nervous system, h for heart, v for vascular, r for respiratory system, and so on. The second letter could be a vowel to indicate the major components of the organ system. Each organ has certain specific disabilities and functional disturbances. A coding system could include a letter designation to cover both organspecific or general pathological processes for each of the major components. The resulting functional disturbances from the specified pathological process could then be designated by the fourth letter in the word. The severity of the ailment could be indicated by the last letter. By such a process, some 40,000 six-letter words could be devised according to a clearly defined system, which would uniquely identify an exceedingly broad spectrum of disease processes with a computer compatible format (16). By alternating vowels and consonants, each of these newly developed words would be pronounceable. By standardizing the pronunciation of each vowel, consonent, and diphthong, there would be no ambiguity regarding how these words should be enunciated when used orally.

This nonconventional proposal is suggested more as an indication that options exist for greatly enhancing and improving medical nomenclature according to some carefully developed schema. It is not intended to indicate a finished product or a discrete solution to a very severe problem. It does, however, serve as a basis for recommending that the role of the National Library of Medicine might well be expanded to undertake the development of new medical nomenclature and new medical coding systems to represent substantial improvements in our ability to organize, analyze, and evaluate biomedical research and clinical practice.

PRESENT PRIORITIES AND PROPOSED ADJUSTMENTS

The present distribution of research efforts among the many and varied health-related topical areas is uncertain for lack of relative data. The mechanisms suggested above are intended to supplement current sources of information as well as to facilitate rationalization of the research and development priorities. The manner in which such an overview could be helpful is suggested in Figure 3-6.

During the mobilization phase, there appeared to be a natural tendency

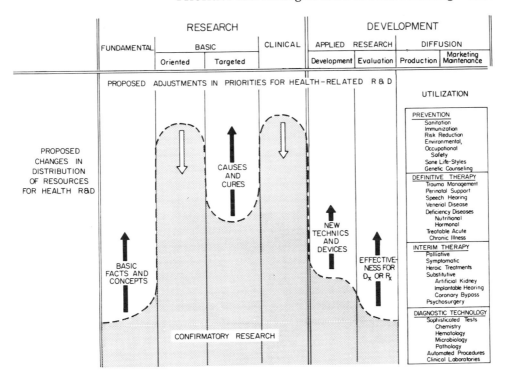

Figure 3-6. An intuitive impression of early priorities would appear to favor functional and clinical categories defined in Table 3-2. The forward-planning process appears to be shifting the distribution of effort toward fundamental research, targeted research, and applied research as indicated by the arrows above. The significance and justification for such changes in emphasis are discussed in the text.

of biochemists, anatomists, and physiologists to concentrate on the structure, function, and control of tissues and organs under experimental conditions (functional research). Pathologists, pharmacologists, and microbiologists focused on causes and cures of disease. Clinicians were naturally interested in the manifestations of disease and their management (clinical investigation). The intuitive impression that these principle thrusts tended to dominate the total effort cannot be proved or discounted by the kinds of data currently available. Assuming this to be the case, there would be merit in giving serious consideration to the desirability of intentionally expanding the absolute and relative distribution of research effort toward fundamental, targeted, and applied research and development as suggested schematically in Figure 3-6. These are trends which are clearly emerging from the forward planning efforts, most particularly those of the National Cancer Program, as described in Chapter 2. This redistribution of effort can be attained in part by diversion of some of the resources currently being directed at the functional research and clinical investigation toward those areas which are believed to have a high level of potential productivity. Of particular importance would be improved mechanisms for the development of new techniques and devices and, even more important, effective mechanisms for determining the effectiveness of new methods for diagnosis and treatment during the process of diffusion into the medical community (see also Chapters 5 and 6). Such judgments are currently based very largely on intuitive impressions with insufficient hard data concerning the extent to which progress has been made toward the various objectives or the magnitude of the current research effort represented by more than 10,000 projects in NIH alone. Clearly, these judgments could be more soundly based if supported by information gathered routinely by mechanisms suggested in previous paragraphs.

The potential significance of deciding to direct greater efforts at both fundamental and targeted research are presented in the next chapter. The impact of technologies on health care are considered in Chapter 5. The methods, motivations, and implications of evaluating health care delivery mechanisms are discussed in Chapter 6.

SUMMARY

1. The ultimate output of research and development is commonly pictured as a sequential progression from the acquisition of new knowledge by experiments in basic science through applied research and development to the production and diffusion of new medical techniques and technologies. A more accurate portrayal presents two processes occurring in parallel with the academic community amassing vast stores of knowledge and experience. Information from the stores of knowledge is selectively employed for the fulfillment of unmet needs.

2. Technical obstacles to progress can be overcome by mounting massive planned attacks (i.e., the NASA approach) when the necessary basic information is at hand. The major diseases and disabilities in modern society are poorly understood, presenting many unsolved questions of causation which must be elucidated by fundamental explorations of intimate etiology and contributing factors.

3. The distinctions between "basic" and "applied" research have been the source of major misunderstandings and controversy between the scientific community and the general public and their representatives in government. Useful distinctions can be drawn by specifying characteristics of several levels of research and development such as fundamental, functional, targeted, clinical investigation and clinical evaluation instead of attempting to make sharp distinctions between only two categories.

4. Very little is known about the process by which new knowledge or key observations are converted into useful technologies, but the sequence can be completed within one year or be delayed for decades for reasons that remain obscure.

5. The priorities used for distribution of resources and effort have been influenced too greatly by mortality statistics and need to be broadened to include additional relevant considerations. One approach is to explore the "burden of illness" of various ailments using factors such as years of

life lost, inpatient days, physician visits, loss of work, limitations in activity, days in bed, and so on.

6. Overlapping areas of responsibility among the various granting agencies and categorical Institutes of Health unavoidably promote repetitive and redundant research efforts beyond those required to conform and complete experimental observations. The magnitude and directions of the national biomedical research effort cannot be adequately assessed on the basis of input (i.e., financial outlays and numbers of projects) but also require additional information about investigator intent, substance of research output, and assessment of current state of knowledge as a rational basis of forward planning.

7. Mechanisms can be envisioned for gaining more insight into the current research effort and evaluating the current state and gaps in knowledge and some representative examples are presented.

REFERENCES

1. Forward Plan for Health, FY 1977-81, DHEW, June 1975.
2. Culliton BJ: Kennedy Hearings: Year long probe of biomedical research begins. *Science* 193:32-35, 1976.
3. *Science Indicators:* 1974 National Science Board Publication NSB 55-1, US Government Printing Office Stock No 3800-00146.
4. Crane LT: Science Indicators—1974 and Basic Research: A partial analysis. Policy Research Division, Congressional Research Service, June 26, 1976.
5. Frederickson DS: The administration's view of basic research and the life sciences. A symposium presented at the Federation of American Societies for Experimental Biology, April 10, 1978.
6. Forward Plan for Health 1978-82, Public Health Service, DHEW, August, 1976.
7. Haeffner EA: Institute for Innovationsteknik. *Technical Review*, Stockholm, pp 18-25, March-April 1974.
8. Comroe JH, Dripps RD: Scientific basis for support of biomedical science. *Science* 192:105-111, 1976.
9. Comroe JH, Dripps RD: The top ten clinical advances in cardiovascular-pulmonary medicine and surgery between 1945 and 1975. Final report, January 31, 1977, Contract 1-Ho-1-2327 from the National Heart and Lung Institute.
10. Comroe JH, Dropps RD: Ben Franklin and open heart surgery. *Circ Res* 35:661-669, 1974.
11. Black DAK, Pole JD: Priorities in biomedical research: indices of burden. *Brit J Prev Soc Med* 29:222-227, 1975.
12. Rice DP, Feldman JJ, White KI: The current burden of illness in the United States, Presented at the Annual Meeting of the Institutes of Medicine, Washington DC, October 27, 1976.
13. Frame JD:, Narin F: The international distribution of biomedical publications. *Fed Proc* 36:1790-1795, 1977.
14. Narin F, Shapiro RT: The extramural role of the NIH as a research support agency. *Fed Proc* 36:2470-2476, 1977.
15. Westbrook JH: Identifying significant research. *Science* 132:1229-1234, 1960.
16. Rushmer RF: Numedcode: a cumulative, compact, computer compatible medical nomenclature is both necessary and feasible. *Dis of the Chest* 56:143-148, 1969.

CHAPTER 4

Targeted Research: Quest for Causes and Cures

In the preceding chapter, distinctions between basic and applied research were explored with a view toward clarifying differences between fundamental (pure), functional, targeted, clinical investigational, and clinical evaluations. Contrary to traditional views, the process of transferring this knowledge and experience into processes, procedures, and devices appears to follow a separate and parallel pathway rather than to proceed in a linear sequence. During the past 30 years, the dominant thrusts of research programs tended to be oriented toward functional research designed to elucidate the structure, function, and control of normal cells and organ systems on the one hand and clinical investigation of overt disease processes in humans on the other. Three categories of investigation have been attacked with less vigor, specifically the very fundamental processes of cell metabolism, genetics, immunology, virology, and enzymology. These issues were relatively neglected in the postwar years, but are now receiving greatly enhanced and concentrated attention.

Targeted research, particularly specific investigation of intimate etiology and detailed pathophysiology, appeared to have received less attention than either functional research or clinical investigation. Experience has indicated that therapeutic mechanisms, evolved on an empirical basis and without specific knowledge of etiology, have proved useful for relieving symptoms and favorably influencing the course of illness to some extent, but have been disappointing with regard to development of effective cures. As a result, there is an increased emphasis on the epidemiology of disease and on the intimate nature of pathophysiology in search of more specific knowledge regarding the causation of the major disease processes. The opportunities and obstacles which are represented by "targeted" research will be considered in this chapter. The problems and prospects of evaluating clinical technologies will be covered in Chapters 5 and 6.

PERSPECTIVES FROM EARLIER PROGRESS

Many of the common, contagious and epidemic diseases, which threatened whole populations in the past, have largely disappeared from the face of the earth. There are lessons to be learned from the sequences that led to successful conquest of killers of former years. It is a peculiar property of health sciences that technical triumphs are marked by disappearance of diseases. Many other forms of human endeavor leave monuments, which are continual reminders of the successful efforts which led to their completion by architects, authors, sculptors, or industrialists. In contrast, the ultimate objective of biomedical research is the creation of voids, namely the absence of disease and disability. Under these circumstances, it is easy to ignore or to forget the sequences and successful strategies that led to the virtual elimination of diseases in the past.

MONUMENTAL TRIUMPHS

A relatively large number of devastating diseases and disabilities is rarely, if ever, encountered by physicians in developed countries. An appropriate monument to these successes would be a void or vaporous cloud to commemorate victories over such conditions as scurvy, pellagra, beriberi, rickets, cholera, plague, yellow fever, smallpox, diphtheria, and many other devastating pandemics. Such conditions have become so infrequent that they no longer represent a significant feature of medical school education, because there are so few patients available to demonstrate the nature of the disease process. These diseases have been demonstrated to have relatively simple, specific, unitary etiology, but each was generally attributed to many diverse and imaginative causes before the underlying process was identified and clarified (Fig. 4-1).

Consider pellagra as an example. In 1902, a case of pellagra was diagnosed in a poor Georgia farmer, and within the next three or four years, the disease was found to be widely distributed throughout the southern states. It is now obvious that pellagra did not suddenly emerge as a new disease that spread rapidly throughout the South, but had existed in this area for a very long time. It is a general phenomenon that a disease "does not exist" for practical purposes until it has been described, named, and recognized. The public was aroused by newspaper and magazine articles describing lurid aspects of this strange and mysterious plague, variously attributed to hereditary, environmental, insect-borne, bacterial, or nutritional origins. If an epidemiological study had been undertaken at that time, a very large number of constitutional and environmental factors would undoubtedly have emerged as potential risk factors in the production of pellagra. The Surgeon General

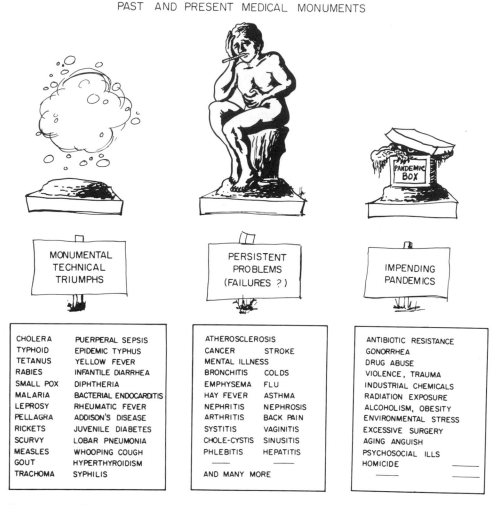

PAST AND PRESENT MEDICAL MONUMENTS

MONUMENTAL TECHNICAL TRIUMPHS		PERSISTENT PROBLEMS (FAILURES ?)		IMPENDING PANDEMICS
CHOLERA	PUERPERAL SEPSIS	ATHEROSCLEROSIS		ANTIBIOTIC RESISTANCE
TYPHOID	EPIDEMIC TYPHUS	CANCER STROKE		GONORRHEA
TETANUS	YELLOW FEVER	MENTAL ILLNESS		DRUG ABUSE
RABIES	INFANTILE DIARRHEA	BRONCHITIS COLDS		VIOLENCE, TRAUMA
SMALL POX	DIPHTHERIA	EMPHYSEMA FLU		INDUSTRIAL CHEMICALS
MALARIA	BACTERIAL ENDOCARDITIS	HAY FEVER ASTHMA		RADIATION EXPOSURE
LEPROSY	RHEUMATIC FEVER	NEPHRITIS NEPHROSIS		ALCOHOLISM, OBESITY
PELLAGRA	ADDISON'S DISEASE	ARTHRITIS BACK PAIN		ENVIRONMENTAL STRESS
RICKETS	JUVENILE DIABETES	SYSTITIS VAGINITIS		EXCESSIVE SURGERY
SCURVY	LOBAR PNEUMONIA	CHOLE-CYSTIS SINUSITIS		AGING ANGUISH
MEASLES	WHOOPING COUGH	PHLEBITIS HEPATITIS		PSYCHOSOCIAL ILLS
GOUT	HYPERTHYROIDISM			HOMICIDE
TRACHOMA	SYPHILIS	AND MANY MORE		

Figure 4-1. The monumental medical triumphs of the past are represented by a wide variety of infections, deficiency diseases, and metabolic ailments having effective therapy, cures, or preventive measures. The many persistent problems include the chronic ailments of an aging population and infections that have not succumbed to current therapy. A large number of ailments with increasing incidence represent impending pandemics for which targeted research is urgently required to overcome either technical or theoretical obstacles.

appointed a staff of 41 men to broaden the assault on pellagra. One of these, Dr. Joseph Goldberger, made a field trip into the South and became convinced that a food deficiency was at the root of the problem. He began a series of relatively simple experiments in which he demonstrated that the disease could be cured by a balanced dietary intake and culminated his work in 1915 by showing that pellagra could be produced in humans by an appropriately inadequate diet (1). This concept was derided and criticized by many physicians, despite evidence that would now appear to be sound and indisputable. Three years later, the Pellagra Commission of the National Medical Association declared that pellagra was a communicable disease resulting from poor sanitation. Some 20 years later, nicotinic acid was discovered as a specific cure for pellagra, and the immediate result was a sharp reduction in the death rate, which had been going down slowly. Pellagra became extremely rare in America within the next few years.

Sequences of this general type can be identified in a wide variety of different diseases and disabilities that have ultimately been controlled. Common characteristics of this process include some or all of the following features:

- Diseases of unknown origin(s) are generally attributed to diverse combinations of an extremely wide variety of factors, generally including:
  - hereditary susceptibility
  - nutritional deficiencies
  - toxic materials in the water or food
  - miasmas in the air
  - infectious agents or contagions
  - unsanitary living conditions
  - unhealthy habits
  - spiritual or supernatural factors
  - degeneration or aging
- Medical management of diseases from uncertain cause(s) is generally supportive and includes some or all of the following:
  - diet
  - healthy habits and living conditions
  - rest or relaxation
  - palliative or symptomatic management
  - rituals, rites, and placebos
- Elucidation of the intimate etiology accelerates progress in:
  - diagnostic criteria
  - definitive diagnostic tests
  - specific therapeutic approaches
  - accelerated reduction of prevalence
  - risk factors relegated to proper perspective

Many of the dreaded diseases that persist in large numbers today are attributed to health hazards from technologies of modern societies. With this prospect in mind, some additional examples of ailments which have been successfully curtailed may merit additional attention.

Beriberi is a disease that has features in common with some of our most critical modern threats to life and health. It was a "new" disease appearing among the populations in Asia and the Philippine Islands resulting from a technological accomplishment. It accompanied the increased use of machines for milling rice, which turned out a product that was more attractive but far less nutritious. In other words, beriberi was a disease that resulted from progress in modern technology. Definitive and effective therapy developed as the importance of vitamins was realized. Vitamin A was discovered in 1913 and vitamin D in 1922. By the late 1930s, virtually all the vitamin deficiencies and similar nutritional diseases were being virtually eliminated, even in pockets of poverty. Clearly, the development of sound concepts of origins and management in one disease opens the door for rapid progress in related ones.

In the centuries before cholera was recognized as a water-borne disease, the calamitous epidemics of this disease were ascribed to a multitude of factors which included hereditary susceptibility, meteorological conditions, dietary deficiencies, poor sanitation, and unfavorable positions of the stars. In the case of yellow fever, miasmas from swamps were prominent among proposed causes, along with a variety of other factors considered to be of great importance. The demonstration of bacterial origin of the disease provided a frenetic search for microorganisms as the cause of this and many other ailments—rightly or wrongly. The advent of prontocil and the more successful antibiotics was followed by intensive use of these materials in all manner of chronic diseases, such as multiple sclerosis, cystic fibrosis, and so forth. There was hope or expectation that these were manifestations of some bacterial disease that might be influenced by an antibiotic. The same phenomenon can be recognized today with the emphasis on virology as an essential part of the research programs in many or most of the Institutes of Health, as indicated in Chapter 3.

The current efforts to prevent or control diseases like cancer, heart disease, chronic pulmonary disease, and others by efforts at eliminating environmental and personal risk factors appears to offer very limited promise of success until the immediate etiology of the lesions is clarified and the causative factors are more distinctly determined.

EPIDEMIOLOGICAL ETIOLOGIES

Many diseases of major importance are characteristic of modern Western civilization and are rare or unknown in primitive communities that still follow traditional ways of life (2). Notable examples are cancer of the lung and cancer of the large bowel, which are common and malignant in Britain and America and relatively rare in primitive peoples (i.e., tribes in central Africa). Ulcerative colitis and diverticular disease are common ailments of the large bowel in civilized communities. Coronary heart disease and gallstones are associated with cholesterol metabolism affected by the fatty content of diet. Obesity and diabetes are also metabolic disturbances which are related to dietary habits. The relative rarity of these diseases in developing countries of Africa and Asia has been amply documented. Furthermore, the prevalence of these diseases tends to increase among persons who move from underdeveloped countries into Westernized communities. They tend to become increasingly frequent in the urbanized communities of Africa and Asia. Recognition of geographical, racial, and cultural association of such diseases stimulated an expanding program of epidemiological investigations designed to discover contributing factors or responsible agents in the development of these chronic and serious illnesses. In contrast to acute infections, the relationships between cause and effect are often obscure when the interval between the appearance of pathological lesions and their clinical manifestation may be years or decades in duration. The potential factors that could be involved tend to include virtually all the environmental, domestic, cultural, and behavioral differences between the groups under study. The vast multitude of diseases which affect human populations poses an extremely difficult choice in the establishment of priorities regarding the most appropriate distribution of resources and effort.

MULTIPLE MECHANISMS ELICITED BY EPIDEMIOLOGY

Experience from the past suggests that virtually all conditions of unknown origin tended to be ascribed to a multiplicity of causes in the quest for elucidation. The search for causal factors frequently centered on hazardous elements in the environment (real or imagined), dietary factors, occupational hazards, hereditary susceptibility, and intangible factors such as meteorological phenomena, astrological signs, and so on. This process might be considered intuitive epidemiology, since it represents an intellectual search for the unknown among multiple factors that might conceivably affect health of the public.

Modern epidemiology is more sophisticated and analytical, providing a more solid basis for judgment about the relative importance of such factors. However, the candidates that emerge as risk factors tend to recur repeatedly in the search for the distinguishing differences between groups of people with high incidence of a particular disease in contrast to other groups with lower incidence. Historically, progress toward the reduction, control, cure, and ultimate prevention of disease virtually always followed the identification of common denominators. For example, recognition that dietary deficiencies were the underlying cause of pellagra, beriberi, scurvy, and rickets, demonstrated nutrition to be the gross common denominator. The individual vitamins later became the specific therapeutic approaches to prevention. The prevalence of cholera was successfully reduced by improving the purity of water without awareness that the intimate cause was bacterial. The difference in mortality between people drinking from the Broad Street Pump and other groups drinking from different water sources was the vital clue perceived by Snow (3). The tortuous paths of medical history disclose numerous examples of diminishing mortality or incidence of diseases without disclosure of their causes. Notable examples include tuberculosis, scarlet fever, mumps, and many other infectious diseases as indicated in Figure 1-2. Similarly, there are other examples of effective therapy being developed without clarification of the etiology of the disturbance.

The discovery that certain populations of World War II draftees entering the army were free of caries led to a specific search for the protective influence. Fluoride in the water supply was found to be significant. The recognition that yellow fever was transmitted by a specific species of mosquito led to effective control by eliminating the common carrier before the microorganism was known. These examples, and many more, provide unwarranted confidence that we can overcome some or most of the persistent problems listed in Figure 4-1 without clarifying underlying causation. Optimism may be ultimately shown to be warranted in some instances, but should not be the basis for a lack of motivation and support for intensive explorations of the immediate etiology of the illnesses and ailments which continue to plague mankind.

The virtual disappearance of many nutritional and acute infectious diseases has confronted the biomedical community with far more challenging problems presented by chronic and resistant illnesses. In acute illnesses where the time relation between the onset of the ailment and the manifestation of the disease was short, the potential causal factors should be identified with greater ease than chronic diseases with protracted courses. Specifically, in 1900, six of the leading causes of death were infectious or related to infection. By 1970, chronic diseases became the leading causes of death, except for respiratory infections (i.e., influenza and pneumonia). In that brief interval, heart disease and cancer increased by 268% and 240% respectively, in terms of deaths per 100,000 people (4). The political pressures for demonstrating progress have impelled the biomedical community to undertake efforts at controlling the modern "epidemics" of cancer, heart disease, and other diseases. The causes of these conditions remain unknown so prevention is being attempted by reducing risk factors that have uncertain relations to the pathophysiology of the lesions. Examples of this phenomenon are discussed below in relation to both atherosclerosis and cancer. With his usual candor, Lewis Thomas indicated the need to face the real possibility that the level of insight into the mechanisms of today's unsolved diseases—schizophrenia, cancer, or stroke—is comparable to the situation for infectious disease in 1875, when the crucial clues were still undiscovered (5). The new era of forward planning (Chapter 2) is designed to identify the essential gaps in knowledge more rapidly and to accelerate acquisition of this knowledge and its translation into effective action.

STAGES OR STEPS TOWARD CURE AND CONTROL (IDEALIZED)

Scientific progress is the result of many contributions, large and small, by a very large number of participants. Relationships that are obvious today were previously mysterious or were overlooked by the biomedical community for years or generations, as illustrated by the long lag-times between discovery and implementation presented in Figure 3-4. Thus, it is misleading to envision progress in research as a series of sequential and logical steps toward clearly-defined objectives. The flash of insight or the "hunch" of an imaginative investigator can suddenly illuminate an issue and produce a surge of progress. An idealized impression of critical phases in biomedical research is presented in Figure 4-2. Retrospective review of progress often results in

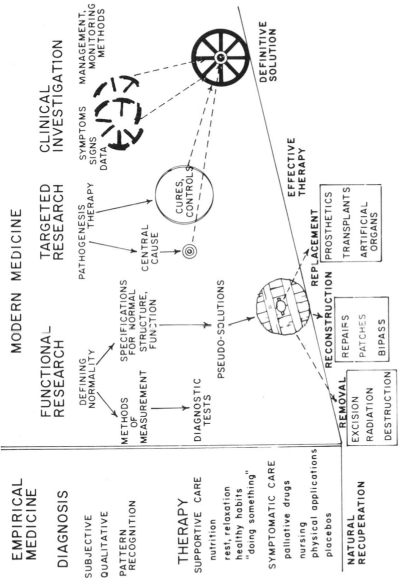

Figure 4-2. An idealized portrayal of biomedical progress displays empirical methods of diagnosis and therapy as utilized in support of the natural recuperative powers against diseases and disabilities for which causes and cures have not been developed. The specification of normality forms the basis for artificial supplements or substitutes for deficient function which must be regarded as primitive "pseudosolutions." Targeted research is designated as a process of exploring pathogenesis of diseases in search of central causes and methods of cure or control. Clinical investigation elicits essential information regarding symptoms, signs, and the course of illness as well as methods of management. The ultimate goal is a functional entity represented by a wheel.

133

descriptions of sequences that can seem like logical progressions along a pathway to success. However, progress toward successful control or cure of ailments rarely if ever evolves in such an orderly fashion. The first stage, common to all diseases and disabilities, is labeled empirical medicine, during which concepts of causes and cures remain uncertain or erroneous.

EMPIRICAL MEDICINE

Empirical medicine can be identified as the intuitive and supportive forms of diagnosis and therapy that physicians have used in all past periods, regardless of depth of ignorance with respect to nature, origins, pathophysiology of ailments, or effectiveness of available therapy. When patients seek medical guidance and help, it is incumbent on the physician to perform to the best of his ability with the tools and methods available and regarded as relevant to the presenting condition. Empirical medicine can be recognized as the reliance on subjective symptoms and qualitative impressions to provide the ingredients for diagnostic pattern recognition (Fig. 4-2). The accuracy and reliability of this process commonly exceeds any reasonable expectations. The attending physician may not be fully aware of the process by which he arrives at a correct diagnosis—the "art" of medicine.

The therapeutic approaches generally available for conditions without known cause or cure take two main forms: (1) supportive measures and (2) symptomatic relief.

Supportive Measures. A common approach to enigmatic conditions in patients includes emphasis on refining nutritional status, improving living conditions, recommending healthier habits, rest and relaxation, reducing stresses, and avoiding risk factors. The implied understanding or unstated contract between a patient and health professional is rarely regarded as complete by either party without "doing something." The active response to a patient's presence may take the form of gathering more data through history, physical examination, laboratory tests, or consultations. With one major exception a patient is rarely told that he is completely healthy and to go home and forget his symptoms. At the conclusion of an annual or periodic checkup, the assurance that the patient has a clean bill of health is a highly acceptable result of the encounter despite the obvious fact that periodic health appraisals are no guarantee that subclinical or undetected disease is absent or not imminent.

Symptomatic Relief. Another common contribution to the care of patients suffering from conditions of unknown origin is the provision of prescriptions for relief of symptoms. The number and diversity of drugs now available at the flick of a pen has greatly expanded in recent years, exceeding the ability of any physician to truly keep abreast of the options. A very large proportion of these drugs has proved useful for the alleviation of symptoms—real or imagined. If no specific medication seems appropriate, it is always possible to prescribe tranquilizers or other mood-altering compounds. The sales volume of these products has increased enormously in recent years as an objective indicator that empirical management is employed for a very large proportion of visits to physicians. Sometimes physical therapy or nursing care can be prescribed to provide contact care for reassurance, relief, and rehabilitation. These measures generally appear to provide favorable responses out of proportion to their effects on the course of illness. The importance of the "placebo effect" produced by the therapeutic efforts indicated above is being increasingly recognized (6). The health professionals are naturally reluctant to admit the extent to which they must rely on the placebo effects of their ministrations. The power and effectiveness of placebos are known to dissipate if the recipient is aware that the ministration is not demonstrably effective. There is also an uncomfortable aura of charlatanism in the use of placebos despite recognition that they are widely, if not universally, used.

It is the long range goal of the biomedical research establishment to lift the very large spectrum of diseases and disabilities currently managed by empirical means into the realm of modern medicine, as illustrated in Figure 4-2.

MODERN MEDICINE

The contributions of various categories of biomedical research (Chapter 3) toward more modern approaches are portrayed in idealized form in Figure 4-2. Functional research provides insight and clarifies the definitions of normality in more specific and quantitative terms. The methods of measurement employed in experimental investigations of "normal" function in animals or humans can be adapted to provide objective and quantitative diagnostic tests. This process is explored in greater detail in the next chapter (Chapter 5). The definitions of normality also represent more specific criteria regarding the functional states toward which the patient should be restored during recovery from disease or disability. These same specifications have also stimulated collaborative efforts by health scientists and engineers to design and develop artificial substitutes or supplements to help bridge the gap when there is no prospect of cure or return to normalcy by available therapeutic regimes. Sophisticated devices employed as substitutes for normal functioning organs have been termed "intermediate technologies" by Lewis Thomas (7). These include many techniques and technologies which are both palliative and useful in improving the quality of life of patients. These might more properly be called "pseudosolutions" when functional substitutes or supplements are provided instead of definitive treatment of the disease. Such pseudosolutions can divert attention and urgency from the unremitting search for central causes and/or effective therapy. Living organisms and organs are so complex that the most sophisticated technologies are extremely crude in comparison with nature's handiwork. This distinction is suggested by representing pseudosolutions as a primitive wheel—it accomplishes a functional objective but is far from an ideal solution (Fig. 4–2).

Technical Triumphs as Pseudosolutions. Definitions of normality are acquired through programs of functional research which specify the structure, function, control, and interactions of organs and systems in both experimental animals and man. Quantitative definitions of normality in terms of chemical, physical, and functional characteristics can also serve as specifications required for the production of substitutes or supplements for organs deleteriously affected by disease processes. These specifications have served to excite the interest of engineers to develop techniques and technologies for removal, repair, or replacement of defective or diseased organs. The patients benefitting from these technical advances may regard the tangible improvements in quality of life as being a godsend. However, to accept these developments as the ultimate answer to medical problems has the effect of distracting attention and possibly depriving future generations of the benefits of definitive treatments, effective cures, or even prevention of ailments that produce the disabilities. A vivid example is the emergence of artificial kidneys or dialysis machines which have proved capable of sustaining the lives of patients with endstage renal diseases for many years. The modern versions of these machines are nothing short of miraculous to the recipients who benefit from prolonged life. Legislation has made it possible for such patients to be covered under Medicare for major coverage of the large expenses ($7,000 to $10,000 per year). These commitments must be honored even though the total annual expenditure has exceeded $500 million per year and estimates range up to $1 billion per year in the next few years. An exceedingly small fraction of such large sums is currently being allocated to the exploration of the immediate causes of chronic renal diseases that ultimately lead to a need for artificial kidneys. Such studies are supported by a small portion of the relatively small budget of the National Institute of Arthritis, Metabolic and Digestive Diseases which obviously has many other important areas of responsibility (see Fig. 2-1). Under existing conditions, the discrepancy between the current massive expenditures for renal dialysis and meager investment on targeted research on the cause(s) of the underlying diseases actually represents a short-term advantage for a few at the expense of patients destined to fall victims of chronic renal disease. The health heritage of future generations is being deprived just as surely as our exorbitant use of the earth's resources will deprive its future occupants of a quality of life to which we would like to be accustomed.

Targeted Research. Investigations of the pathophysiology of diseases affecting organs or systems occupies the borderland between traditional "basic science" and clinical investigation. It most commonly involves pathophysiological, pathological, and microbiological studies of patients with diagnosed diseases or the responses of animals in which abnormal states are induced or simulated. An important thrust is to elicit improved understanding of the immediate causes of the malfunctions. Another branch of the research is devoted to identifying and exploring drugs, devices, or procedures which might serve as definitive therapy of the underlying causes. Such objectives are distinguishable from the more traditional approaches to supportive and symptomatic therapy of conditions of unknown or uncertain etiology. Specific investigations directed at causes and cures have been relatively neglected in the allocation of resources and efforts in the past. The development of forward plans includes opportunities for concentration of talent on the elucidation of immediate causes of important categories of disease because past history has shown that identification of intimate causation has frequently initiated a surge of progress toward definitive therapy and ultimate cures or prevention.

Clinical Investigation. Physicians engaged in clinical investigation deal with subjective symptoms, objective signs, laboratory data, and other sources of information leading to diagnoses with increased specificity and reliability. Clinicians are particularly interested in acquiring relevant information regarding the diagnostic patterns and the course of illness along with evaluation of the response to various modes of management. They are also engaged in applications and evaluations of methods of management. Empirical approaches are employed for conditions of doubtful origin or pathophysiology. New and improved techniques for arriving at definitive diagnoses and more effective therapy are generally the result of collaborative efforts among physicians and basic medical scientists, often aided by engineers of various types.

THE ULTIMATE GOAL: DEFINITIVE THERAPY OR PREVENTION

The forward-planning efforts, which are assuming increased importance in all aspects of the biomedical research enterprise, represent a far more rational and studied approach to biomedical research than could be expected from spontaneous investigator-initiated projects of the past (see Chapter 2). The comprehensive plans developed by the various Institutes of Health have much more clearly defined goals, objectives, and strategies. This process is epitomized by the massive exploration of alternatives in the evolution of the National Cancer Program. One consequence is much greater emphasis on current consensus regarding the factors of importance in carcinogenesis, including molecular and cellular biology, mutagenesis, and factors of heredity, immunology, spreading factors, and metastatic mechanisms (see Fig. 4–4).

If the ultimate objective be schematically portrayed by a unified functional wheel, specific knowledge about the etiology can be represented as the hub around which all the other component parts can be arranged. The rim of the wheel represents definitive therapy, serving to integrate and support the entire structure, as illustrated in Figure 4-2.

PRESENT PRIORITIES AND PRIME TARGETS

The categorical Institutes and corresponding voluntary agencies are tangible evidence of the priorities ascribed to the various kinds of diseases and disabilities affecting mankind. These priorities were established by political process rather than scientific rationale as described in Chapter 1. Cancer and cardiovascular diseases have consistently "stolen the scene" from the many other serious sources of disease and disability. The financial investment in biomedical research into these common killers dominate all other categories and notable progress has been made without question. Premature pronouncements that "breakthroughs" are either here or imminent have created a distorted impression that the theoretical obstacles have been virtually overcome and the technical obstacles that lie ahead can be surmounted on the basis of current knowledge and experience. A critical examination of our present position casts some questions on the validity of such impressions. A closer look at the theoretical obstacles to ultimate control of cancer and atherosclerosis reveals wide gaps in our understanding which must still be bridged before coming to grips with the immediate cause of these dread diseases. On this basis, it seems desirable to explore in greater depth the current status and future prospects of targeted research oriented toward elucidation of carcinogenesis and atherogenesis.

CANCER AND NEOPLASTIC DISEASES: CURRENT STATUS

Cell division is a process that occurs normally under a variety of circumstances. Embryological development involves the progressive cell division from a single cell to the billions of specialized cells comprising a newborn child. Cell division proceeds continuously in bone marrow, stomach lining, and many other tissues, including the dermis of the skin. The mechanisms which stimulate body cells to divide remain unclear. Conversely, the mechanisms which tend to inhibit cell division are equally mysterious. When a single cell divides into two daughter cells in the replacement mode, one of the daughter cells retains the ability to continue dividing, while the other may indeed become specialized and lose this ability. The distinguishing features between these two types of daughter cells arising from the same source constitute key issues which will ultimately be resolved only through fundamental research. Examples can be found in the reparative processes of connective tissue forming scar tissue, in the regrowth of endothelial cells denuded from the lining of blood vessels, and possibly in atherogenesis, as indicated below.

CANCER CHARACTERISTICS

In common usage the term *cancer* is employed as though it were a single entity. This tendency obscures the fact that a wide variety of cell types become neoplastic in many different tissues and organs representing a wide variety of cellular environments. The diversity of sites and tissues which can be involved in cancer production are indicated in Figure 4-3. Cancer can originate in or invade virtually all tissues of the body. Not only are many different cell types involved in neoplasms of different degrees of malignancy, but the environments in which they exist differ widely. For example, the

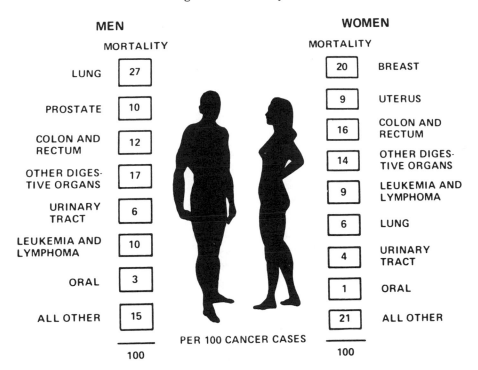

Figure 4-3. The leading causes of death due to cancer in various organs are displayed for both men and women according to sites of origin. Skin cancer is not included. Neoplastic cells of many different types emerge in a wide variety of anatomical relations and environmental circumstances. Thus, the term "cancer" probably encompasses an extremely large number of different diseases or conditions under the influence of a variety of environmental risk factors.

skin and lungs are far more exposed to noxious elements in the atmosphere than solid organs in the abdomen. The lining of the intestine is more exposed to ingested material than are muscle, bones, or brain. Ultraviolet light affects the skin but is almost completely absorbed in the outermost layers. In contrast, x-rays tend to penetrate the entire body and are more completely absorbed in radiodense tissues such as bone. The immediate environment of cells within the body tends to be maintained fairly uniform by the circulating blood and body fluids, but the concentration of hormones and other materials may vary considerably. Furthermore, the response of cells to hormones and to environmental factors must be discretely different. The tendency toward mutation by various cell types may vary significantly in different anatomical locations and among individuals with different genetic heritage. The diversity of cells and sites that may be involved in cancer have led some investigators to believe that this term may cover as many as 150 distinguishable diseases.

Epidemiological Risk Factors. Epidemiological exploration in search of clues regarding causes of cancer have tended to focus on conditions encountered in the environment, in occupation, and in personal health habits. Lung cancer has increased in incidence more rapidly than any other type of cancer, leading to suspicion that materials in the atmosphere and cigarette smoking may be contributing significantly. Similarly, the high incidence of cancer in the gastrointestinal tract directs attention toward ingested food and fluids as potential sources of carcinogenic influences. Ionizing radiation is known to increase the frequency of mutation and is encountered in many forms, including not only x-rays but also cosmic rays and nuclear energy. Skin cancer is believed to stem in part from exposures to ultraviolet light. In modern society, there are increased opportunities for exposure to chemical substances capable of producing mutations or cancer, as indicated in Figure 4-4. Current efforts tend to be directed toward attempting to reduce the risk of exposure to such materials, controlling their commercial use, and encouraging people to avoid exposures unnecessarily. A prime example is cigarette smoking, which is increasingly regarded as responsible for cancers not only of the lung, but in other parts of the body. The broad-scale effort to reduce the threat of lung cancer by encouraging the public to give up the habit of smoking is familiar to all.

Reviewing the trends in cancer mortality for a committee of Congress, Dorothy Rice (9) disclosed evidence indicating that cancer deaths are rising at alarming rates, considering the population as a whole. The death rate for white men is higher than for white women. The rates are even higher in the black population than in the white population. There is evidence that death rates from certain types of cancer are declining (i.e., prostate, stomach, and rectum), while others are continuing to climb. The types of cancer with increasing death rates are even more numerous and diverse in black than in white men. Interpretation of these trends is extremely difficult and subject to varied perceptions. For example, the geographic distribution of death rates from lung cancer, assembled county by county, illustrated "interesting peculiarities," including unexpected prevalence in some regions. Most lung cancer is ascribed to cigarette smoking, but research maps do not seem to correlate closely with cigarette-smoking patterns. High rates were encountered along the southeast coast of the United States, suggesting the need for research into industrial correlates in addition to cigarette smoking (10). Data such as these indicate how widespread is the common tendency to regard epidemiological risk factors as "cause" rather than factors or associations with the ailment under consideration.

SMOKING: CULPRIT OR CONTRIBUTORY FACTOR

The studies that led to a widespread conviction that smoking is *the* important risk factor in production of lung cancer also elicited a large number of other factors that were not so obviously relevant. The Hammond Report (11) was a three-year investigation of some 422,094 men over a period of nearly three years to explore the relationship between smoking and mortality. The study disclosed consistently higher death rates among cigarette smokers than nonsmokers. In addition, coronary artery disease appeared to

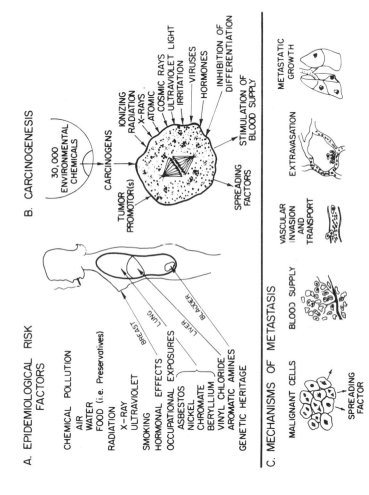

A. EPIDEMIOLOGICAL RISK FACTORS

CHEMICAL POLLUTION
  AIR
  WATER
  FOOD (i.e. Preservatives)
RADIATION
  X-RAY
  ULTRAVIOLET
SMOKING
HORMONAL EFFECTS
OCCUPATIONAL EXPOSURES
  ASBESTOS
  NICKEL
  CHROMATE
  BERYLLIUM
  VINYL CHLORIDE
  AROMATIC AMINES
GENETIC HERITAGE

BREAST
LUNG
LIVER
BLADDER

B. CARCINOGENESIS

30,000 ENVIRONMENTAL CHEMICALS

CARCINOGENS

TUMOR PROMOTOR(s)

IONIZING RADIATION
X-RAYS
ATOMIC
COSMIC RAYS
ULTRAVIOLET LIGHT
IRRITATION
VIRUSES
HORMONES
INHIBITION OF DIFFERENTIATION

STIMULATION OF BLOOD SUPPLY

SPREADING FACTORS

C. MECHANISMS OF METASTASIS

MALIGNANT CELLS

SPREADING FACTOR

BLOOD SUPPLY

VASCULAR INVASION AND TRANSPORT

EXTRAVASATION

METASTATIC GROWTH

Figure 4–4. (*a*) A wide variety of "risk factors" have been associated with various kinds of cancer elicited by epidemiological studies. The differences in incidence of various forms of cancer among peoples and cultures disclose many factors which might predispose to cancer. (*b*) Carcinogenesis at the cellular level could be attributed to many different etiological factors, including a large number of chemical agents in the environment, various forms of radiation and hormonal and hereditary influences. The diversity of possible causes strongly suggests that the major obstacles to progress are mainly theoretical rather than technical at the present time. (*c*) The metastatic spread of cancer cells to other anatomical sites is an important complication involving spreading factors for tumor growth, invasion of blood or lymph channels, arrest and escape in distant organs, and metastatic growth.

141

be related to cigarette smoking as well. This study, subsequently confirmed by others, formed the foundation of the nationwide program to discourage smoking by the American people and citizens of other countries as well. The data indicated the extreme complexity of attempting to sort out relevant factors from untold numbers of distinguishing features of individuals living in our complicated society.

The Hammond report produced some results that were neither anticipated, explained, nor widely publicized (12). Specifically, Table 7 of that report presented relationships between age-standardized death rates and a variety of other factors. A notable example was the data among both non-smokers and smokers (20+ per day). There are data indicating a lower death rate among those men who ate more fried food. This is somewhat unsettling, because fried foods are believed to contain lipids commonly regarded as being associated with atherosclerosis (and with cancer, by some investigators). People with more education also tended to have lower death rates. Taller men (up to 73 inches) had lower death rates than shorter men. Additional examples included support for the notion that married men are less likely to die. Sleeping seven hours a night appeared to be healthier than either more than nine or less than five. There appeared to be a higher death rate among bald people and circumcised people than others. These data indicate the extreme complexity of attempting to sort out relevant factors from untold numbers of distinguishing features of people living and dying in our complicated society. The intensive antismoking campaign has created confusion by implying that smoking is a *cause* or even *the cause* of lung cancer rather than one potential risk factor. Smoking is frequently associated with cancer and is probably a contributing factor, but if smoking were completely eliminated, would either cancer or heart disease disappear? The fact that such confusing statistics can be elicited in such a careful and comprehensive study indicates caution must rule in interpretation of epidemiological data. Restraint is particularly important when the relations between "risk factors" and intimate cause(s) of lesions are obscure.

CARCINOGENESIS

The relationships are extremely vague among the many risk factors statistically associated with cancer deaths and the immediate causes of uncontrolled cellular proliferation (Fig. 4-4a). Many different factors have been incriminated as direct causes of cell proliferation and tumor production. Prominent among them are spontaneous mutation, viral effects, x-rays, other radiations (i.e., ultraviolet light), mechanical irritation, and chemical carcinogens. The discovery that certain tumors in mice are viral in origin promoted a flurry of interest in cancer virology, which appears to be subsiding at present. The factors that inhibit cell proliferation are also of great interest but are poorly understood. Major emphasis is currently focused on chemical carcinogens as key causal factors. At least a dozen specific chemicals have been identified as causes of some forms of human cancer, mostly from industrial exposures. Tars and extracted petrochemicals have long been known to produce skin cancers in experimental animals repeatedly exposed to them. The number and variety of chemicals that might be involved in carcinogenesis are so great as to render impractical a broad-scale effort at evaluating them individually. Clearly, a major effort is fully justified for "targeted research" designed to bring order out of the chaos represented by many thousands of candidates as tumor-producing chemicals.

Targeted Research Results. The number and variety of "chemical carcinogens" have increased so rapidly, there is recognized need to identify types or categories with common characteristics. Data have accumulated indicating that some chemicals producing mutations have strong electrophilic reactivity. This is important in helping predict both metabolic effects and also highlight the kinds of chemicals most likely to be carcinogenic. Some agents produce tumors at sites remote from the point of administration. One important clue stemmed from evidence that certain chemicals were activated by metabolism to become carcinogenic. The binding properties of certain proteins appeared to indicate a mechanism by which their anatomic localization might be rendered more specific.

Carcinogenesis is increasingly considered to be at least a two-stage process involving two different types of materials. The chemical carcinogens indicated above can be applied for long periods without inducing malignancy. However, another type of chemical (i.e., the phorbol esters) have been shown to greatly accelerate development of epidermal tumors after application of small "initiating" doses of chemical carcinogens (see Fig. 4-4b). The applications of these "promoters" apparently result in increased synthesis of phospholipids, RNA, protein, and DNA, along with an increased mitotic rate. Such observations have led to exploration of various enzyme systems that might be involved.

Despite some impressive progress in understanding various aspects of carcinogenesis, it is apparent that the ultimate objectives of definitive therapy based on knowledge of cause still eludes us. The linkages between the "risk factors," the chemical carcinogens and the intimate etiology of malignancy remain obscure.

Relations Between Cancer Cells and Their Hosts. The defenses that the body uses to resist invasion of foreign microbes, proteins, or other foreign bodies may not successfully challenge or combat the incursions of cancer cells. It is known that immune reactions cause rejection and destruction of implanted tissues derived from an unrelated donor. The search for features distinguishing cancer cells from normal cells has included intensive exploration of tumor-specific antigens. These were demonstrated in mice belonging to highly inbred strains (13). An attractive aspect of immune reactions in either diagnosis or therapy lies in the extreme specificity that can be demonstrated in antigen-antibody reactions, although immunology has not yet attained a definite place in management of cancer. Some regression in neoplasms has been reported in association with nonspecific potentiation of the immune system through an intercurrent infectious process. Infections that appear to potentiate the immune systems are reported to produce regression of cancers.

Such observations hold out interesting and exciting prospects of more direct approaches to cancer control.

Metastasis. The growth, invasion, and spread of malignant neoplasms involves interactions between cancer cells and the host organism. Cancer cells can multiply only to a certain size before they extend beyond the viable blood supply. Thus, the mechanisms by which tumors stimulate the expansion of blood supply is an important basic issue in tumor growth (Fig. 4-4C). The spread of cancer cells is generally believed to require penetration of either lymphatics or the microcirculation (probably through thin-walled venules) and then transported through the blood (or lymph) to distant organs. They may be destroyed in passage through the reticuloendothelial system in unknown numbers. Some are arrested through the filter action of the lungs and may then penetrate into the lung parenchyma and produce metastases at that (or other) sites (14), as illustrated schematically in Figure 4-4C. Current knowledge about the intimate details or mechanisms involved in stimulating blood supply and metastasis of cancer is no further advanced than our understanding of the fundamental mechanisms in its initiation.

ATHEROSCLEROSIS

For more than 50 years, heart and blood vessel diseases have been the major cause of death in this country as the life expectancy of the American public became progressively longer (see Fig. 1-1). Vital statistics identify 10 leading causes of death, with 3 intimately related to atherosclerosis as the principal pathological process [i.e., heart disease, cerebrovascular disease, and atherosclerosis (Table 4-1)]. The combined mortality from these three items greatly exceeds that of cancer as the second most common cause of death. Atherosclerosis is characterized by thickening of the inner layer of arterial walls by cellular and fatty deposits (atheromatous plaques). It is generally believed that virtually all adult individuals have significant amounts of atherosclerosis, as indicated by post mortem examinations on young soldiers killed during the Korean conflict. It is a slow and progressive disease that may start in childhood and progress without symptoms for 20 to 40 years or longer. The local protrusion into the vascular channels progressively obstructs blood flow to organs beyond the lesions. Thus, atherosclerosis is an obstructive disease process, progressively impeding blood flow to the heart, brain, and/or lower extremities.

Before World War II, atherosclerosis was generally regarded as a degenerative process associated with aging and therefore not susceptible to medical management. The discovery of relationships between occlusive vascular complications and high blood lipid levels suggested that altered fat metabolism was involved and might provide opportunities for medical management.

"The direct biological chain of events which produces the atherosclerotic lesion has not been completely established, and the reasons are not entirely understood for precipitation of its sequelae—a blocked artery, a heart attack,

TABLE 4-1. Ten Leading Causes of Death in the United States, 1974

Cause of Death	Number of Deaths	Percentage of Deaths[a]	Rate per 100,000 Population
Total	1,934,388	100.0	915.1
1. *Diseases of the heart*	738,171	38.2	349.2
2. Malignant neoplasms	360,472	18.4	170.5
3. *Cerebrovascular diseases*	207,424	10.7	98.1
4. Accidents	104,622	5.4	49.5
5. Influenza and pneumonia	54,777	2.8	25.9
6. Chronic obstructive lung disease[b]	39,303	2.0	18.6
7. Diabetes mellitus	37,329	1.9	17.7
8. Cirrhosis of the liver	33,319	1.7	15.8
9. *Arteriosclerosis*	32,239	1.7	15.3
10. Certain causes of early infancy deaths	28,786	1.5	13.6
All other causes	297,946	15.4	141.0

[a]Percentages do not total 100 due to rounding.

[b]This includes deaths from emphysema, bronchitis, and chronic obstructive lung disease. This grouping is not on the official National Center for Health Statistics (NCHS) list of 10 leading causes, but it will be beginning in 1979. The total shown does not reflect deaths from related diseases—asthma and bronchiectasis—that bring total deaths to 41,942.

Monthly Vital Statistics Report, Vol. 24, No. 11, U.S. Department of Health, Education and Welfare, The National Center for Health Statistics, 1976.

or a stroke." (15). With these words, the Director of NHLBI frankly acknowledged the extent of the mystery that still envelops the process by which atherosclerosis develops. Epidemiologic studies have convinced many that atherosclerosis is related to certain lifestyles and habits, of which smoking is a notable example. High blood lipids, high blood pressure, obesity, diabetes, and stress are factors believed to predispose to atherosclerosis. Studies are currently underway to identify other risk factors that may exist in the environment or result from modern lifestyles. A wide variety of risk factors have now been identified and supported with masses of epidemiological data (Fig. 4-5). These risk factors represent potentially valuable clues related to the development of atherosclerosis. However, the causal relationships between these factors and the development of pathological lesions remain obscure. Specifically, these risk factors tend to affect all parts of the cardiovascular system. The chemical composition and the blood pressure are similar in all arteries of corresponding sizes throughout the entire vascular system, so the risk factors might be expected to affect all parts of the arterial tree more or less equally. On the contrary, atherosclerotic plaques are generally located in strategic sites, specifically thoracic aorta and coronary arteries, the branches of the cerebral vessels, and arteries extending into the legs. The arteries of the arms are essentially spared, as are the smaller branches of the

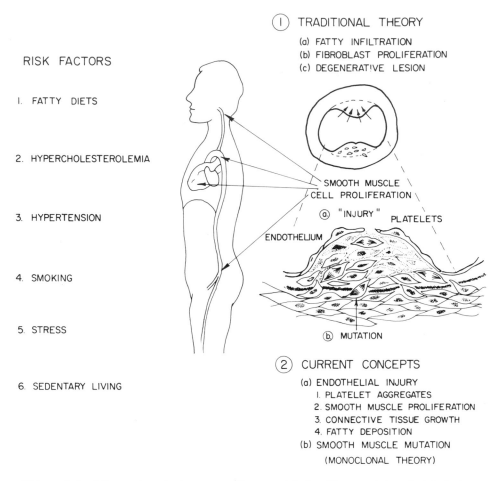

Figure 4-5. Atherosclerosis is apparently associated with a variety of risk factors, some of which are common to those encountered in carcinogenesis. Migration and proliferation of smooth muscle cells are attributed to repeated injury or mutation in contemporary concepts (see text).

arterial tree. The discrepancies between the general character of the risk factors and the intimate pathophysiology of localized lesions in the arterial walls represents an unresolved problem, which can be elucidated only by improved understanding of the disease process at the sites of the lesions.

ATHEROGENESIS

Two basic concepts dominated the biomedical perceptions of atherosclerosis for nearly a hundred years. Rudolph Virchow (16) interpreted pathological appearances as indicating a process of infiltration of fatty substances from the blood stream into arterial walls. The resulting deposits of cholesterol were believed to act as irritants, causing inflammation and cell proliferation in the inner layers of the wall. According to this concept, the characteristic cellular material was attributed in part to migration of fibroblasts into the arterial wall. The subsequent association of atherosclerosis with high fat diets and elevated blood lipids appeared to support this durable and dominant concept of Virchow.

Since World War II, the electron microscope revealed evidence that the cells within the atherosclerotic lesions were not fibroblasts, but probably smooth muscle cells that normally occupy the media of the arterial walls (Fig. 4-5). Current concepts revolve around mechanisms designed to explain the proliferation of smooth muscle cells and their accumulation in the intima of arteries, predominantly in the locations indicated in Figure 4–5. Presumably, the smooth muscle cells in the media proliferate and migrate toward the inner layer of the arterial wall, and this process is accompanied by the accumulation of substances such as connective tissue, proteins, and lipids. The current thrust toward elucidating atherogenesis is directed toward mechanisms that could account for proliferation of smooth muscle cells in arterial walls. Many imaginative concepts have been proposed. Recently two competing hypotheses have emerged, with quite different explanations and conclusions (17–19).

Recurrent Injury. Recurrent injury is regarded as one central theme that is an extension of Virchow's concept. The proponents of the response to injury concept have elicited evidence that lesions like those in human atherosclerosis can be produced by a wide variety of endothelial injuries in experimental animals. Damage to endothelial lining of arteries has been demonstrated to result from trauma due to mechanical abrasion or injury produced by immunological or chemical insults. These injuries are believed to disrupt the continuity of the endothelial layer, which permits infiltration of the various chemical constituents of the blood into the underlying layers of arterial wall. This process is reminiscent of the older fatty infiltration concept, since lipids of the blood are still believed by some to be potential factors in stimulating smooth muscle cell proliferation.

A platelet-dependent serum factor has been demonstrated to stimulate the proliferation of arterial smooth muscle cells in tissue cultures by Ross and his colleagues (17,18). Proliferating smooth muscle cells are believed to secrete proteins and other macromolecules, both in vivo and in vitro. Connective tissue and lipids accumulate if the endothelial injuries are sustained or repeated, and these lesions then resemble advanced atherosclerotic plaques in humans. Additional types of "injuries" include high blood pressure and other nonspecific types of insult. None of these proposed injurious elements focuses on the localized distribution of the atherosclerotic lesions in coronaries, aorta, cerebral, or leg arteries. For this purpose it has been necessary to invoke hemodynamic or other factors. It can be demonstrated that liquids flowing rapidly through branching channels may exhibit flow separation and added stresses on the walls at locations that roughly correspond to the development of lesions in some parts of the arterial tree.

The recurrent injury concept can be summarized by the following sequence (17):

1. Focal desquamation of endothelial cells
2. Adhesion and aggregation of platelets to the exposed subendothelial connective tissue
3. Local release of platelet constituents, including a platelet "factor" that stimulates cell division or mitosis of smooth muscle cells
4. Passage of plasma constituents into the underlying arterial wall
5. Migration of smooth muscle cells through gaps in the internal elastic lamina and into the intima
6. Proliferation of the smooth muscle cells invading the intima in response to a platelet factor.
7. Formation of a connective tissue matrix by smooth muscle cells elaborating and excreting collagen, elastic fiber proteins, and glycosamineoglycans
8. Accumulation of lipids both intracellularly and in the extracellular spaces.

It has been noted that in animals experiments, the injured endothelium may be completely regenerated if the insults are discontinued. When the endothelial lining of the blood vessel is fully repaired, the subendothelial lesions may regress and virtually disappear. This observation is taken as support of the concept that endothelial injury is the initiating event that leads to atherosclerosis. A key question arises regarding the intimate causes of smooth muscle cell proliferation when arterial endothelium is injured. In humans and in animals with elevated blood lipids, low density lipoproteins might cause smooth muscle cell proliferation as in tissue culture. Other substances in the blood that might cause smooth muscle cell proliferation may be released from platelets that aggregate at the site of injury. A growth stimulating factor is postulated as being released from platelets when blood clots form (i.e., at the site of "injury"). Factors from platelets can be demonstrated to induce smooth muscle cell proliferation, which is not present in cell-free serum. It is assumed that in the absence of endothelial damage, such materials are confined to the blood and do not enter the arterial wall in quantities sufficient to induce cell proliferation.

The response to injury hypothesis is based mainly on studies of animals with supportive indirect evidence from clinical examples. The initial events in human atherosclerosis are nearly impossible to identify and follow. According to some investigators, the lesions of injured arteries in animals are not necessarily comparable to the human atherosclerotic plaques observed at postmortem examinations. A competing theory avoids this controversy, based on data derived primarily from studies of atherosclerotic plaques removed from human cadavers.

Mutation (Monoclonal Concept). Dissatisfied with existing theories of atherogenesis, Benditt (19) conceived that one cell or possibly a few could migrate from the media and proliferate in a slowly developing mass of cells in the intima, without involvement of lipids in the early lesions. In later stages, degenerated or dead cells would contribute intercellular debris and fatty deposits.

A different hypothesis was considered and explored: namely, that the proliferation of smooth muscle cells might result from the sequential reproduction of a single smooth muscle cell through mutation. Under these conditions the daughter cells from a single origin would have the same genetic and enzymatic characteristics. Evidence for this concept was derived from the fact that samples of smooth muscle from normal segments of human arterial walls could be demonstrated to contain mixtures of at least two different kinds of cells based on sensitive tests for enzymes. Samples of cells derived from individual atherosclerotic plaques were reported to have but one type of enzymatic pattern. On this basis it was postulated (19) that atherosclerotic lesions were the result of smooth muscle cell proliferation from single mutant cells corresponding to "benign tumors." The permanence of genetic mutations as opposed to the more transient effects of irritation is a principal distinction between these two contemporary views of atherogenesis.

The postulate that atherogenesis stems from abnormal cell proliferation forges a very strong link between atherogenesis and carcinogenesis (see Figs. 4-4, 4-5). Among the possible initiating factors are intrinsic genetic susceptibility that may favor mutations. Some factors that lead to mutation in cancer might have relevance to atherosclerosis. The administration of "mutagenic" materials has been reported to have increased the number of plaques in the aorta of experimental animals. Epidemiological relationships between death rates from cancer of the colon and atherosclerotic heart disease have been reported. Breast cancer rates have been found to correlate with dietary fat intake resembling relations found for deaths from heart disease.

The monoclonal theory fails to explain the anatomical distribution of the lesions, since there is nothing obvious about various sites that would cause mutation of smooth muscle. However, there is evidence that cells from different arteries undergo aging at different rates: cells from segments of the aorta, where lesions are prone to occur seem to age more rapidly. This might be a factor contributing to the concentration of lesions in discrete anatomic locations.

Senescence Hypothesis. One of the most obvious risk factors in the development of atherosclerosis is advancing age. The smooth muscle population in the arterial wall is believed to be maintained by proliferative activity of a few scattered "stem" cells in both the media and intimal layers of arterial walls. Their reproduction is envisioned as controlled by inhibiting factors called *chalones* secreted by the newly formed smooth muscle cells. Martin and Sprague (20) postulated that the control or feedback system of smooth muscle proliferation deteriorates with age, allowing persistent proliferation in the intima to occur with the resulting production of atherosclerotic lesions. These three hypotheses can be characterized as postulating "stimulation" of cell proliferation, or "mutation," to produce uncontrolled proliferation.

The three concepts pretty well cover the main mechanisms that might be envisioned. Such a brief discussion fails to do justice to the masses of data that have now been assembled in support of the various concepts of atherogenesis. Our current concepts of pathophysiology fail to suggest courses of therapy that might be particularly effective. Our base of knowledge does not elucidate the relationships between the development of lesions in the arterial walls and the common risk factors that have been disclosed through epidemiological studies. Serious deficiencies in our understanding of causes and cures impede progress toward definitive therapy. Instead, reduction of risk factors is the basis for nationwide programs designed to "control" cardiovascular disease. The major thrust of therapy is toward the alleviation of complications (i.e., pain and occlusive infarcts) by widespread applications of various pseudosolutions.

THERAPEUTIC APPROACHES

Despite some notable advances in our understanding of pathophysiology, the ultimate origins of atherosclerosis are not sufficiently advanced to provide a basis for definitive therapy. The many and varied components of our knowledge cannot be integrated into an effective whole, pending the elucidation of the central hub (see Fig. 4-2). A surge of progress toward the development of effective therapy, cure, and ultimately prevention of atherosclerosis should follow elucidation of the key issues—the etiology of smooth muscle proliferation, according to current concepts. Although the pace of progress is deliberate and frustrating, ultimate rewards are so great that continued efforts by the most imaginative and skilled investigators is warranted with extremely high priority, despite the temptations to proceed prematurely toward the applications of available therapeutic modalities.

Reduction of Risk Factors. Widespread atherosclerosis can develop gradually to advanced stages without producing signs or symptoms. Reduction in risk factors requires heavy dependence on the willingness of susceptible persons to comply with dietary and therapeutic regimes that are believed to be effective in reducing the probability of complications. It has proved remarkably difficult to encourage or to cajole changes in behavior, even with the mobilization of the major mass media. Avoidance of high cholesterol diets, sensible health habits, and adequate control of diabetes and hypertension have proved surprisingly difficult to sustain in persons at risk of atherosclerosis, but without symptoms of the disease. However, progress is demonstrable in the reduction of smoking incidence among the older age groups, despite an increased incidence among the young. The 10 million people who are engaged in jogging for health is a notable accomplishment, but its ultimate contribution to health status is still conjectural. Reduction in the incidence of death from cardiovascular disease is reported to be faster than the decline of noncardiovascular death rates. Such results are not the basis for complacency, because cardiovascular diseases remain the leading burden of illness on the American public by a variety of criteria (see Fig. 3–5).

Care of Complications. Two of the most frequent and feared complications of atherosclerosis are angina pectoris and myocardial infarction. Development of sophisticated monitoring devices and techniques for defibrillation have undoubtedly prolonged the lives of many persons who have suffered what might otherwise have been fatal heart attacks. The enthusiasm with which coronary care units have been developed across the nation has provided improved access to expert management of this critical illness. There are reasons to suspect that the numbers of coronary care units emerging in certain geographic locations probably exceed actual need. This possibility is accentuated by evidence from abroad, that the death rates from myocardial infarction may be remarkably similar among patients who are treated either at home or on general hospital wards instead of in these highly sophisticated, expensive coronary care units. This issue is considered in more detail in Chapters 5 and 6.

Surgery for Angina Pectoris. The intolerable pain that develops on exertion among so many patients with coronary insufficiency is a powerful stimulus to the development and use of measures promoting symptomatic relief. Medical measures often fail to provide the results desired and surgical interventions of many types have been proposed, used widely, and then discarded. The most recent example has been the enthusiastic acceptance of coronary bypass surgery, which has virtually swept across the nation in a remarkably short time.

The concept of improving the blood supply to the myocardium through surgical intervention has a long and interesting history. One of the most vigorous proponents of coronary surgery was Claude Beck (21), a surgeon in Cleveland, Ohio. Beck noticed that the adhesions between the pericardial surface and the surface of the heart contained blood vessels that bled actively from both cut surfaces. This was interpreted to mean that coronary blood supply might be supplemented by the development of adhesions to the heart surface, with ingrowth of new blood vessels connecting up with the preexisting coronary circulation. Many and varied means were used to produce adhesions, including abrasion of the pericardial surface by means of a mechanical burr, installing bone dust as an irritant, suturing pectoral muscle to the surface of the heart, or the introduction of chemical irritants such as powdered asbestos and talc. Additional interventions included ligation of the coronary sinus to impede venus outflow from that channel, believed to stimulate creation of intercoronary channels and blood supply to ischemic areas. Additional modifications of these basic procedures were carried out by many other prominent surgeons over a period of some 25 years. The usefulness of these procedures was evaluated in experimental animals by comparing mortality after experimental ligation of the anterior descending coronary artery, and in man by the reported reduction in angina pectoris among these patients. The underlying concepts and the results of many efforts were reviewed in a Symposium on Coronary Artery Disease in 1957. Oddly enough, objective methods were regarded as having little value for evaluating the medical and surgical treatment of coronary insufficiency. Instead, reliance was placed on each patient serving as his own control, with reports of subjective relief of symptoms as the principal sign of success (21).

Some additional efforts at enhancing the coronary blood supply included the ligation of the internal mammary artery, in the belief that this would shunt blood into the coronary circulation. Another approach involved the introduction of the cut end of mammary artery into a tunnel formed in the wall of the heart (22).

This varied assortment of surgical approaches was applied to an extremely large number of patients, running into the thousands. The initial results of the different procedures were enthusiastically reported as being extremely good. For example, Brotman (23), reporting on 100 consecutive patients who were alive and could be evaluated after six months to five years, noted that 90% had symptomatically excellent results. (Forty-two percent were able to work with no limitations, while 48 were better able to work with some limitations). Thus, 90% were reported to be "economically productive," in contrast with 45% who had been able to work only half time or less. These results are particularly remarkable in view of the fact that there is now a widespread consensus that these operations could have little or no functional effect in reinforcing the blood supply to the myocardium. For example, ligation of internal mammary artery was subjected to a pair of critical evaluations by Cobb et al. (24) and Diamond et al. (25). In these evaluations, the results of actual ligation were contrasted to simulated operations consisting of incisions of the skin, sewed up without ligation of mammary arteries. By chance, a better statistical result was disclosed among the "sham" operated patients than among those in whom the mammary artery had been ligated as the "experimental" group. There is now a general consensus that all these efforts at producing increased coronary blood supply through pericardial adhesions and occlusion of coronary sinus or mammary arteries were based on faulty concepts of hemodynamics and were functionally useless except for psychological or "placebo" effects.

Coronary Bypass Surgery. A far more physiologically sound approach originated with Murray (26), who directly joined mammary arteries to coronary arteries beyond obstructions to provide supplemental blood flow. From 1954 until the mid 1960s, various types of bypass channels were installed between the aorta or its central branches to the coronary arteries of experimental animals. The first reported arterial anastomosis to a coronary artery in humans was by Kolessov (27) in 1966. Clinical applications of vein grafts to connect the aorta with coronary arteries was begun in 1967 with the work of Favaloro (28). By 1977, coronary artery bypass surgery had gained such widespread acceptance (29), that some 65,000 operations were being performed annually in the United States, at an approximate cost of at least $10,000 per procedure. Reports indicate some 70 to 80% of such patients professed partial or complete relief from their angina in the early years after their operation. There have been reports of improved functional status as a result of the procedure, but this claim remains somewhat controversial. For example, Barnes et al. (30) found no improvement in work status or hours worked after surgery in 350 patients evaluated. There is corresponding uncertainty regarding the extent to which surgical measures add to the longevity of patients.

Preston (31) marshalled evidence on the possibility that much of the beneficial effects of these heroic surgical efforts stem more from a placebo effect than from a physiological or functional improvement. This important issue is currently under intensive study as one of the clinical trials being carried out by the National Heart, Lung, and Blood Institute. Initiated in fiscal year 1970, critical evaluation of coronary bypass surgery has been undertaken as a collaborative study among 18 prestigious institutions. The choice of institutions will tend to bias the results, since most favorable outcomes are to be expected from fully equipped and exceptionally talented teams engaged in very active cardiac surgery. The volume of coronary bypass surgery has become so great in institutions large and small, that the data derived from such a study may not be safely extrapolated to the rest of the nation. These issues will be considered further in relation to the impact of technologies, as discussed in Chapter 5.

Transplants and Implants of Mechanical Hearts. Development of interim technologies, or pseudosolutions, is one response to the incessant demands of patients for relief from painful and life-threatening ailments. Even more dramatic examples were represented by the flurry of heart transplants that caught the imagination of the world over a period of two or three years. The enthusiasm for heart transplants was relatively rapidly dissipated by the rather frequent appearance of the rejection phenomenon, indicating that the basic research into immune reactions had been inadequate for wide-scale success of heart transplants.

Still another contemporary technical pseudosolution is the development of a fully implantable mechanical heart. The basic idea of constructing an artificial heart as a substitute for the natural one is relatively old. John Gibbon reported success in keeping cats alive for nearly three hours using a mechanical apparatus as a heart-lung substitute in 1939. Specifications for circulatory assist devices emerged with the advances in cardiovascular physiology and surgery along with the proliferation of many mechanical heart-lung devices. The artificial heart program of the Heart Lung Institute has four major categories:

· Emergency systems
· Temporary cardiac assist systems (both implanted and external)
· Permanently implantable assist systems
· Total artificial heart replacement, substituting mechanical pumps for the heart as a long-range goal

At the outset, the projections as to need for implanted mechanical hearts ranged as high as 200,000 per year. This figure has been revised downward to a range of 16,000 to 50,000 per year. The tendency for blood to clot when in contact with foreign surfaces has been a major problem. Substantial progress has been made in development of pumping mechanisms through improved design and materials. Even more serious is the difficulty in developing a compact power source to meet high energy requirements of the circulation. The heart muscle is such an efficient energy converter that artificial substitutes are gross and clumsy in comparison. It is technically possible to insert into the body a storage battery of reasonable weight and size that could power an artificial heart with four recharging periods per day over a two-year period. Alternatively, the use of nuclear power would provide greater longevity but also increases the hazards of radiation to patients and to people with whom they might come in contact under a wide variety of undesirable circumstances. Legal, social, ethical, medical, economic, and psychological implications of the totally implantable heart have been carefully considered by the Artificial Heart Assessment Panel in June of 1973. This is one of the first comprehensive technology assessments in the biomedical area, and will be discussed in additional detail in Chapter 5.

TOP PRIORITIES IN ATHEROGENESIS AND CARCINOGENESIS

The foregoing discussion disclosed a remarkable commonality of basic issues in current concepts of etiology of cancer and atherosclerosis. Both of these dread diseases appear to stem from a common or closely related origin; namely, the inappropriate or uncontrolled proliferation of cells. In atherosclerosis, the smooth muscle cells are believed to proliferate and migrate into the intima, producing local lesions which protrude into arterial channels. This proliferation is attributed to stimulation of cell division or mutation of individual smooth muscle cells. Neoplasms are also characterized by abnormal replication of cells by mutagenic processes of unknown nature attributable to either carcinogenic stimulation or mutation. The metastatic tendency of some malignant tumors might be regarded as an extreme manifestation of the process rather than a fundamental difference in the basic etiological proprocesses.

The fundamental mechanisms leading to cell mitosis and uncontrolled cell proliferation clearly represent a target of the greatest importance in the genesis of the two most dreaded diseases besetting mankind. The importance of mounting a large scale and coordinated targeted research effort directed at elucidating the common causes of these two health hazards can hardly be overestimated. The potential rewards for successful efforts along these lines would appear to justify a very large scale effort of the magnitude currently proposed by the Institutes of Health. However, answers to these enigmas will not come readily and may emerge from totally unexpected sources. Meanwhile, the attractive prospects from such an effort must not be allowed to divert too much attention from the very large number of other sources of disease and disability as represented by the other components of the NIH and other granting agencies.

OTHER LEADING CAUSES OF DEATH, DISEASE, DISABILITY, AND DISCOMFORT

The preeminent position generally awarded cancer and heart disease has tended to overshadow the many other hazards to health that occur with great frequency among the American people. The uncertainties surrounding the causation of these important maladies obscure the prospects or probabilities of overcoming theoretical obstacles. Large investments are also warranted in support of targeted research into some of these other kinds of diseases and disability. Such efforts might return even richer rewards from more reasonable investments. The number of options is so very great that they cannot be encompassed in a limited publication such as this one. The limited space devoted to some selected examples of common complaints should not be interpreted to indicate anything about their relative importance. The potential rewards of successful targeted research in any one of them would certainly warrant a major investment and relatively high priority. In addition, there are hordes of additional ailments that could have been mentioned with equally persuasive reasons.

The priorities implied by the 10 leading causes of death include trauma on the highway, home, and occupation with homicide and suicide as related items (Table 4-1). An essential requirement for dealing with injuries stemming from accidents or violence is emergency care—a traditional role of the physician and surgeon from earliest times. However, modern technology is capable of materially reducing both the incidence and severity of these injuries to a significant degree (i.e., seat belts, home and occupational safety measures), but use of these mechanisms requires the cooperation of people. The ability to modify human behavior has proved to be a greater challenge than we are prepared to meet with existing concepts and approaches. The origins of these threats to life and health are social and behavioral and beyond the scope of the present discussion of "targeted" research in biomedical research. However, these areas are ripe for investigation at the more fundamental levels in disciplines such as sociology and behavioral sciences. In contrast, influenza and pneumonia appear as the fifth most common causes of death and the number one as causes of bed disability and limitation of activity (Table 4–2).

BED DISABILITY AND LIMITATION OF ACTIVITY

The numbers of persons afflicted with conditions that require care in bed greatly exceed the causes of mortality (Table 4-1). At the top of the list are influenza and pneumonia, believed to involve some 250 million days of bed disability (Table 4-2). Upper respiratory diseases, particularly head colds, are next in line but are not responsible for so many persons with chronic limitations. In contrast, the number of people affected by heart disease is substantially smaller than either of the respiratory disease categories but accounts for more than 4.5 million persons with chronic limitation in activity. Three categories of interim solutions are listed for heart disease, specifically pacemakers, coronary bypass operations, and mechanical hearts for temporary use or engineered for implantation. Arthritis is an exceedingly mysterious condition, causing excruciating pain to huge numbers of persons. The current modes of therapy are largely symptomatic, with artificial joint replacement serving as an interim technology until more definitive therapy can be devised. Mental disorders are also extremely common and the most common therapy is by means of various mood-altering drugs. Pharmaceuticals could be classified as pseudosolutions, and psychosurgery is rather heroic and extreme example of an interim technology that is being phased out in most centers.

Examining the list of chronic conditions producing limitations in activities creates an impression that most of them have etiologies that are either unknown or controversial. Most of the diseases are treated primarily by symptomatic and support mechanisms and/or by pseudosolutions. These conditions clearly need and deserve sustained efforts at basic research at all levels, fundamental, functional, and targeted, to enhance the prospects of more definitive therapy emerging in the future.

INFLUENZA AND PNEUMONIA

Influenza is familiar to all as a common affliction that tends to appear in epidemics sweeping across the nation. To the young and fit, "flu" is a self-limiting ailment of considerable discomfort, but to the aged or the chronically ill, it is a life-threatening illness too often terminating in pneumonia. Influenza and pneumonia together are the fifth leading cause of death in the United States. The antibiotics that have proved so valuable in combating bacterial infections have little effect on viruses. Three types of influenza virus have been identified (A, B, C). The genetic make-up of respiratory viruses have been found to consist of continuous strands of nucleic acid (RNA or DNA). However, the influenza viruses are different, consisting of seven or eight discrete pieces contained within an envelope, studded with two antigens that play an important role in the attack on cells. The fragmented nature of the virus is believed to account for the strange ability of the influenza virus to undergo periodic changes which render useless vaccines from previous epidemics so the population is vulnerable to the next one. The rapidly growing bank of knowledge regarding genetic manipulation provides promise of mating virulent viruses with less virulent strains to produce effective vaccines. Extensive experience with an anti-viral agent—interferon—has given hope that persistent efforts will succeed in developing or stimulating the material in sufficient quantity to be effective (i.e., in common colds—see below).

Immunization against influenza is uncertain in its effectiveness and potentially hazardous as displayed in the massive application of swine flu vaccines. The therapy for influenza is generally supportive, symptomatic, and palliative rather than definitive. The use of bed rest, aspirin, fluids, and temperature control has not differed significantly from the ministrations of grandmothers or maiden aunts of previous generations. The pneumonia that often complicates the disease in the aged or infirm most commonly involves pneumococci, staphylococci, streptococci, or *Hemophilus influenzae.*

Pneumococcal pneumonia is just as common today as it was before the advent of the "wonder drugs" (i.e., some 200,000 to 400,000 instances with about 45,000 deaths per year). Pneumococci account for nearly 80% of all

TABLE 4-2. Bed Disability and Limitation of Activity Due to Selected
Conditions in the United States, 1974

Diagnostic Condition	Days of Bed Disability	Number of Persons Chronically Limited	Interim Technologies (Pseudosolutions)	Estimated Need for Basic Research
Influenza and pneumonia	275,573	???		++
Upper respiratory	149,490	478,000		++++
Heart disease	108,141	4,753,000	Pacemakers Bypass Mechanical heart	++++
Arthritis	76,412	4,258,000	Joint replacement	++++
Mental disorders	51,154	2,111,000	Psychosurgery	++++
Fractures, dislocations	45,100	???		+
Malignant neoplasms	42,906	633,000	Excision Radiation Chemotherapy	++++
Cerebrovascular disease	39,719	793,000		++++
Diabetes	30,426	1,448,000		++
Back and spine	29,855	2,051,000		+++
Hypertension	29,732	1,976,000		++++
Paralysis	29,000	974,000	Powered extremities	++++
Asthma	27,550	1,434,000		+++
Emphysema	25,166	822,000		++++
Lower extremities	20,274	1,889,000	Powered wheelchairs	++
Hernia	19,078	690,000		++
Bronchitis	17,968	293,000		+++
Gallbladder	15,887	179,000		+++
Ulcer	15,533	550,000		+++

Basic Data relating to National Institutes of Health (1976), Office of Program Planning
and Evaluation

acute bacterial pneumonias. The gelatinous capsule composed of polysac-
charides surrounding the diplococcus protects the organism from engulfment
by leukocytes. The characteristics of the capsules distinguish more than 80
types, of which about 14 account for about 75% of the infections in man.
Like other types of illness, pneumococcal pneumonia is most prevalent in
people with certain risk factors, such as:

· Viral upper respiratory infections
· Chemical irritation of the respiratory tract
· Patients who are "chronically ill"
· Infants
· Patients with asthma

· Diabetic patients
· Patients in heart failure
· Chronic bronchitis
· Emphysema
· Debilitation from cancer
· Cultural and environmental conditions (i.e., in American Indians)

Despite the availability of effective antibiotics, the mortality has risen during the past decade. This is attributable in part to the aging population. Even more important is the appearance of strains of organisms that are increasingly resistant to antibiotics from indiscriminate use of these antibacterial agents by the health professions. For this reason, there is an urgent need for an effective vaccine against these pneumococci for use on high-risk groups of patients. Worth noting is the firm foundation and vast experience in the area of control and prevention of infections that could be mustered for an attack on this problem. The obstacles to be confronted in development of a vaccine are inherently technical rather than theoretical and could be the basis for mobilizing a major sustained attack on the problem. Unfortunately, the resources have not been allocated for this purpose, partly because of the distribution of available resources to conditions in which the obstacles are fundamentally theoretical (see Figs. 4-4 and 4-5).

Common Acute Conditions. The conditions that threaten life or produce chronic disability are not among the most common afflictions of mankind. Surveys have disclosed the predominant place of common colds, influenza, accidents, gastrointestinal disturbances, and so forth in the roster of ailments that beset the common man. For example, colds and upper respiratory infections eclipse bronchitis and pneumonia so far as incidence in concerned. "Flu," with or without gastrointestinal symptoms, is reported to be the next most frequent. It is much easier to mobilize sympathy, support, and resources for conditions which threaten lives than for conditions that merely cause misery. We have no yardsticks for relating the relative importance of death or chronic disability in a few patients as opposed to self-limited misery of the many.

COMMON COLDS

There appears to be little sense of urgency for the development of a cure or preventive measure for the common cold. However, the significance of the ailment is not trivial, by humanitarian or economic standards. Common colds are believed to account for some 35% of acute illnesses resulting in some 400 million work-days lost. The dollar cost of pills and formulas for runny noses is estimated at more than $550 million per year (32).

More than 100 different viruses are believed to be able to produce the symptoms of a common cold, but only about 30% to 50% of the infestations can be related to specific viruses. In the others, no infectious agent can be isolated. Rhinoviruses were the first important group to be associated with colds. More recently, coronaviruses have received attention as causing these symptoms during December through February when rhinoviruses are less common. Numerous other infectious agents have been associated with common cold symptoms. One promising area of research is directed toward means of stimulating antiviral activity in the body of the host. One such antiviral substance is interferon, a part of the body's natural defense mechanism against viruses.

Interferon: An Antiviral Agent. Since viruses are true parasites, it has proved very difficult to develop drugs that would be effective against the virus particles while sparing the host cells in which they reside. Viral interference—the capacity of one virus to inhibit or interfere with the growth of another—has been known for many years (33). For example, influenza viruses infecting chick embryo cells have been shown to release into the culture medium a material that can make other cells resistant to infection by a different virus. The quantity of material produced by such a process is extremely small, so that quantities sufficient for utilization in man have not been produced. However, there is some prospect of finding ways by which the host cells can be induced to create interferon in response to some attenuated virus or other stimulus. The cellular production of interferon is currently regarded as a rather complicated process involving at least two steps (Fig. 4-6). According to this theory, the genetic material of the host cell contains the necessary instructions for the production of the protein known as interferon. The host cell does not undertake this synthesis until stimulated by the entrance of a virus. An antiviral protein is synthesized by part of the cellular DNA. The interferon produced by the reaction may not be confined to the originating cells but is believed to invade adjoining cells, contributing to the process of developing antiviral proteins. This process is theoretical and presented schematically, but it contains the essence of an approach to control of virus infections that currently resist available antibiotics. Interferon has been shown to have effect against the common cold, hepatitis, and other viral infections. Current efforts are being directed toward the development of substances capable of exciting host cells to produce endogenous interferon, rather than attempting to develop quantities of the material sufficient for injection into patients.

Notable successes in providing definitive therapy for both bacteria and viruses must not be permitted to cloud our perception of the targeted research directed toward infectious disorders of the gastrointestinal tract, urinary tract, skin, and so forth. The enormous background of experience in the development of antibiotics and immunity provides added assurance that massive attack on the technical problems should be rewarded.

Impending Pandemics. Impending pandemics include increasing incidence of microorganisms for which effective therapy is currently available (i.e., venereal diseases). Thus, the development of definitive therapeutic modalities is not always a final answer. It is also necessary to overcome social, psychological, cultural, and other obstacles to complete the process. For this reason, the added emphasis on behavioral and social sciences in the forward plans for NIH seems particularly timely and appropriate (Chapter 2).

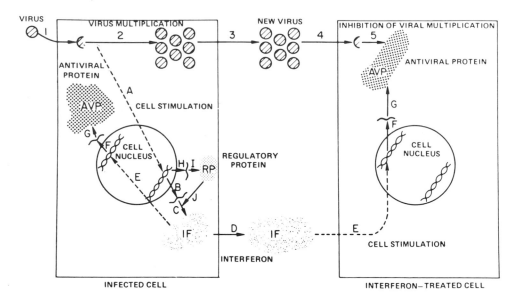

Figure 4-6. Interferon is produced when a virus enters into a body cell, releases its genetic material, and replication occurs, according to current concepts. Stimulation of a gene in the DNA of the host cell releases messenger RNA, leading to development of the interferon protein. Interferon is then released into perivascular fluid and enters other cells where it stimulates production of an antiviral protein (AVP). In this way, interferon may help to protect cells from subsequent invasion of viruses (From NIAID [34]).

SUMMARY

1. Many and varied health problems are persistent threats to the health of the American public. Targeted research into immediate and intimate etiology of such ailments must have high priority in the programs of health-related research. Elucidation of cause(s) is an essential element in the development of more definitive diagnosis and effective therapy.

2. Interim technologies employed for conditions of unknown origin take the form of drugs or devices that serve as supplement or substitutes for normal function, instead of being directed at the underlying pathological processes. Such pseudosolutions may be very beneficial but inordinately expensive, diverting attention from the need to actively pursue more definitive methods of management.

3. The forward-planning effort of the National Cancer Program includes major efforts directed at "risk factors," causative factors, and funda-

mental relationships between neoplastic cells and the host organism. Many different etiological mechanisms are postulated—chemical carcinogens, viruses, radiation, among many others. The multiplicity of proposed causes clearly indicates that the main obstacles to progress are theoretical, not technical (see also Chapter 3).

4. Current concepts of atherogenesis are focused on factors believed to induce proliferation and migration of smooth muscle cells from the media into the intima in the production of characteristic lesions.

5. A very large proportion of common ailments, life-threatening or self-limited, are deserving of major targeted research efforts. The current state of knowledge regarding the origins of persistent infections (i.e., colds, "flu," pneumonia, and others) is sufficiently advanced that some of the technical problems could be surmounted, using past experience and knowledge. More intensive research and development efforts directed at these conditions might provide rich rewards in improving the health of the American public.

REFERENCES

1. Duffy J: *The Healers; The Rise of the Medical Establishment* New York, McGraw-Hill Book Company, 1976.
2. Burkitt DP: Some diseases characteristic of modern western civilization. *Brit Med J* 1:274-278, 1973.
3. Hunter D: *The Diseases of Occupations*, ed 4., Boston, Little, Brown and Company, 1969.
4. Glazier WH: The task of medicine. *Scientific Am* 228:12-16, 1973.
5. Thomas L: Planning of science. Notes of a biology watcher. *N Engl J Med*, 289:89-90, 1973.
6. Bourne HR: The placebo—a poorly understood and neglected therapeutic agent. *Ration Drug Ther*, 5:1, 1971.
7. Thomas L: Guessing and knowing; reflections on the science and technology of medicine. *Saturday Review, Science* 55:52-57, 1972.
8. Kolff WJ: Artificial organs and their impact, in Kronenthal RL, Oser Z, Martin E (eds): *Polymers in Medicine and Surgery*, vol 8. New York, Plenum Publishing Corporation, 1975, pp 1-27.
9. Rice D (Director, National Center for Health Statistics): Statement before Intergovernmental Relations and Human Resources Subcommittee, Committee on Government Operations. House of Representatives, June 14, 1977.
10. National Cancer Program, 1976 Annual Plan for FY 1978-1982, National Cancer Institute, December, 1976.
11. Hammond EC: Smoking in relation to mortality and morbidity. Findings in the first thirty-four months of follow-up in a prospective study started in 1959. *J US National Cancer Institute* 32:1161-1188, 1964.
12. Morowitz HJ: Hiding in the Hammond Report. *Hospital Practice* 10:35-39, 1975.

13. Old LJ: Cancer immunology. *Scientific American* 236:62-79, 1977.
14. Fidler IJ: Tumor heterogeneity and the biology of cancer invasion and metastasis. *Cancer Research* 38:2651-2660, 1978.
15. Fourth Report of the Director, National Heart, Blood Vessel, Lung and Blood Program, DHEW Pub No (NIH) 77-1171, March 1, 1977.
16. Virchow R: *Gesammelte Abhandlunger zur Wissenshaftlichen Medicin* XIV: 1024 (3), Frankf am, Meidinger Sohn U Comp, 1856.
17. Ross R, Harker L: Hyperlipidemia and atherosclerosis. *Science* 193:1094-1100, 1976.
18. Ross R, Glomset JA: The pathogenesis of atherosclerosis. *N Engl J Med*, 295:369-377 and 420-425, 1976.
19. Benditt EP: The origin of atherosclerosis. *Scientific Am* 236: 74-85, 1977.
20. Martin GP, Sprague CA: Symposium on in vitro studies related to atherogenesis; life histories of hyperplastoid cell lines from aorta and skin. *Exp Mol Pathol*, 18:125-141 (cited in Ref 18), 1973.
21. Beck CS: Symposium on coronary artery disease, blood supply to ischaemic myocardium distal to the occlusion of a coronary artery. *Dis Chest* 31:243-252, 1957.
22. Vineberg AM, Niloff PH: The value of surgical treatment of coronary artery occlusion by implantation of the internal mammary artery into the ventricular myocardium. *Surg Gyne and Obst* 91:551-558, 1950.
23. Brofman GL: Surgical treatment of coronary artery disease; medical management and evaluation of results. *Dis Chest* 31:253-264, 1957.
24. Cobb L, Thomas GK, Dillard DH et al.: An evaluation of internal mammary ligation by a double-blind technique. *N Engl J Med* 260:1115-1122, 1959.
25. Dimond EG, Kittle CF, Crockett JE: Comparison of internal mammary artery ligation and sham operation for angina pectoris. *Am J Cardiol*, 5:483-486, 1960.
26. Murray G, Porcheon R, Hilario J, et al: Anastomosis of a systemic artery to the coronary. *Can Med Assoc J* 71:594-597, 1954.
27. Kolesov V: Mammary artery-coronary artery anastomosis as method of treatment for angina pectoris. *J Thorac Cardiovasc Surg* 54:535-543, 1967.
28. Favaloro RG: Saphenous vein graft in surgical treatment of coronary artery disease. *J Thorac Cardiovas Surg* 58:178-185, 1969.
29. Mundth ED, Austen WG: Surgical measures for coronary heart disease. *N Engl J Med*, 293:124-130, 1975.
30. Barnes G, Ray MJ, Oberman A, et al: Changes in working status of patients following coronary bypass surgery. *JAMA* 238:1259-1262, 1977.
31. Preston TA: *Coronary Artery Surgery: A Critical Review.* New York, Raven Press, 1977.
32. Common Cold: Infectious Diseases Research: National Institute of Allergy and Infectious Diseases. DHEW Pub No (NIH) 77-167, 1977.
33. Antiviral Substances (including interferon). Infectious Diseases Research, National Institute of Allergy and Infectious Diseases. DHEW Pub No (NIH) 77-1047, 1977.

Part Three

Assessment of Health Technologies and Services

Life and health have always been regarded as so inherently valuable that justification of health services has never been deemed necessary. Benevolent extravagance on the part of physicians was realistically regarded as appropriate thoroughness when the number and diversity of diagnostic and therapeutic choices was very limited. The vast array of available clinical tests and treatments can no longer be used indiscriminately without serious escalation in costs beyond prospects of benefit to the patient. Attention is increasingly focused on the importance of appraising health technologies and on evaluating processes by which health care is provided to the population.

The rapid expansion of biomedical research was accompanied by the emergence of a very large assortment of sophisticated devices for acquiring, recording, storing, and analyzing data from various kinds of experiments on animals and human subjects. One response to the pressures for payoff has been to convert such new technologies into diagnostic instruments. In this process, the kinds and quantities of clinical data have expanded exponentially. Automation and computer technologies have increased the speed with which the data can be collected, assembled, and analyzed. New and innovative instruments permit direct vision of virtually every hollow organ while energy probes conveniently produce images displaying many different features of internal organs. Arrays of diagnostic tests can be used at great expense to identify many different diseases for which effective therapy is lacking. Important causes of escalating health care costs include the enormous expansion of health personnel, now numbering some 13 people in support of each physician on the average. The discrepancies between diagnostic capability and therapeutic effectiveness account in large measure for the relatively slight improvement in health status of the public that can be reasonably ascribed to improved health care delivery. Assessment of health technologies in terms of contributions, costs, consequences, and complications is recognized as an important new activity for which methods have not been fully developed.

Evaluation of health service is growing in importance along with the need for technology assessment and for the same reasons. The methods

163

employed are largely derived from other disciplines such as sociology, psychology, and biostatistics, but are still in a relatively primitive state when applied to health program evaluation. The difficulties and obstacles are so ominous that a very large proportion of evaluation projects have been directed at rather simple and superficial problems. A substantial majority of projects underway are directed at processes or procedures to determine if they are being handled smoothly and efficiently. The greatest difficulty lies in assessing the extent to which patients have derived benefit from the health services they receive. The relationships between costs and benefits defy analysis to a considerable degree and may be approached by considering the "value added" by various levels of therapy.

CHAPTER 5

Impact of Health Technologies:
Contributions and Consequences

During the past 30 years, a technical revolution has drastically altered virtually every aspect of the health care delivery system of this country. Increasingly sophisticated devices have been adopted by medical school faculties in both basic science and clinical departments. New recording and analytical techniques have been developed to provide objective and quantitative information regarding the functional characteristics of various organ systems in health and disease. They provide greater precision and more detail than could have been conceived a few decades ago. Many of these research techniques have been converted into expanding arrays of diagnostic equipment. In addition, life support systems now permit surgeons to invade virtually any organ of the body to remove, repair, reconstruct, or replace components that have been distorted or destroyed by disease processes (see Chapter 4). Engineering technologies have been successfully employed to provide functional substitutes and supplements for many of the most important bodily functions. Such profound changes in the fabric of the health care system have necessarily involved major changes in its organization and operational mechanisms.

The traditional family physician, conducting medical practice out of a little black bag, has been largely replaced by highly trained specialists and subspecialists, new health professionals, practitioners, and technicians required to use effectively the increasingly complex equipment available for management of diseases of the various organ systems. As costs have escalated, the government has become increasingly involved in the details of health care far beyond the support of the research enterprise. Government has assumed roles in the safety and effectiveness of new devices (Food and Drug Administration) and in the financial support of health services for the military, the

165

veterans, the aged, and the poor. The entire population will be covered if comprehensive national health insurance ultimately becomes a reality.

This chapter is intended to review briefly the impact of modern technological achievements, some of the contributions to health care, and the unpredicted consequences and complications from their applications.

CONVERSION OF RESEARCH TECHNOLOGIES INTO DIAGNOSTIC DEVICES

At the turn of the century, physicians were highly dependent on their own five subjective senses for gathering diagnostic data. They were aided to a degree by the newly developed x-ray and electrocardiograph machines, and a limited number of laboratory examinations on samples of blood, body fluids, and excreta. During the first half of the century, the private practice of medicine was little affected by the surges of technical progress in other parts of society. Specifically, the equipment in the average doctor's office was altered less than the average housewife's kitchen. Expanding laboratory facilities tended to be concentrated in hospitals, but at a relatively slow rate.

BASIC BIOMEDICAL RESEARCH TECHNOLOGIES

Before World War II, the traditional approaches to basic medical research continued to be leisurely, scholarly, subjective, and intuitive. Anatomical components were explored by gross dissections and microscopic observations. The concepts of function and control were based largely on direct observations supplemented by crude records to show time relations between events. Two related functions exhibiting changes at the same time were commonly regarded as implying cause and effect relationships. After World War II, attention was focused on basic medical research by James Shannon and others as an essential ingredient for attacks on the diseases affecting mankind (see Chapter 1). The primitive types of research equipment generally employed throughout the basic medical science departments was recognized as totally inadequate for more rigorous or "scientific" approaches to biomedical investigation. There was obvious need for more quantitative measurements and more rigorous analytic approaches to biology and medicine. Instrumentation and analytical techniques commonly used in physics, chemistry, and engineering, were progressively adapted to the study of living organisms and organ systems.

Electron microscopes provided enormously enhanced magnification and resolution as compared with traditional light microscopes (Fig. 5-1). The subjective interpretation of images by the operator can now be reinforced by increasingly sophisticated techniques for recording and analyzing images. The precision and reproducability of the chemical determinations were greatly improved by conversion from laborious manual procedures into direct reading or automated chemical analysis. Chromatography, spectro-

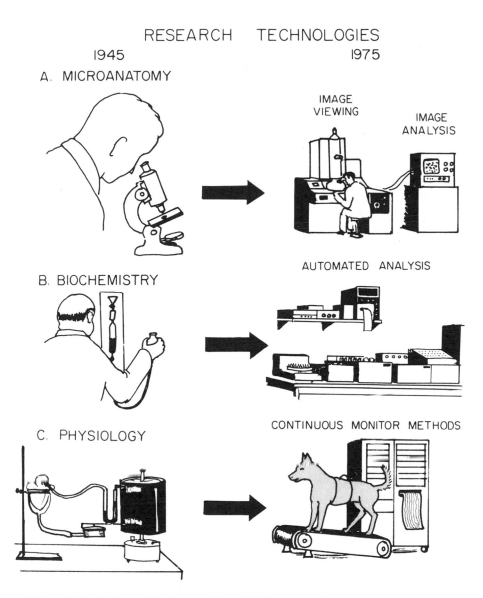

RESEARCH TECHNOLOGIES

1945   1975

A. MICROANATOMY

IMAGE VIEWING

IMAGE ANALYSIS

B. BIOCHEMISTRY

AUTOMATED ANALYSIS

C. PHYSIOLOGY

CONTINUOUS MONITOR METHODS

Figure 5-1. Basic medical research methods were still extremely primitive by the end of World War II. The impetus provided by NIH resulted in rapidly expanding research technologies. (a) Direct vision of microscopic specimens has been enhanced by electron microscopes. (b) Chemical tests have been converted from crude manual operations into increasingly sophisticated direct-reading or even automated chemical testing processes. (c) The simple mechanical and hydraulic systems employed for physiological investigation were replaced by small responsive sensors, amplifiers, and recorders. Special sensors could be implanted chronically to continuously monitor the changing functions of internal organs during a variety of responses by healthy, active animals.

photometry, isotope detectors, and a host of other methods entered into routine use in biochemical laboratories. Primitive mechanical levers and smoked drums used for recording the functions of exposed or isolated organs in physiology laboratories were progressively replaced by a growing array of sensors, amplifiers, and responsive recorders (1). Such measuring equipment could be applied to exposed organs or chronically implanted in animals to study the function of internal structures. Specifically, new sensors were developed to provide accurate information regarding the mechanical function of internal organs. Tiny devices designed to continuously register the changing dimensions, blood pressures, and blood flow velocity in the heart and major blood vessels could be implanted for investigating cardiovascular responses in healthy, active animals during spontaneous and experimentally induced changes (2). Such techniques provided data for continuous analysis of cardiovascular functions in the same quantitative terms that engineers employ for analysis of hydraulic systems. By such techniques, simultaneous recording of many relevant variables could be obtained during various kinds of activity, under stresses, or during delivery of drugs and hormones. Functional disturbances associated with disease states that beset humans could be simulated and studied. Devices capable of gathering such detailed information from healthy experimental animals could have obvious value as diagnostic tests for use on patients in clinical settings. The growing pressures for payoff accelerated conversion of research tools and technologies into new clinical tools with astonishing results.

ADAPTATIONS FOR CLINICAL APPLICATIONS

New developments in optics made it possible for physicians to inspect directly many tissues deep within the body. Long fiberoptic catheters were developed for direct inspection of the larynx, the trachea, and the bronchi, or alternatively, the esophagus and the stomach (Fig. 5–2a). Other similar devices proved useful for inspecting the bladder and the ureters or the rectum and the colon. Just as the electron microscope enhanced the vision of the anatomists, imaging techniques using energy sources permitted exploration of various internal organs of the body. X-rays can be employed to display on plates, screens, or cathode ray tubes the position, size, shape, and movement of internal organs (see Fig. 5–2b). Beams of ultrasound can also be used to create images of structures within the various portions of the body.

The energy emitted by radionuclides contributes additional information of value to the diagnosis of certain ailments. Injected intravenously, certain isotopes accumulate selectively in specific organs (i.e., iodine in the thyroid) as an indicator of function. The spatial distribution of isotopes can be displayed to indicate the blood flow or blood content in various internal organs. Arrays of isotope emission detectors (gamma cameras) can produce images illustrating the geometrical distribution of radionuclides in specific locations in organs and can be interpreted to indicate the position of blocked blood vessels in the lung or heart.

Infrared cameras, commonly used to display geographical characteristics of the ground from high flying aircraft or satellites, can also be employed to record the temperature distribution over the surface of the body. Such thermographs once excited much enthusiasm as a means of detecting pathological processes (cancer or infection) under the surface of the skin (1). The diagnostic value of thermography has not been fully realized.

The chemical analysis of samples which have previously been performed laboriously by hand can now be carried out by new and sophisticated machines capable of detecting a wide variety of chemical constituents, enzymes, and trace elements. The gas content of exhaled air or blood can be measured or estimated directly. Automated mechanisms for analyzing both the blood cells and the blood chemistry have been introduced into hospital laboratories with 12 to 20 or more different determinations of blood chemistry carried out automatically on each specimen (Fig. 5-2c). The cellular and chemical composition of blood, body fluids, urine, and stools can be examined in great detail.

The intrinsic energies that are developed within the body can be analyzed and recorded in the form of electroencephalograms, electrocardiograms, and electromyograms, as illustrated in Figure 5-2d. Continuous displays of the electrocardiogram, arterial pressures, and other vital signs have been incorporated into consoles for monitoring the conditions of patients requiring intensive care. Such equipment is now being widely used during and following high risk surgical operations (i.e., intracardiac surgery). Similar systems are also used in the care of patients after heart attacks—the familiar coronary care units. Such sophisticated facilities for continuous surveillance have been enthusiastically incorporated at great cost into hospitals, large and small.

Nuclear magnetic resonance has demonstrated great usefulness in analyzing chemical constituents by changing the spin of protons (H^+) with strong magnets and in analyzing the responses. The resonance of protons is different depending on their position in relation to other elements in molecules. Excitement has developed in many quarters over the prospect of engaging in indirect biochemical analysis of internal tissues by computerized imaging technologies. These techniques are at the earliest stages of development as a continuing process of converting sophisticated physical, chemical, and engineering technologies into the biomedical research tools.

METAMORPHOSIS OF CLINICAL LABORATORIES

The newly developed basic research tools greatly expanded the diagnostic capacity of clinical medicine. For example, the electron microscope has opened new vistas in the study of subcellular elements in both fundamental and clinical investigation of virus infestations, cancer, genetic disturbances, and many other central issues. The growing diversity of laboratory tests for the chemical and cellular composition of blood, body fluids, and

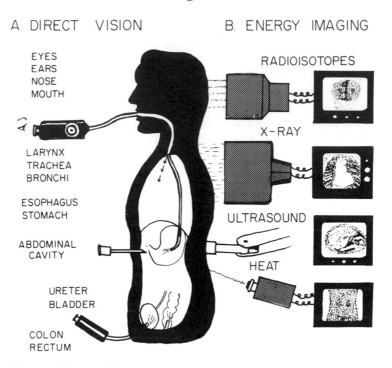

A. DIRECT VISION

EYES
EARS
NOSE
MOUTH

LARYNX
TRACHEA
BRONCHI

ESOPHAGUS
STOMACH

ABDOMINAL
CAVITY

URETER
BLADDER

COLON
RECTUM

B. ENERGY IMAGING

RADIOISOTOPES

X-RAY

ULTRASOUND

HEAT

Figure 5-2. (a) Direct visual observations can be made on eyes, ears, nose, mouth, and linings of all accessible hollow organs of the body by means of fiberoptic fibers and modern optics. (b) Various forms of energy probes (i.e., isotopes, x-ray beams, ultrasound, and heat) can be used to produce images. Such images provide vast quantities of useful data with great convenience and little or no discomfort or hazard to patients (see also Fig. 5–3). (c) Some examples of clinical testing techniques include direct analysis of the composition of exhaled air, automated blood cell counts, auto-

tissue samples have utterly transformed laboratory procedures. Automation of testing sequences provides batch processing of small samples to provide multiple simultaneous test results at greatly reduced unit costs. Thirty years ago, most hospital laboratories routinely performed only ten or twenty different types of tests. Today, larger hospital laboratories provide a selection of more than 300 tests.

EXPANDING MEDICAL ELECTRONICS

The escalating costs of sophisticated equipment have been reported in a special market study published in 1975. The early examples began with electrocardiographs and x-ray systems, but the major advances became prominent only after 1950 with the advent of large-scale cardiac monitoring, cardiac catheterization, scintillation cameras (gamma cameras), medical computers, and other complicated equipment. Worthy of note was the

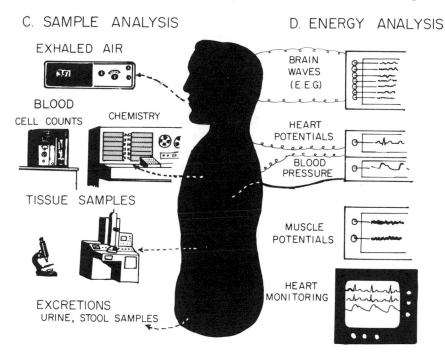

C. SAMPLE ANALYSIS

EXHALED AIR

BLOOD
CELL COUNTS   CHEMISTRY

TISSUE SAMPLES

EXCRETIONS
URINE, STOOL SAMPLES

D. ENERGY ANALYSIS

BRAIN
WAVES
(E.E.G)

HEART
POTENTIALS

BLOOD
PRESSURE

MUSCLE
POTENTIALS

HEART
MONITORING

mated determination of multiple chemical constituents from single samples and greatly extended observations on samples of body fluids and tissues. (d) Various forms of energy generated by the brain, heart, or muscles within the body can be detected at the skin surface and analyzed to provide valuable diagnostic data. Simultaneous measurements of electrical potentials, blood pressures, and other vital signs can be monitored continuously during intensive care of life-threatening illnesses.

projection that the domestic market for diagnostic, therapeutic, and monitoring medical electronic reach $840 million in 1974 and was estimated to exceed $1.4 billion in 1979. The actual figures probably surmounted these estimates.

APPLICATIONS OF ENERGY PROBES

Energy probes of various types are used to elicit information about the internal structure, position, movements, and function of internal organs by directing beams of energy into the body and analyzing the energy as it emerges. Immediately after the discovery of x-rays in December 1895, scientists in the United States began to carry out experiments with them. Roentgenography was largely limited to shadowgrams on photographic plates, or the moving of images on dimly illuminated fluorescent screens. After World War II, motion pictures of x-ray images were created, first with standard cameras and later with image intensifiers and television monitors (Fig. 5-3). The applications of roentgen rays are not limited to the presentation of size, shape, position, and movement of internal organs, but can be extended to the analysis of the function of internal organs through additional operational procedures. Injecting or ingesting radiopaque materials provides information of the function of the liver, kidney, or gastrointestinal tract. By taking roentgenograms from two positions at 90-degree angles, it is possible to calculate the volume of internal organs, such as the chambers of the heart, and to display such information as a three-dimensional presentation on an oscilloscopic screen. Sophisticated image reconstruction processes have now been developed using computers to produce a refined type of tomography, which has rocketed into widespread use trailing clouds of currency (4).

Computerized Axial Tomography (CAT Scanners). *Tomography* is a term applied to the development of x-ray images of various planes in the body by specialized techniques. For example, an x-ray tube programmed to move in one direction, while the x-ray plate is transported in the opposite direction, will produce an image of a single plane that appears to remain stationary and unblurred. The application of high-speed computers to this relatively simple mechanical process has produced costly but versatile instruments that have attracted widespread attention among physicians and public alike. The basic principles of image reconstruction have been recognized since 1917. In application, a very narrow x-ray beam penetrates the body from many different angles and positions to provide an enormous amount of data, which is collected and processed to reconstruct an image of a plane transecting the body perpendicular to its long axis (5). Repeated, this process provides an infinite number of views of the body that cannot be obtained using directly penetrating beams in the traditional manner. The equipment is illustrated schematically in Figure 5-3a. In early versions, an x-ray tube was mounted on one side of a large housing and a sensitive x-ray detector was positioned on the opposite side and was coupled to the x-ray tube so that they moved together. The tube and detector scanned back and forth across the portion of the body positioned within the circular orifice. The intensity of the x-ray beams that reach the detector was recorded at each of 160 positions along each scan. The housing then rotated one degree and another series of scans ensued. The process was repeated 180 times to produce some 28,000 values for x-ray intensities of beams penetrating from all these positions and angles. They were stored and analyzed in the computer and were reproduced

Figure 5-3. (*a*) Diagnostic imaging techniques have become increasingly sophisticated and costly as indicated by the progression from image intensifiers to computerized axial tomography (CAT scanning), or isotope imaging. (*b*) Ultrasound can be used to provide images and recordings distinctly different from those produced by x-ray beams, opening whole new vistas of clinical diagnostic techniques, indicating the location, size, shape, displacement, and velocity of various tissues and organs in the body (see text).

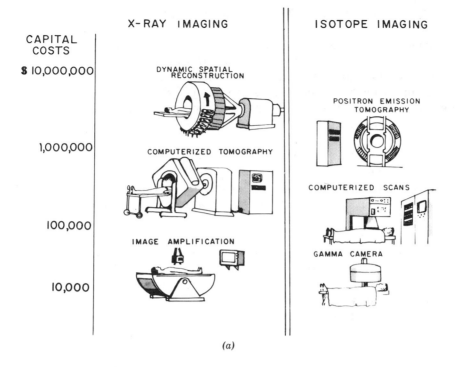

X-RAY IMAGING

ISOTOPE IMAGING

CAPITAL COSTS

$ 10,000,000

DYNAMIC SPATIAL RECONSTRUCTION

POSITRON EMISSION TOMOGRAPHY

1,000,000

COMPUTERIZED TOMOGRAPHY

COMPUTERIZED SCANS

100,000

IMAGE AMPLIFICATION

GAMMA CAMERA

10,000

(a)

B. ULTRASOUND

A. ULTRASONIC HOLOGRAM

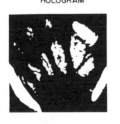

B. ECHOENCEPHALOGRAPHY

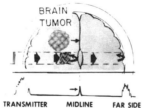

BRAIN TUMOR

TRANSMITTER PULSE   MIDLINE ECHO   FAR SIDE

C. ULTRASONIC SCAN

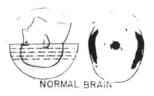

NORMAL BRAIN

D. ULTRASONIC SCANS (A and B)

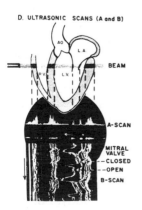

AO

LA

PV LV

BEAM

A-SCAN

MITRAL VALVE
—CLOSED
— — OPEN

B-SCAN

E. PULSED DOPPLER

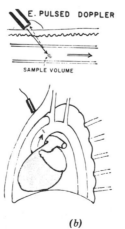

SAMPLE VOLUME

F. DUPLEX SCAN

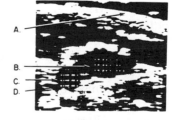

A.
B.
C.
D.

A. SKIN SURFACE
B. JUGULAR VEIN
C. CAROTID ARTERY
D. FLOW POINTS

(b)

173

as an image of some 6,400 to 25,000 tiny areas (pixels) in the plane of the scan. Very subtle differences in x-ray absorption delineate both normal and pathological structures with different radiodensity. In more recent models, the scanning time has been reduced to about 4.8 seconds to produce a complete image through the use of fan-like x-ray beam penetrating the body and impinging on an array of some 288 detectors on the opposite side of the housing.

CAT scanners have displayed rapid technological changes with the development of three generations of models since the early 1970s. The unbridled enthusiasm with which the equipment was adopted produced a demand that outran the supply. With each new generation, the older versions became obsolete. A report by the Institute of Medicine provided the following information on the costs of CAT scanners (6). Purchase price and installation charges range from $300,000 to $700,000. Annual operating costs range from $259,000 to $371,000 (average about $285,000). These high costs can be amortized only with high-volume use of equipment, such as 2,500 patient examinations per year as a minimum. The enthusiasm with which hospitals aspired to obtain this equipment exceeded reasonable bounds. Restraints are being considered or imposed by health service agencies or third-party payment sources. The uninhibited demand for these devices seems decidedly premature, because their clinical effectiveness is not yet fully established.

Just over the horizon is a superscanner being developed at the Mayo Foundation. This Dynamic Spatial Reconstructor (DSR) incorporates 28 separate x-ray tubes arrayed around the outside of a huge drum (15 feet in diameter), which can rotate four times per second (Fig. 5–3). The 28 x-ray tubes fire in rapid succession within a hundredth of a second, repeated 60 times a second. Twenty-eight image intensifiers are mounted on opposite sides of the huge housing, and these are scanned by special image television cameras. Data for 250 cross sections are collected each time the 28 x-ray tubes fire. These data are fed into a huge computer to analyze and to reconstruct all the accumulated information to rapidly provide huge numbers of images, which ultimately will be viewed in three dimensions. The extent to which this enormous technical achievement will be useful remains to be seen, but the accomplishment of such an ambitious project is noteworthy in itself.

Other energy probes (such as ultrasound) have been shown to produce whole new vistas of diagnostic information including dimensions, displacements, velocities, and acceleration of movements, variations in tissue characteristics as well as images corresponding to the x-ray scanning devices. These new and highly complex diagnostic devices are rapidly emerging and promise to exacerbate enormously the costs of clinical testing, perhaps to an exorbitant extent unless evaluation and restraints are accomplished in time.

Diagnostic Ultrasound. The normal hearing range extends to only about 20,000 hertz (cycles per second). Very high frequency sounds can be readily generated by electrically pulsing certain types of ceramic crystals at frequencies in excess of 1 megahertz (1 million cyles per second). Sonar is a familiar use of ultrasound for detecting the location and distance of ships and underwater ojbects. Ultrasound waves penetrate the tissues and are absorbed and scattered by tissues to different degrees than are x-ray beams. Thus, ultrasound can be used to extract entirely different information from the internal organs than is revealed by x-ray techniques. A common example is the application of modified sonar techniques to measure the time required for pulses to traverse the brain substance and be reflected from a midline structure and from the far side of the skull (Fig. 5–3b). A displacement of midline structure of the brain may indicate a developing brain tumor.

Ultrasonic images can be derived by scanning techniques corresponding to those described above for x-ray beams. By moving the source and receiver of ultrasound through different positions and angles, an image of internal organs can be effectively painted on the surface of a screen like a television image. Detailed transverse images can now be obtained of the brain, eye, abdomen, uterus, and other organs of interest. The process promises to be rendered more effective and faster by current developments in arrays of ultrasound transducers and receivers—ultimately coupled to dedicated high speed computers to improve both resolution and efficiency.

Ultrasound waves have unique backscattering properties that help to provide extremely valuable information. For example, a wave of ultrasound traversing the heart (Fig. 5–3b) is backscattered (reflected) from the walls of the chamber and from the valve leaflets. The movements of these various internal structures of the heart can be continuously observed on the face of an oscilloscope (A scan) or recorded on moving paper (B scan) for future analysis. Abnormal positions or dynamic movements of the various structures of the heart can be detected by such mechanisms. Ultrasound waves are also backscattered from blood cells, providing a means of registering changes in blood flow velocity by the familiar Doppler shift principle. (This is the physical mechanism causing a change in pitch of whistle on a moving train as it passes by.) The changing velocity of blood ejected from the heart can be continuously indicated by placing an ultrasonic probe at a strategic location just above the sternum (breast bone).

A combination of ultrasonic imaging and flow detection provides a means of deriving information about the blood flow velocity directly on the ultrasonic image of vascular channels in the body at various accessible locations. It is even possible to create images of all locations where blood is flowing faster than some predetermined velocity when this is of interest. The many and varied applications of diagnostic ultrasound are emerging in increasing numbers of clinical laboratories providing a whole new spectrum of clinically useful information.

DIAGNOSTIC IMPERATIVE

The breathless speed with which whole new diagnostic batteries have been made available to the medical profession has resulted in a veritable deluge of new clinical data. The medical markets for new and ever more sophisticated diagnostic technologies have stimulated rapid expansion of industrial production. The swelling flood of techniques and technologies tends to be concentrated in hospitals and independent laboratories. Most diagnostic devices have emerged long after most physicians graduated from medical school, so their applications and limitations must be learned "on the job," through medical meetings and literature or from sales representatives. The impacts of technologies on medical practice have occurred at such a rapid rate that there has been little time to adapt or control the consequences.

Physicians are prompted by powerful incentives to use the new diagnostic technologies fully, not only to clarify the sources of symptoms but also to seek evidences of pathological changes before signs or symptoms appear. With increasing numbers of persons being covered by various forms of insurance, there are few incentives to exhibit restraint in the use of these modern diagnostic technologies. This is particularly true of those sophisticated imaging devices that derive large amounts of data without pain or hazard. Potentially wasteful duplication of these costly devices has already developed at a disquieting rate. Equally disturbing is the prospect that correspondingly sophisticated instruments can and probably will be developed to take advantage of the additional information that can be presented by other wave energies such as ultrasound, isotopes, microwaves, positron emission, nuclear magnetic resonance, and others unannounced.

THERAPEUTIC PROGRESS

The diagnostic data available to modern physicians have far outstripped their ability to provide therapy for many of the conditions they discover. Some deficiencies of medical therapy were considered in the preceding chapter (Chapter 4). Despite enormous investments and demonstrated progress in the development of devices, drugs, and procedures, a very large proportion of the common persistent clinical problems (mild, moderate, chronic, and severe) are managed symptomatically or by supportive measures. The array of available drugs is so huge that it is always possible for a physician to "do something" for the benefit of almost any condition that a patient may bring to him. The most common uses of drugs are symptomatic or supportive; many are "mood altering," and some function as placebos. Surgical techniques, formerly limited to removing or repairing malfunctioning organs, have now been extended to reconstructing or replacing organs by transplants or artificial substitutes. All these developments combine to give the impression that the health professions have progressed to the point that they can favorably affect the course of virtually any disease to which humans are subject. This impression is misleading and requires clarification to understand the nature of the dilemmas that confront the health enterprise of the country. For this purpose a schematic summary of recent progress is presented for a selected sample of significant diseases and disabilities. The extent of therapeutic effectiveness can be divided conveniently into two main categories, namely (1) management methods and (2) definitive treatment (see Fig. 5-4). The management methods include diagnosis,

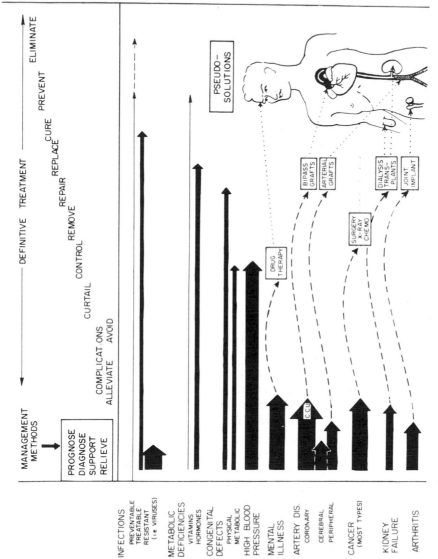

Figure 5-4. Advances in effectiveness of therapy can be considered in two main categories. Management methods include empirical, supportive, and symptomatic methods for conditions lacking truly effective therapy. Definitive treatment involves alleviation or avoidance of complications, curtailing or controlling progress of disease processes, removal, repair, or replacement of defective organs, and finally cure, prevention, and ultimate elimination of diseases. The current status of advances in therapy is represented by the horizontal arrows extending toward the right. The thickness of the arrows is intended to indicate the relative prevalence of the various ailments.

177

prognosis, general supportive treatment, and relief of symptoms. These steps conform to the schema presented previously in Figure 4-2.

Both patients and physicians are impelled to use available therapy even if it does not change the course of illness. Alleviation of complications can be regarded as management, while avoidance of complications is listed under definitive treatment because it represents a potential change in the course of illness. The corrective benefits that can be provided by physicians can be listed in ascending order of importance as follows:

1. *Curtailing* illness refers to methods of therapy that shorten the course of illness.

2. *Control* of disease processes implies suppression of abnormal function (i.e., blood pressure) without affecting the underlying process.

3. *Removing, repairing*, or *replacing* tissues and organs are the essence of surgery. Removal of a diseased organ by surgical escision is a time honored means of therapy (appendectomy, amputation, etc.). Similar effects can be obtained by other forms of destructive mechanisms such as radiation or chemotherapy (i.e., in cancer therapy). The repair of damaged or malfunctioning tissues and organs may be achieved by suturing lacerations, by plastic restoration or by reconstruction of con- genital deformities of many types. Replacement of diseased or defective parts can be accomplished by transplantation of organs from one individ- ual to another or by installing artifical tissues and organs to substitute for structural or functional deficiencies or defects (see also Chapter 4).

4. *Cure* is intended to represent elimination of cause of disease or disabili- ties such as the effective use of antibiotics to eliminate infections.

5. *Prevention* of disease can result from immunization, risk reduction, or anticipatory types of management. In recent years the concept of preven- tion has been popularized and extended to embrace such diverse aspects as immunization (primary prevention), improved nutrition and sanita- tion, avoidance of risk factors, moderation, and healthy lifestyles. In Figure 5-4, the term *prevention* is intended to imply "primary" preven- tion, or avoidance of disease by active efforts.

6. *Elimination* implies eradication of diseases, usually the result of large scale programs of immunization, often coupled with contemporary im- provements in nutrition, hygiene, environmental living conditions, and other factors discussed in Chapter 1 (see Fig. 1-2).

The comparative effectiveness of medical and surgical therapy for various ailments can be schematically represented as progress according to these criteria, as illustrated in Figure 5-4. The length of the horizontal arrows suggests the extent to which modern medicine has attained success in the progression of steps from management toward elimination of diseases. The width of the arrows indicates roughly the relative incidence of the various conditions. Thus, there are certain infections that are essentially eliminated as indicated by the long thin arrow at the top (see also Fig. 4-1).

Progress in the treatment of many infections is extremely impressive, resulting in virtual eradication of quite a large number. Cholera, plague, smallpox, diphtheria, polio, typhoid fever, yellow fever, malaria, and many other diseases have become absent or rare in the American scene. Antibiotics can "cure" certain kinds of infections, such as those involving streptococci, pneumococci, and others. However, there remain large numbers of infections that persist with little sign of cure or control, such as colds, flu, hepatitis, certain parasitic infections, etc. These resistant diseases remain a problem and a challenge for the future and are represented by the thick short arrow in Figure 5-4. Some can be classed as "impending pandemics," such as venereal disease or antibiotic resistant organisms (Fig. 4-1).

Many metabolic deficiencies have been clarified and resolved to the point that vitamin deficiencies are now quite rare and former problems of rickets, scurvy, pellagra, and others are largely eliminated by adequate nutrition. Hormonal deficiencies can be alleviated by appropriate replacements, as in the case of diabetes, hypothyroidism, and adrenal deficiencies. The underlying processes are not remedied by the therapy, but the patients' life quality and life expectancy are returned toward normal.

Congenital defects are numerous—about one baby in 60 is born with one of the common defects. Many of the physical defects of heart, gastrointestinal tract, or urinary tract can now be corrected surgically in infancy, converting "hopeless cases" of the past into children with very favorable outlooks, both in duration and quality of life. Similarly, certain of the metabolic defects can be countered or corrected, sometimes with amazing results. For example, the metabolic defect known as PKU can lead to mental retardation if undetected. Prompt dietary restriction can avoid this complication and provide a normal life expectancy.

High blood pressure can now be controlled to a major extent by using drugs and relaxation techniques. However, there remains some uncertainty regarding the extent to which the underlying pathological processes are suppressed (i.e., the factors that may lead to stroke).

Some forms of mental retardation can be avoided (i.e., PKU), but most types defy therapy. Traditional forms of mental illness remain mysterious as to origin. Therapy is protracted and outcome is uncertain. Mood-altering drugs have assumed an important place as interim therapy but do not solve the underlying problems in most instances. Developing drug dependence is an increasing complication of such therapy.

The immediate etiology and the role(s) of risk factors in the most common killer diseases have continued to resist intensive investigation as indicated in Chapter 4. Pressures have mounted for "payoff" for the years of generous investments in research on such conditions as atherosclerosis, cancer, chronic kidney disease, and other chronic diseases such as arthritis (see Chapter 4). One consequence has been the emergence and widespread application of interim technologies or pseudosolutions such as coronary bypass operations, destructive cancer therapies, artificial kidneys, or hip replacements (Fig. 5-4).

There is some danger that the huge expenditures being channeled into pseudosolutions could divert efforts from the longer range goal of developing effective cures or controls of these important illnesses (see also the section on technology assessment, below).

COMPLICATIONS OF TECHNOLOGICAL TRIUMPHS: DIRECT AND INDIRECT

The typical American approach can be characterized by the phrase: "It may be possible—let's do it!" This exuberant attitude pervaded our entire society before the last decade. Only recently has the realization dawned that we are fully capable of developing technology much faster than we can learn to use it wisely and effectively.

The most pressing problems of modern societies can be attributed to unexpected complications of technological triumphs. Notable examples include the population explosion, urbanization, unemployment, depletion of resources, and deterioration of the environment. In medicine a profusion of new and novel diagnostic methods has emerged with increasing complexity, sophistication, and capabilities. More comprehensive and reliable information for purposes of diagnosis is generally regarded as a triumph of unquestioned value to the public, the profession, and society as a whole. However, consideration must be given to the "price of progress" in terms of two central issues:

1. The ability to gather clinical data has proceeded so rapidly that it has greatly outdistanced our ability to treat many of the conditions which can now be recognized with confidence.
2. Diagnostic technologies are major contributors to the soaring costs of health care delivery due in part to pervasive pressures toward overuse with inadequate incentives for restraint on the part of either physicians or the public.

Overuse of diagnostic technologies is not due solely to excessive zeal on the part of physicians. It is also a natural response to many other converging forces such as increased patient demands and expectations, third-party payments, peer review mechanisms, standards of quality based on thoroughness, "scientific medicine," and the ubiquitous underlying threat of malpractice litigation.

DIAGNOSTIC OVERSHOOT

The roles of physicians have been greatly affected by the availability of advanced technologies for diagnosis and therapy. The doctor-patient relationship is no longer limited to face-to-face encounters but is diluted by shuttling patients to many different health services. The modern physician serves as a professional purchasing agent, selecting services deemed appropriate to the conditions presented by his patients. The role of purchasing agent is a new relationship between doctors and patients, for which health professionals are ill prepared and inadequately trained (see Chapter 6). Both the patients and the physicians' peers expect a full use of available resources for many cogent reasons. The traditional criterion of quality medical care has been *thoroughness* implying comprehensive coverage of the probable alternative diagnoses. There are many incentives for physicians to avoid short-cuts and to cover all contingencies, particularly in situations where third-party payment mechanisms are covering all or most of the costs. Economic incentives also promote overuse of technologies by the average physician. Consider the time and effort involved in a complete history and physical examination that might require 45 minutes and bring in $40. In contrast, the time required to order and later interpret an electrocardiogram or an x-ray film may be only 2 to 10 minutes or so and charges are $25 or $30. The objectivity of the tests and the permanence of the records also add to the attractiveness of technology. The same considerations apply to the generous use of the many tests that can be quickly ordered in various combinations from clinical and chemical laboratories. The patient and the physician tend to derive benefits in the form of reassurance that diseases or disabilities are either correctly identified or not overlooked in the process. Thus, many powerful incentives encourage full utilization of available health services, and restraining influences are weak or virtually absent.

There is growing awareness that long-established routines may not warrant their consistent use or even provide unwarranted reassurance. Third-party payments may be denied for the routine tests for nonsurgical hospital admissions. Skull x-ray films are taken semiautomatically on patients with head injuries, without much regard for severity. Evaluation of the consequences of omitting this examination in some 1,500 patients on the basis of a preliminary clinical examination disclosed relatively small benefit to patients from the rather large expenditures involved (7). Yet both patient and physician are prone to feel uneasy or dissatisfied at the thought of discriminative deletion of this ritual.

PROLIFERATING PERSONNEL

In the first part of this century, the practice of medicine was primarily a solo operation such that each physician was supported on the average by one additional person (nurse/secretary/receptionist). A large proportion of physicians, particularly the specialists, have now assumed the role of team leader with responsibilities extended to a substantial group of persons, all contributing to the welfare of the patient. The number of persons employed in health occupations has expanded enormously in the past 30 years to reach a total number of more than 4.5 million. On the average, 13 health personnel support each physician. The number and distribution of these people in the health fields are illustrated in Figure 5-5. This tabulation ignores the large number of people employed in the manufacture of drugs and devices and many other peripheral health functions, such as the provision of health insurance, the health roles of police and firemen, and many other contributors to the health and welfare of the population. The labor costs that support these many vital services are fundamentally responsible for the greatly increased costs of health care (see Figure 5-6).

Fragmenting Effects of Diversification. The country doctor or the family physician early in the century carried most of what was needed for a diag-

PROLIFERATING PERSONNEL

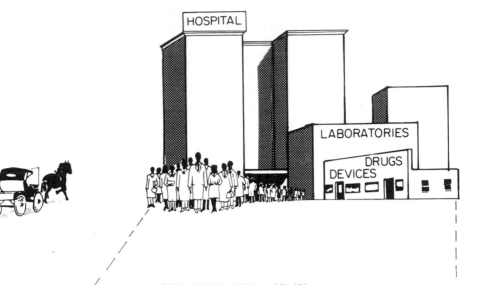

TOTAL NUMBERS (1974) 4,672,850

DIRECT PATIENT SERVICES		SUPPORT SERVICES	
MEDICINE AND OSTEOPATHY	362,700	BIOMEDICAL RESEARCH	
DENTISTRY AND ALLIED SERVICES	269,800	BASIC MEDICAL SCIENTISTS	60,000
NURSING AND RELATED SERVICES	2,319,000	BIOMEDICAL ENGINEERING	12,000
REGISTERED NURSES	857,000	ANTHROPOLOGY, SOCIOLOGY	1,700
PRACTICAL NURSES	492,000	MEDICAL ECONOMICS	400
NURSING AIDES, ETC	936,000	ADMINISTRATION OF HEALTH SERVICES	48,200
HOME HEALTH AIDES	34,000	MEDICAL RECORDS MANAGEMENT	60,000
MIDWIVES	4,300	SECRETARIAL SERVICES	300,000
PHARMACY	132,000	SOCIAL WORK	38,600
OPTOMETRY	25,300	LIBRARY SERVICES	10,300
PHYSICAL THERAPY	26,100	HEALTH COMMUNICATIONS	10,500
REHABILITATION: SPECIAL SERVICES	13,250	HEALTH EDUCATION	23,000
PSYCHOLOGY	35,000	VITAL STATISTICS	1,350
DIETETICS AND NUTRITION	72,700	OPTICIANS	12,000
PODIATRY	7,100	ORTHOTISTS, PROSTHETICISTS	3,800
OCCUPATIONAL THERAPY	14,500	FOOD AND DRUG PROTECTION	47,900
SPEECH THERAPY	27,000	VETERINARY MEDICINE	33,500
CHIROPRACTICS	16,600	ENVIRONMENTAL SANITATION	20,000
HEALTH SERVICE TECHNICIANS		SYSTEMS ANALYSIS AND DATA PROCESS	5,000
RADIOLOGY	100,000	FUNERAL DIRECTORS, EMBALMERS	50,000
CLINICAL LABORATORIES	172,500		
EMERGENCY MED. TECHS	260,000		
RESPIRATORY THERAPY	19,000		
OPHTHALMIC ASSTS	20,000		
SURGICAL TECHNICIANS	12,000		
PHYSICIAN ASSTS	2,000		
ELECTROCARDIOGRAPHIC	9,500		
ELECTROENCEPHALOGRAPHIC	4,000		

Figure 5-5. Practice of "modern" medicine has been largely transformed from individual care by solo physicians to "scientific" medicine administered by teams of physicians, health professionals, and support personnel numbering more than 4.5 million people. The various categories of personnel are presented in two subgroups: namely, provision of direct patient services and support services.

182

nosis and treatment within a small black bag. For this reason, it was possible for a patient to get the limited available medical care at one place, very often at home. The greatly expanded complexity and sophistication of modern medicine has produced dispersion of facilities and services. Physicians commonly find it necessary to send patients to several locations to obtain the more specialized tests or to seek consultation or special treatments. A common complaint by the general public is the fragmentation of medical care, which results largely from inadequate coordination. Delays are common between each of the steps and the patient may be inadequately informed of the reasons or results of the procedures. As a consequence, many patients feel they are treated by their physician and the cohorts of health personnel as a bundle of symptoms rather than a living person. The impersonal attitude of many doctors toward their patients may be in part due to their changing roles and excessive work load, but the fact remains that the public is highly critical of the depletion of the person-to-person element in the practice of medicine.

Dehumanization. The increasing accuracy and reliability of sophisticated diagnostic technologies do not entirely make up for a loss of warm, sympathetic doctor-patient relationships. The technologies that provide information without either pain or hazard to the patient are typically very complex and costly. To many patients who are already worried or frightened, massive equipment must seem menacing. There is little warmth in arrays of devices which are used for obtaining images using energy probes such as x-ray, ultrasound, or radionuclides. Many therapeutic instruments have equally ominous appearance. It is common experience that increasing dependence upon sophisticated technologies and complicated organizational relationships have generally been associated with impersonalization, frustration, disenchantment accompanying expansion of services, and improved "efficiency," but complicated access to health services.

The use of high technologies and sophisticated devices does not *necessarily* result in dehumanization or preclude very personal types of interaction. There are many opportunities for health professions to reestablish warm and sympathetic relationships between the myriad health workers and the patients, but such changes will require a reversal of current trends toward specialization.

PROFESSIONAL SPECIALIZATION

The combination of an explosion in biomedical information and proliferation of ever more sophisticated technologies has made it increasingly difficult for physicians to maintain high levels of competence in all the fields of medicine. Keeping up-to-date with advances in medicine would be virtually a full-time occupation for a general practitioner whose attention is intensively occupied by seeing 20 to 50 patients a day. One price of progess in medicine has been the major shift out of general practice and into the various specialties and subspecialties of medicine in metropolitan areas.

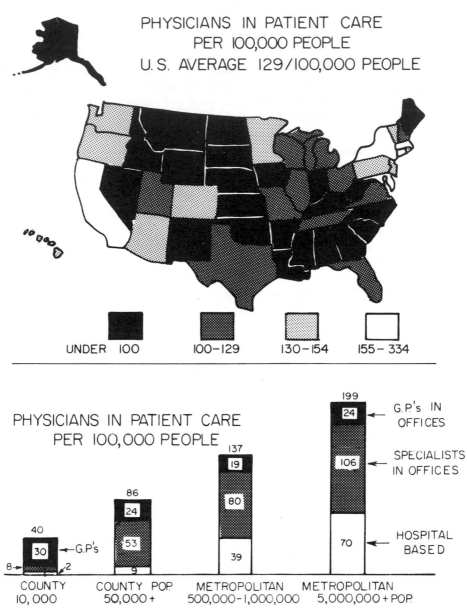

Figure 5-6. Progressive specialization of both physicians and facilities has led to heavy concentrations in populated states like California, New York, and Massachusetts in response to many attractions described in the text. The number of physicians (per 100,000) and of specialists is far greater in metropolitan areas in contrast with counties with populations of 10,000-50,000.

In 1950, well over half of the nonfederal physicians were in general practice. The subsequent growth of the total physician population and the great enlargement of the medical, surgical, and other specialties are phenomenal. General practitioners have shrunk to about 16 to 24% of the total physician community, a number which is totally inadequate to take care of the first contact, or primary care, of patients. The migration of physicians into the specialties has occurred in excessive numbers, particularly in metropolitan and suburban areas. One result has been that highly trained and expert specialists often serve as first-contact physicians, playing the role of a general practitioner at very inflated costs. Specialists in pediatrics and internal medicine have always served as high level primary care physicians. However, it is now becoming ever more commonplace for orthopedic surgeons, obstetricians, and family practice specialists to supplement the short supply of general practitioners. This is an extremely expensive mechanism for providing the primary care requirements of the general population.

Maldistribution. The medical and surgical conditions that actually require the complicated equipment and procedures described in previous sections are not very common in the general population. Sufficient patient flow to justify the existence of such facilities tends to require that large hospitals be located in metropolitan centers, where large numbers of people are concentrated. Obviously, a small rural hospital of 25 to 100 beds is in no position to support the kind of costs that are implied by such sophisticated technologies. Similarly, the highly trained specialists who are prepared to use this equipment fully also tend to gravitate to metropolitan and suburban areas. Cities and suburbs hold such great attractions for physicians, that many of the different specialties are to be found in surplus quantities in metropolitan areas, particularly in rich suburbs where the demands for highest quality health care are heaviest (Fig. 5-6). In 1973, nearly 87% of all physicians were clustered in metropolitan areas, averaging more than twice the number of doctors per capita in cities compared with the regions containing mostly smaller cities, towns, and farms (Fig. 5-6). Physicians gravitate to the wealthier districts of metropolitan areas. For example, wealthy sections of Chicago have about 210 physicians per 100,000 residents, while deprived areas in the same city have only about 25 physicians per 100,000. Certain states appear to have unusual attractions for physicians, as exemplified by California, New York, and Massachusetts, which lead the nation in the number of physicians (see Fig. 5-6). The unequal distribution of physicians also mirrors the unequal distribution of hospital facilities. For example, at the end of World War II, more than half the counties in the United States lacked hospitals, a deficiency which was the target for the Hill-Burton legislation. Hundreds of small hospitals in all parts of the country have been built with federal support. In addition, several programs have been introduced to encourage physicians to locate in underserved areas (i.e., National Health Service Corps). Some medical schools have been actively recruiting students from remote and rural areas, with particular efforts directed at attracting minorities. These efforts, while well conceived, have had little impact on the shortages to date. Indeed, the problem has worsened in some areas during the last decade. For example, 50 of 100 counties in Kansas lost physicians between 1963 and 1973. The number of doctors in inner cities or ghetto areas is also decreasing. In rural pockets of poverty, the problems are particularly acute. The principal problem areas in this country are represented by the blackened areas in Figure 5-6.

Complicated Access. The enormous expansion and diversification of health personnel and services have failed to meet some of the essential needs of the general public. A common complaint is the inability of patients to gain access to the services of a physician at time of need. Consider the problem of a distraught mother, desperately concerned about her squalling baby in the middle of the night and unable to contact a physician who will render service. The public regards these circumstances as justifying a house call by a physician. However, the percentage of house visits by physicians has diminished from 10.2% in 1957 to 1958 to about 1.1% in 1974. Before World War II most medical practice was conducted in doctors' offices or patients' homes. During the war years, large numbers of physicians were drafted into the army, where most of them were in charge of large groups of very healthy soldiers. Most of the soldiers' common problems were taken care of by medical corpsmen at sick call. Many military doctors discovered how pleasant and rewarding medical practice could be without being continuously on-call and rarely needing to get up at night for a house call. The few physicians remaining at home were clearly overwhelmed by the demands for service, and were easily justified in refusing to make house calls under those circumstances. Both of these segments of the physician population discovered the personal advantages of more regular working hours. Since a very large proportion of requests for nighttime services are for conditions which are greatly improved in the morning, it is not too difficult for physicians to rationalize deferral of many problems until the next day. However, this does not really solve the problem confronting the terrified patient in the darkness of the night.

One result of the decline in house calls has been the increasing utilization of both the telephone and the emergency rooms in hospitals. These emergency rooms were designed to take care of patients who have suffered accidents or life-threatening incidents. They are not really set up for the managment of standard or self-limited clinical problems.

It is not always easy to obtain health services, even under the best of circumstances. Many physicians have closed their practices at current levels and are unwilling to accept new patients. This poses a problem in a population as mobile as that of the United States, since every move to a different location requires reestablishing contact with a different physician or facility. Even when a physician has been selected, it is often necessary to wait for days for a scheduled appointment, and then to spend frustrating periods in the waiting room beyond the appointed time. It is hardly necessary to mention the fact that there is little or no provision in medical education for the training of physicians in the management of practices, or the development of smoothly running organizations (see Chapter 7).

Apparent Physician Shortage. To the patient who is unable to find a physician in times of crucial need, there is clearly a shortage of physicians. However, this is a misleading impression. The total number of physicians in this country is substantially greater than is actually needed to provide adequate "sick" care, if there were sufficient numbers of family physicians with necessary support personnel, equitably distributed across the country. The number of medical school graduates has doubled in the past 10 years. The total number of physicians will have increased to more than half again between World War II and 1980. The continued training of physicians will not necessarily solve the problem of access if the current tendency toward specialization at the expense of general practice is not reversed. It is also necessary to develop effective incentives that will encourage physicians to set up practice in remote and rural areas or provide alternative mechanisms (Chapter 6). It was mentioned above that there is a net loss of physicians in both rural areas and in central cities. The current tendency to continue to produce highly trained specialists in surplus numbers is contributing enormously to the overall costs of health care in this country. An eminent economist, Eli Ginsberg, has estimated that the net addition of one physician adds approximately $250,000 to the annual operating costs of the health care enterprise. In recognition of these factors, Joseph Califano, former Secretary of DHEW, has publicly announced at the meeting of the Association of Medical Colleges a new policy that would encourage medical schools to gradually reduce the size of the medical classes, discourage the development of new medical schools, and oppose admission of foreign medical graduates (8).

HOSPITAL CENTERED PRACTICE

The modern hospital is a response to the need for concentrating the complex new technologies and competent professional personnel in a unitary organizational setting. Modern hospitals are designed to avoid some of the fragmentation mentioned above. They have become the doctor's indispensable workshops and are expressly organized and designed to meet the needs and to cater to the desires of the staff physicians. The staff physicians exert a great influence in hospitals they use, representing the sole source of patients and necessary revenue to keep the institution running. The nurses, technicians, and other hospital staff members are responsible for carrying out the orders of the doctors, almost as if they were his employees, but he has no obligation to provide their salaries or little responsibility for the maintenance of the facilities and services they bring to his patients. Hospitals are in heavy competition with each other trying to provide the most modern equipment and services to entice physicians to join the staff, and to encourage admission of their patients.

Physicians benefit greatly by having patients conveniently grouped and well-served in central locations. Since their own professional services are supplemented by those of the hospital staff, they can take care of many patients efficiently and with little time wasted. In addition, they can order a bewildering array of tests or procedures at the flick of a pen with assurance that the hospital staff will carry out orders. Obviously, hospitals are organized to "save peoples' lives, not their money." In his role as a professional purchasing agent, the physician is continually confronted with the need to balance off the potential advantages to the patient (and to himself) of

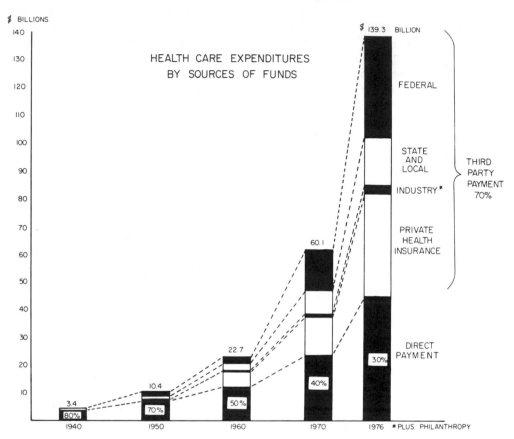

GROWTH OF THIRD PARTY PAYMENTS

HEALTH CARE EXPENDITURES
BY SOURCES OF FUNDS

Figure 5-7. The expenditures for health care have escalated rapidly since 1940 and the proportion of these costs defrayed by third parties (particularly federal and insurance sources) have increased from 30% to 70% during the intervening period (From PHS Forward Plan for Health, FY 1978-82).

ordering more tests and treatments than are absolutely necessary, and the balance is almost always tipped toward extravagance.

SOARING COSTS OF HEALTH CARE

According to long-standing tradition, the inherent value of life and health are so great that we rarely count the cost of protecting them. Many people feel the need for assurance that "everything is being done that can be done" when health is at stake. The overall costs of health care are high and ascending rapidly, as indicated in Figure 5-7. Physicians influence the magnitude of the bills for health care, since they uniquely determine the size and scope of both diagnostic and therapeutic efforts. However, they are not entirely free agents in making these decisions, because they are under a wide variety of intense pressures from several sources. The general public is constantly being bombarded by promises or prospects of new and exciting technologies touted by mass media as the solution to various diseases and disabilities. The pharmaceutical industry is continuously presenting persuasive prospects of instant relief from all kinds of signs and symptoms. The insurance industry offers ever-expanding coverage of health care costs. The governmental involvement has become huge and threatens to become even more universal through some form of national health insurance. As the third-party payments have escalated, costs of health care paid directly by patients diminished from 80% in 1940 to 30% in 1976.

There are really no villains in this scenario, because each member of the cast is functioning in accordance with his individual training and experience, supremely confident of acting in the best interests of society in general and specific patients in particular. Doctors and other health professionals are dedicated to prevention, cure, and alleviation of ailments in accordance with traditions and training that encourage full utilization of available resources. John Q. Public is insisting on more and more health care. Expanding insurance policies and federal subsidies encourage excesses and discourage restraint. Labor negotiations often emphasize the provision of health services as a part of fringe benefits for employees. The costs of drugs and devices have been increasing, from the point of view of both quantity and diversity. People pay a premium for materials used by health professionals. For example, nylon fishing line costs a small fraction of the same material used as surgical sutures. Stimulated by public demand, the federal government is contributing to the expenditure of funds nationwide by generous appropriations. Health and health care are such popular political issues that national health insurance of some sort seems inevitable. The experiences of all the countries of Western Europe have demonstrated that total expenditures for health are greatly increased by government-supported health programs. The huge influx of federal funds without adequate alteration in the basic health care delivery mechanisms inherently inflate costs (see Chapter 9).

The judicial system of the country has a major impact. The upward surge in malpractice insurance rates is directly reflected in bills paid by patients and by third parties. When the judgments are paid by malpractice insurance, physicians' resources are not depleted directly, and the population as a whole shares in the greatly increased cost from two sources: (1) by increased charges to cover malpractice insurance and (2) by intense pressures to reduce the likelihood of malpractice suits by covering all conceivable contingencies. The practice of defensive medicine to minimize the possibility of malpractice litigation is greatly increasing the total overall cost of health care in this country. Since all the participants in the health care delivery process are individually contributing to the rising costs, the upward surge will not be moderated or reversed until most or all of them exhibit a degree of restraint which is not now currently visible. On the contrary, there is every indication that all of the pressures for increased expenditures are becoming more intense. Experience in other countries has indicated that when the total health care costs reach levels of about 10% of the gross na-

tional product, a functional ceiling tends to be reached with intense economic pressures for realignment of priorities. Expenditures for health care
are now approaching 9% of the gross national product for health, and can be
predicted to reach a level or limit within the next few years. The total economic costs of illness extend far byond the direct expenditures for health
services (9).

Former Secretary Califano predicted that current trends would elevate
health care costs to $1,000 billion (about 12% of GNP) by the year 2000
(8). The escalating costs of expenditures for health care are undoubtedly
based on an assumption that they will demonstrably improve the health
status of the American public. There is growing suspicion that expenditures
for health are not necessarily reflected in improved status of the public's
health using traditional yardsticks.

COMPARATIVE RETURN ON INVESTMENT

The United States is a wealthy country, and its citizens are generous
when it comes to health. Few people will begrudge their neighbors opportunities to avoid or eliminate disease or disability. The voluntary contributions to health and social agencies (i.e., the United Way) are large and widely
supported. The health enterprise has achieved the level of the third largest
industry in this country. It seems timely to inquire whether or not the results
achieved are commensurate with the magnitude of the resources being expended. It is very difficult to assign a value or to develop a meaningful scale
for the benefits derived from the new health personnel, facilities, and technologies (see Chapter 6). The traditional guidelines have been based largely on
age-adjusted death rates and estimated life expectancies. Death rates in the
United States and in industrialized countries have been declining at a fairly
steady pace over many decades. Between 1900 and the 1930s, the death
rates were decreasing at a rate of approximately 1% per year, and diminished
further during 1930–1950, apparently from the introduction of sulfa
nomides and antibiotics. A plateau appeared to develop in the mid-1950s,
and persisted until the late 1960s (Fig. 5-8a). The cause of this plateau and
the apparent resumption of the declining death rate are not well understood.

The falling death rates in the United States have been encouraging but
have been even more pronounced in other countries. The United States
spends more per capita than virtually all other governments but ranks below
many nations of the world in combined mortality according to statistics
from the World Health Organization (10). Similarly, among the countries
with the highest life expectancies, the United States also ranks below 18 or
19 others, depending on the age selected for comparison (Fig. 5-8b).

It seems reasonable to assume that there should be some relationship
between the magnitude of the investments in health care and the overall
result, in terms of the nation's health status. One of the first to critically
examine this assumption was William Forbes (11). He contrasted the growing expenditures for health from less than $50 billion to more than $180

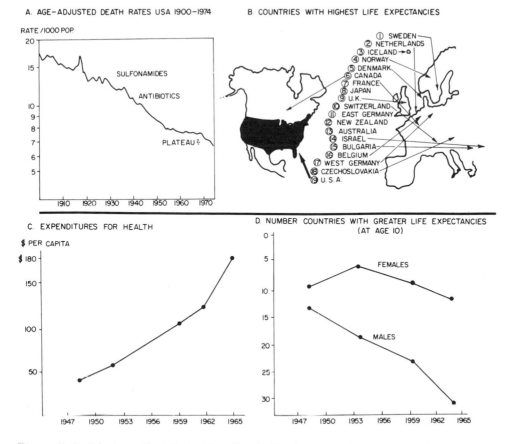

Figure 5-8. (a) Age-adjusted death rates declined progressively in the United States during this century with a temporary plateau occurring during the 1960s for unknown reasons. (b) Despite a very large expenditure per capita for health care, this country ranks 19th in life expectancy (at age 10) and about the same level in other vital statistics. (c) Despite progressive increase in expenditures for health, the ranking of the United States in life expectancy and other vital statistics has fallen in comparison with other countries, many of whom spend less than we do (see also ref 11).

billion between 1947 and 1965, while the ranking of the United States with relation to other countries was declining. In other words, no relationship was evident between the quantity of money spent on health and the results achieved on a comparative basis with the experience of other countries. This impression has been subsequently reaffirmed by other authors (12,13,14). Mortality rates or life expectancies may not be the most ideal criteria of benefits from health services. The ease and certainty of counting dead people does not make up for their deficiencies as indicators of quality or efficacy of health care.

Improvements in death rates and life expectancies should not be attributed solely to improved health care delivery, as discussed in Chapter 1. More equitable comparisons might be achieved by the use of criteria such as the years of productive life, the number of days in bed, the incidence of illness of various categories, or the economic loss due to disease and disability (Fig. 3-5). In any case, it is clear that there is widespread discontent and disenchantment among the general public with the current health care delivery mechanisms despite the enormous progress which has been achieved during the past 30 years.

UNREALIZED EXPECTATIONS

The mounting criticism of modern medicine is not attributable solely to lack of progress. It is a peculiar phenomenon that the rapidly rising competence of physicians and their teams to diagnose and manage disease effectively should be accompanied by a precipitously falling image in the minds of the general public. One reasonable explanation for this phenomenon is that the expectations of the public have greatly exceeded the ability of the physicians to meet their demands. Benevolent extravagance due to overuse of facilities and services also causes concerns and complaints.

These complex issues must be more objectively and critically analyzed for purposes of developing sound decisions and wise policies for the allocation of public moneys for both biomedical research and health services. One manifestation of these concerns has been the rapid growth of new approaches under the general title of Technology Assessment.

HEALTH TECHNOLOGY ASSESSMENT

The processes involved in device development follow recognition of an unmet need and a concept of ways to solve the problems. A key factor at the outset is the prospect of benefits accruing to the public in addition to profit motivation. Virtually any decision by corporations or government is likely to provide gains for some and losses for others. There is growing awareness that preoccupation with short-term gains has led to serious long-term losses, including risk factors and new hazards to health (Fig. 4-4 and 4-5). Obviously, inadequate attention has been directed toward anticipation of undesirable complications from technological achievements during the early stages of development. Growing concerns in Congress gave rise to a bill introduced by Representative Emilio Q. Daddario, Democrat from Connecticut and Chairman of a Subcommittee on Science, Research, and Development, establishing a Technology Assessment Board to provide "a method for identifying, assessing, publicizing, and dealing with the implications and effects of applied research and technology." In pursuit of these objectives, panels were established by both the National Academy of Sciences and the National Academy of Engineering to explore the problems of assessing technology (15). The rates at which new technologies are adopted have often exceeded the most enthusiastic projections, producing rapid changes that are difficult or impossible to reverse. A notable example was the diffusion of television sets, which numbered 100,000 in 1948, 1,000,000 in 1949, and 50,000,000 in 1959. Such exuberant growth might seem unlikely in the health field, but corresponding examples include the explosive adoption of technologies such as the CAT scanners or procedures like coronary bypass surgery.

Wenk (16) proposed that society should be the "keeper of its technology," requiring evaluation processes as early warning systems. The possible consequences of new developments need to be identified before technical enterprises have developed high momentum—otherwise, reversal becomes costly or impossible. There is obviously need for new approaches and procedures by which relevant data can be collected and analyzed to reduce the degree of uncertainty in decision making, to maximize the possible gains, and to minimize eventual losses in much broader perspective.

A series of seven steps has been proposed (17):

1. Definition of the assessment task (scope and depth)
2. Description of relevant technologies and alternatives
3. Exploration of the key societal assumptions—both technical and social
4. Identification of areas of potential impact (such as values, goals, environment, economics, social factors, etc.)
5. Making a preliminary impact analysis including controllability, priority, effectiveness, cost, obstacles, and degree of uncertainty.
6. Identification of possible options and actions
7. Completion of impact analysis by identifying the extent to which the alternatives might affect, in a desirable way, the impact of the technologies on society.

Such approaches are clearly as relevant to new developments in health care technology as in other segments of society, but progress along these lines has been extremely limited. Despite the obvious desirability of systematically considering the ultimate advantages, complications, and uncertainties about the many health technologies, few comprehensive health technology assessments had been completed as of August 1976 (18,19). The Office of Technology Assessment has examined the *need* for assessing social impacts and the kinds of questions that should be asked with reference to nine selected medical technologies.

1. Continuous flow-blood analyzer (see Fig. 5-2)
2. Computerized axial tomography (see Fig. 5-3)
3. Polio and rubella vaccines
4. Radical mastectomy for breast cancer
5. Anticoagulants for acute myocardial infarction
6. Renal dialysis (see Fig. 5-4)
7. Cardiac pacemaker
8. Cortical implants to provide "vision"
9. The totally implantable heart

These examples were selected as representative of a broader spectrum of techniques, drugs, equipment, procedures, and diagnostic devices among the many and diverse advances that have appeared in recent years. The exploration was directed more to the opportunities and approaches to assessment rather than undertaking any definitive analysis.

RENAL DIALYSIS AS A PROTOTYPE

Chronic renal dialysis for patients with end stage renal disease is now supported by Medicare under the Social Security Amendments of 1972. The implications of this act were addressed by a panel of the Institute of Medicine and released by the National Academy of Sciences. From the medical standpoint, hemodialysis and kidney transplants are effective life-extending technologies. According to initial estimates, 8,000 to 10,000 patients per year were expected to need dialysis, reaching some 60,000 by the tenth year. With a $10 billion annual budget for Medicare, $135 million appears relatively inexpensive. Catastrophic insurance coverage has attracted substantial support in Congress and renal dialysis can be viewed as a dramatic example. However, questions have been raised with reference to the annual cost of hospital dialysis (believed to range from $10,000 to $40,000 per patient). In contrast, home hemodialysis can be carried out at costs as low as $3,719/patient/year, and averaging below $5,000/year. These economic considerations seem important in view of annual costs of dialysis now exceeding $500 million.

In 1976, this program provided care for 21,500 eligible patients at a cost of $448 million. The cost is expected to reach $1 billion by 1984 and perhaps cost $1.7 billion by 1990 (covering some 70,000 patients). There is no question of withdrawing this kind of support from patients who would die without it. However, it seems desirable to query what alternatives are being neglected by virtue of this large allocation of resources for the benefit of a relatively small number of patients. For example, kidney transplants are recognized as preferable to the continued enslavement to dialysis machines. The common rejection of kidney transplants can be avoided only by greater understanding of the underlying immune reactions. The scientific community has an obligation to carefully consider whether the huge expenditures for dialysis are diverting efforts away from solving the immune reaction problems or the fundamental origins of the kidney disease process. If this is the case, we could be sacrificing the potential benefits of much preferred treatment, cure, or prevention for future generations in exchange for limited benefits for a relatively small number of patients today. These considerations apply to varying degrees to all of the present pseudosolutions but the artificial heart exemplifies the breadth and depth of the fundamental issues.

TOTALLY IMPLANTABLE HEART

The National Heart and Lung Institute sponsored two assessments of prospective cardiac technologies: "The Totally Implantable Artifical Heart" (20) and "Left Ventricular Assist Device" (21). The study of implantable artificial hearts was conducted by a seven-member multidisciplinary panel on the basis of nine two-day meetings. The evaluation was conducted holistically but without rigorous analytical techniques. It was an exercise in technology appraisal rather than a full scale technology assessment.

The concept of substituting an artificial pumping device for the heart appeared realizable in 1939 when John Gibbon succeeded in keeping cats alive for nearly three hours with a mechanical apparatus that substituted for both the heart and lungs. The life support systems that opened wide the thorax and the heart chambers for surgical repair and reconstruction were the direct result. By the late 1950s heart "assist" devices had reached a stage that encouraged some investigators to push for a totally implantable heart. Congress earmarked appropriations for such a development in 1965. Most of the technologies, essential materials, and successful implantable pump systems have been developed, but methods of meeting the power requirements remain elusive.

Animals have been kept alive for weeks with implanted pumps but external power sources. Advances to date indicate that successful prototypes could be ready for implantation in man within a decade. Estimated numbers now are in the range of 17,000 to 50,000 people per year (judging by the spread of coronary bypass operations, this estimate seems extremely conservative). The implications for various components of society include the following examples (20):

Patients. Recipients of artificial hearts could be expected to lead a fairly active life but the anxieties and uncertainties could have serious psychological effects. Monitoring of patients may be required to keep track of the radioactive materials incorporated into nuclear power packages. This could lead to some loss of freedom. Quick and relatively comfortable death from heart disease may be relinquished in favor of a more prolonged and lingering existence.

Patients' Families. The benefits to the family may be significant, particularly if the patient were the breadwinner. The enormous costs must be borne by some third party—otherwise the family's financial stability would be permanently jeopardized. The personal and psychological impacts on the family are difficult to evaluate.

Society. Many of the candidates for implant will be elderly. This will further increase the absolute number and relative proportion of the older age group in the population. The natural tendency for society to preserve the lives of people "at any cost" indicates that the government must become the source of funding. The demand may well become so great that sufficient numbers of devices cannot reasonably be produced to meet all the requirements. Under these conditions, the rationing of such life-sustaining equipment becomes a difficult or impossible task for the government of a democratic society.

Health Care Delivery System. The requirements for extensive and expensive surgical facilities for implantation of hearts would need to be supplemented by many adjunct services including intensive care, monitoring stations, and social and psychological counseling services. The total cost of each implant device would probably be in the range of $250,000 not counting ancillary services that could mount to $50,000 to $100,000. The diversion of major financial resources toward heart implants would necessarily deplete funds required for many other types of health services.

Legal System. The judicial system would undoubtedly be involved whenever there were insufficient numbers of artificial hearts to satisfy the real or perceived demand. Liability for failure would fall on the manufacturers, physicians, and perhaps government.

Economic Implications. The minimum expected costs of artifical hearts would be at least $500 million per year (assuming 20,000 eligible recipients per year). This figure neglects enormous potential costs from ancillary services or much larger demands than can easily be visualized. It is worth noting that the annual costs of artificial kidneys already exceeds that figure by a substantial margin and renal disease is relatively rare compared to heart disease.

The time has come when these and many related considerations must be explored with relation to the ultimate impact of current pseudosolutions and new ones that are emerging every year or so. For example, the same kinds of analysis are urgently needed to assess the efficacy, economy, and outcome benefits from such sophisticated diagnostic equipment as the CAT scanners and subsequent generations of equipment employing the various energy probes and automated equipment (see also Chapter 6).

The need for multidisciplinary evaluation of the ultimate impact of health technologies is just now becoming more widely apparent. Technology assessment is a concept whose time has come—perhaps too late to avoid mistakes of the past, but absolutely essential for avoidance of even worse problems in the future.

SUMMARY

1. Many tools developed for accelerated biomedical research were readily converted into extremely versatile diagnostic devices and equipment of increasing sophistication. As a consequence, the sources of clinical data multiplied rapidly, providing direct visual access to internal organs, comprehensive information regarding the chemical and cellular composition of blood and body fluids, energy probes producing images and records of the geometry and function of many internal organs, conveniently and painlessly.

2. The progress in diagnostic technologies outstripped the therapeutic mechanisms so that a very large number of ailments can be accurately recognized but cannot be curtailed or cured by available treatments.

3. The impact of health technologies has affected all components of both the health care delivery system and the general public's relation to it.

Health professionals have become increasingly dependent on health technologies. One consequence has been the progressive specialization of physicians, health practitioners, and technicians. A corresponding decrease in general practitioners has depleted the ranks of primary care physicians.

4. Impacts of medical technology include growing specialization of doctors and teaching hospitals (see Chapter 7) and growth in numbers and diversity of health personnel. These trends are accompanied by larger investments in hospitals through Medicare, Medicaid, Health Insurance, and Hill-Burton Legislation. The resulting emphasis on sophisticated secondary and tertiary care has contributed to maldistribution of doctors. All these factors have escalated health care costs. The natural reactions to these effects have been increased government regulation, trends toward cost controls, extended insurance coverage with growing emphasis on HMO development, and other forms of group practice.

5. There is growing evidence that the advances in health technologies have developed too far, too fast, and with exuberant enthusiasm by the health professionals. The outcome for the public in terms of their actual health status has been recognized in the improved management of life-threatening ailments, but many common malfunctions and chronic complaints that depress the quality of life have gone essentially unchallenged. A realignment of priorities seems timely in support of the health status of children and the productive population, even if it requires a reduction in the relative resources devoted to prolonging both life and death of the aging population. The process of technology assessment must be developed and progressively refined to permit crucial evaluation of current and future priorities. The single most important requirement for effective technology assessment is the consideration of the broadly interdisciplinary impacts on the social, economic, legal, and political components of modern society.

6. The dramatic changes in health care delivery systems have created growing interest in developing mechanisms for assessing the effectiveness, efficiency, cost/benefit and outcome for the patients receiving health care in the extraordinarily complicated health services. Some approaches to assessment of health services delivery will be considered in the next chapter.

REFERENCES

1. Ray C: *Medical Engineering.* Chicago, Year Book Medical Publishers, 1975.
2. Rushmer RF: *Cardiovascular Dynamics*, ed 2. Philadelphia, WB Saunders Co., 1976.
3. Rushmer RF: *Medical Engineering; Projections for Health Care Delivery.* New York and London, Academic Press, 1972.
4. Williams S (ed): *Health Services and Medical Care.* New York, John Wiley and Sons (in press).
5. Gordon R, Herman GT, Johnson SA: Image reconstruction from projections. *Sci Amer* 233:56–71, 1975.

6. Computed Tomographic Scanning; a policy statement, Institute of Medicine. National Academy of Sciences, Washington DC, April 1977.
7. Bell RS, Loop JW: The utility and futility of radiographic skull examination for trauma. *N Engl J Med* 284:236-239, 1971.
8. Califano to Med Schools: Cut back class size. *Science* 202:726, 1978.
9. Cooper B, Rice DP: The economic cost of illness revisited. Social Security Bulletin, US DHEW, DHEW Pub No (SSA) 76-11703, February 1976.
10. Haughten JG: *Health in America 1776-1976*, DHEW Pub No (HRA) 76-616, 1976.
11. Forbes WH: Longevity and medical costs. *N Engl J Med* 277:71-78, 1967.
12. Burger EJ: Health and health services in the United States; a perspective and a discussion of some issues. *Ann Int Med* 80:645-650, 1974.
13. Cochrane AL: *Effectiveness and Efficiency; Random Reflections on Health Services.* London, Nuffield Provincial Hospital Trust, 1972.
14. McNerney WJ: The quandary of quality assessment. *N Engl J Med* 295:1505-1511, 1976.
15. Brooks H, Bowers R: The assessment of technology. *Sci Am* 222:13-18, February 1970.
16. Wenk E: Technology assessment in public policy; a new instrument for the social management of technology. *Proc IEEE* 63:371-379, 1975.
17. Jones MV: The methodology of technology assessment. *The Futurist* 6:19-26, 1972.
18. Development of Medical Technology, Opportunities for Assessment. United States Congress Office of Technology Assessment, Government Printing Office Stock Number 052-003-00217, August 1976.
19. Arnstein SR: Technology assessment; opportunities and obstacles. Paper presented at a staff seminar of the National Center for Health Services Research, May 12, 1976.
20. The totally implantable artificial heart; legal, social, ethical, medical, economic, psychological implications. A report of the Artificial Heart Assessment Panel of the National Heart and Lung Institute. DHEW Pub No (NIH) 74-191, 1974.
21. Report on the Left Ventricular Assist Device, TECO-models VII and X, National Heart and Lung Institute, DHEW Pub No (NIH) 75-626, 1975.

CHAPTER 6

Appraisal of Health Services

The preceding chapter presented vivid examples of startling new technical and procedural innovations that have been rapidly developed and widely dispersed throughout the health care delivery system. Therapeutic pseudo-solutions have been adopted and diffused throughout the country with unbounded enthusiasm. Once there is widespread acknowledgment that a particular therapy might have value, it becomes difficult or impossible to retard its further distribution. Clinical trials are widely regarded as unethical if they deprive patients of potentially effective treatment while determining whether the therapy will do more good than harm. Clearly, there is pressing need for the development of effective mechanisms disclosing the efficacy of diagnostic and therapeutic methods in terms of the outcome for the patients, the family, and the fabric of society. The soaring health care delivery costs make mandatory the inclusion of cost/effectiveness and cost/benefit in such evaluations.

Sources of diagnostic data have also been enormously expanded through the advent of increasingly sophisticated technologies providing objective recordings of the chemical composition of blood, body fluids, tissues and other samples. Electrical potentials, pressures, sounds, and other intrinsic energies developed within the body are subject to recording, measuring and monitoring in clinical diagnostic laboratories and in intensive care units. Various forms of energy are increasingly used as probes to provide images of internal organs, notably x-rays, radionuclides (isotopes), ultrasound, infra-red radiation, and others. Socio-economic consequences of such technological triumphs are only now being critically considered by a process called "technology assessment" (see Chapter 5).

The revolutionary changes induced in the health care delivery system by technologies have vastly increased its magnitude, diversity, scope, and complexity. The organizational frameworks and operational mechanisms of this huge enterprise are poorly understood and very little studied. These deficiencies become acutely manifest when key decisions must be made regarding major additions or modifications by decision makers groping unsuccessfully for the information and understanding required for rational courses of action. Only recently has this crying need for reliable, valid, and relevant information been recognized and expressed in the growing programs of health services research, both here and abroad.

It is no longer considered adequate to address these complex issues intuitively or by trying to interpret the public will. The costs and consequences of misguided judgment have become too great and too visible to rely on expediency and educated guesses in the absence of more extensive and valid data. As a consequence of these pressures, new approaches to program evaluation in the health field have been developing relatively rapidly beginning at ground zero. New "basic" approaches are required for objective and quantitative exploration of socioeconomic factors involved in health care delivery.

The evaluation of health services is a totally new enterprise of very recent vintage for which the necessary methodologies are having to be developed, validated, and utilized under extremely great urgency and pressures. Health services research is expected to provide the necessary data on which to base rational and defensible decisions at a time when the overall objectives of the health care delivery system have not been clearly spelled out. In its initial efforts, the principal focus has been directed toward assessing ways by which relatively simple health services can be delivered more efficiently as implied by the term cost/effectiveness. Many key issues regarding the relationships between costs and benefits must await new methods of assessment. A plethora of new health status indicators are emerging from many different centers in hopes of identifying more quantitative or valid indicators of health in individuals or groups of individuals.

In general, mechanisms of appraisal have been adopted from established disciplines such as statistics, epidemiology, sociology, anthropology, and psychology. This process is reminiscent of the manner in which the techniques, technologies, and concepts of engineering were converted for biomedical research and practice during the past 30 years. The following discussion deals with current status and some future opportunities in this newly developing field of health services research as a vital and essential movement affecting all elements of health and health care. The National Center for Health Services Research is a tangible manifestation of a need for mechanisms to develop soundly based data and concepts regarding health services, present and proposed.

THE NATIONAL CENTER FOR HEALTH SERVICES RESEARCH

Public law 93–353 (1974) contained new provisions for the National Center for Health Services Research, the National Center for Health Statistics, and the National Library of Medicine. The program in Health Services Research established a substantial intramural effort accounting for about one-fourth of its research budget, but the programmatic priorities made no distinction between in-house and extramural projects. The principal areas of research have been developed on the basis of an issue-oriented framework, as a means of assuring explicit relevance. Categories such as technology development and demonstration projects are not included. Eight priority issues were identified for intensive research efforts in 1976 (1) with significant modifications projected for FY 1979–80 (2), as follows:

Priorities (1976)	Projected Priorities 1979–80
Quality of care	*Technology assessment:* Analysis and evaluation
Inflation, productivity, and costs	of new technologies
Health care and the disadvantaged	*Health Insurance:* Analysis of various National
Health manpower	Health Insurance proposals
Health insurance	*Cost Containment:* Incentives which can modify
Planning and regulation	costs of health services
Ambulatory care and emergency	*Planning and Regulation:* Methods for cost-
medical services	effective decision-making
Long term care	*Health Manpower:* Economic and behavioral
	aspects in education; requirements and resource
	development

Additional details have been published, particularly with reference to quality of care (3) and cost containment (4). In view of the enormous expenditures in providing health care to the American people, the magnitude of the effort in assessing its effectiveness is grossly restricted by a very limited budget (5). The change in emphasis represented by the two sets of priorities listed above specifies a shift toward more immediate and "practical" problems facing the nation. The pressures for immediate relevance appear to gain dominance over issues such as quality of care, care of the disadvantaged, emergency care, and long term care for chronically ill and aging populations. The following discussion is oriented toward considerations affecting priorities for evaluating health services and health care delivery.

DEFINITIONS AND DISTINCTIONS

The overall objective of health services research is to develop and use procedures designed to provide necessary information to facilitate rational decisions regarding feasibility, efficacy, and efficiency of various aspects of delivery of health services. The organizing concept makes use of "evaluation" experiments, to be distinguished from "scientific" investigations. The scientific method typically takes the form of rigorous investigations designed to improve *understanding* of natural phenomena. In contrast, health services research and analysis are generally directed toward the acquisition of information to be used for arriving at rational *decisions*. The number and diversity of decisions regarding health services defies imagination, since they are being made daily at all levels from private practice to major governmental agencies and involving virtually all aspects of the health care delivery system.

Before World War II, very few of the health programs had been subjected to critical evaluation of any sort. Acceptance was often based upon biased sources, untested and frequently erroneous assumptions, and inherently unreliable and sometimes irrelevant measurements. It was only in the mid-1960s that significant progress began to appear in efforts to remedy such shortcomings in the methods of evaluation research. At the outset, very few people had the training, experience, and skills required to engage in soundly based experimental designs, data acquisition, and analysis as applied to health services.

Program evaluation is rarely afforded the luxury of a prospective experimental design in a newly developing enterprise. In contrast, most program evaluation necessarily deals with procedures, processes, or technologies that are already in place and functioning, thereby exhibiting inherent resistance to change or critical questioning. The greatest deficiency in such assessments is a lack of reliable and valid measures which can indicate the outcome for patients manifesting various disease states and encountering health professionals, facilities, and services. Outcome criteria (or signs of success) of programs are vitally needed for decision makers and policy makers who are required to consider the need to expand, to cut back, or to abolish programs. Since this is a relatively new field of endeavor, it is important to make some distinctions between different types of activities embraced by the term *health services assessment.* A useful and timely description of evaluation processes has recently been presented by Shortell and Richardson (6).

Process Evaluation. The extent to which an organizational component is functioning smoothly and efficiently can be evaluated by methods commonly employed in industry to assess the efficiency of processes. The time devoted to various aspects of the procedures, the waiting periods, time and motion studies, costs of supplies and capital expenditures all represent objective data which can be collected and analyzed. The extent to which the training of personnel is appropriate to the assigned tasks can be evaluated. Mechanisms for improving the flow and efficiency of the procedures tend to emerge from such analytical efforts. The extent to which improvements have favorably influenced the effectiveness of an organization can be assessed by controlled comparisons, employing the same objective measurements. It is far more difficult to estimate the value added to a patient's health by virtue of a specific procedure than it is to explore the process by which that service was delivered.

Program Evaluation. The extent to which a program, consisting of a set of planned activities, reaches the desired and intended objectives can be approached by many mechanisms for the purpose of providing necessary information for the participants, administrators, and decision makers in a program. To an increasing degree, efforts are being made to develop the rigor employed by the scientific method or approximations to this approach. Such analysis requires identification and definition of relevant objectives, the distinction between short-term and long-term effects, the magnitude and nature of the effort, identity of the group to be served, the relationships between the objectives and processes being employed to reach them, and the outcome in terms of both intended and unexpected consequences.

Outcome Evaluation. Assessment of the outcome of programs in terms of tangible benefits to patients is exceedingly important but rarely attained for lack of measurable consequences, which are unequivocally the result of a specific procedure or health service. A commonly cited example would be the effectiveness in the control of high blood pressure through a major screening and educational effort applied to large populations. As part of its research program, the NCHSR supported a study by the Rand Corporation for development of disease-specific outcome measures for eight medical and surgical conditions.

1. Asthma
2. Breast masses and breast cancer
3. Cholecystectomy
4. Diarrhea and dehydration in children
5. Ischemic heart disease
6. Osteoarthritis
7. Otitis media in children
8. Tonsillectomy with or without adenoidectomy

These conditions were selected to serve as prototypes for a broader spectrum of health problems. The findings of the study and the outcome measures suggested for each of these conditions are featured in a publication available on request from NCHSR (3). Such studies represent the early faltering steps in the development of more consistent and valid measures of outcome of health services as an essential ingredient to more rational decisions regarding cost-effectiveness and priorities for program development and resource allocation (7). Another evidence of great interest in this general area is the development of a "Clearing House on Health Indexes" comprised of annotated bibliographies published four times a year containing methods or criteria for evaluating various composite measures of health status (8). These cumulative annotations are designed to serve as reference guides for investigators engaged in assessing health status of individuals or groups. Such indices appear to be essential ingredients in assaying the efficacy and cost efficiency of health services. Clear-cut and well-defined criteria for judging outcome is remarkably rarely encountered as a direct result of either health care or preventive measures. The enormously expanded sources of objective and quantitative diagnostic devices (see Chapter 5) have not been utilized sufficiently in controlled experiments for evaluating outcome of treatment. Attractive alternatives are presented in a subsequent section.

ELEMENTS OF PROGRAM EVALUATION

A wide variety of investigations, analyses, and assessments are encompassed by the theory and practices of health services research. For convenience, the most common types can be considered under three main headings:

1. The assessment of *need, demand,* and *utilization* of services.
2. The evaluation of the services rendered.
3. The effects of alternative resource allocation.

The concept of *need* for health care is difficult to define, depending on the perspective. The perceived needs for health care may be vastly different for individual patients, physicians, or a community. Epidemiologists can measure the prevalence and incidence of various disease conditions (9). Their colleagues in social science and psychology can facilitate identifying the behavioral consequences of these and employ analytical tools for expressing and interpreting such "needs" (see Fig. 6-1).

The methods for estimating *demand* require the development of techniques by which the requests for service can be measured, accumulated, and analyzed. The underlying explanation for discrepancies between the prevalence of the complaints of obvious disease states and the demand for their care is an important aspect of the problem. Factors which influence demand for medical care include age, sex, social class, occupation, educational status, and more complex sociological and psychological variables.

Utilization or *usage* is indicated by data from records, surveys or local and national samples, data provided by health institutions, and many other sources. One contribution of epidemiology is to assess the accuracy and validity of the information and the interpretations derived from it.

Evaluation of Services Provided and Alternative Options. Information of the sort outlined above is the essential ingredient for decision makers faced with the need for assessing the effectiveness of existing procedures and programs, the relative priorities of alternatives, and desirability of implementing new processes or programs. The intelligent allocation of limited resources is far more difficult and complex than appears on the surface. The situations in all cases are complex, variable, and to some degree uncontrollable. Furthermore, most decisions must take place in institutional or organizational environments established through long tradition and solidified by prior decisions.

FORCES IMPELLING EXPANDED
EVALUATION RESEARCH

The practice of medicine at any particular stage in history is a composite representing the remnants of past traditions and beliefs, supplemented by more recent additions. Literally thousands of "new" treatments have been introduced over the past centuries. Many of these now seem risky, crude, or heartless but once were deeply ingrained in the fabric of medical therapy over decades or centuries. For example, bleeding was routinely used over many centuries for ridding the body of bad humors (10). Purging persisted into the present century with the concept of "intestinal autointoxication."

A surgical folklore, based on the mistaken concept that many ailments resulted from "foci of infection," led to the removal of millions of teeth, hundreds of thousands of tonsils, and uncounted gallbladders and vermiform appendices. Tonsillectomies remain the most common surgical operation in the country, despite the weight of authority that most of them are unwarranted. (See the section on surgical surpluses.)

Thousands of stomachs and uteri have been resuspended into positions regarded as "more normal." Misguided therapeutic enthusiasms were shared widely in the form of bland diets for peptic ulcer and fat-free diets for infectious hepatitis, which probably accomplished little for the patient (10). Patients have been put to bed unnecessarily for prolonged periods of time for a wide variety of ailments.

There can be little doubt that a vast number of currently popular and expensive home remedies, medical therapies, and surgical operations are equally overrated or overused. Cochrane (11) emphasized the critical importance of randomized control trials (RCT) for assessing efficacy of treatment, because "recent publications using this technique have given ample warning of how dangerous it is to assume that well-established therapies, which have not been tested, are always effective." He cited numerous examples, such as evidence casting doubt on the value of oral antidiabetic therapy, insulin, and diet in the treatment of adult diabetics. Insulin appears to have little advantage over diet with respect to outcome in adult (not juvenile) diabetics. The value of iron administered to nonpregnant women with lowered hemoglobins is questionable. Ergotamine tartrate may have little effect as a treatment of migraine. (11)

Obviously, there are many drugs and devices which have such manifestly favorable results that they are not seriously being questioned; however, there are many common treatments that have never been subjected to a critical evaluation. Some of these are in urgent need of assessment. It seems significant that a large and growing number of well-entrenched diagnostic and surgical procedures have proved to be controversial or ineffective when subjected to rigorous testing under controlled conditions. Notable examples include radical mastectomy, or skull x-rays in head injury. Even the efficacy of intensive coronary care units has been thrown into question by controlled experiments in Britain (see the section on avoiding exorbitant use of available technologies.)

From these examples it becomes apparent that many or most elements of the health care delivery process deserve some critical evaluation. The crucial requirement is to develop more effective methods and priorities to address the most pressing needs from the immense array of medical practices. The evaluation of health service programs bears striking resemblance to the process of forward planning, for obvious reasons. They are both activities designed to develop rational bases for decisions regarding the expansion or contraction of programs, the implementation of new approaches, and the distribution of resources as a result of a decision-making process. By far the most important step in both forward planning and program evaluation is the clear definition of the ultimate aims, the objectives, the strategies, and the criteria of success with provisions for followup and feedback.

THE EVALUATION PROCESS

The initial step toward program evaluation is the selection of a target or an objective toward which the effort should be directed. Strangely enough, this initial step is frequently the weakest element in the subsequent sequence. The most rigorous and soundly based process directed at an ill-conceived or poorly defined objective has little prospect of ultimate utility. All too often, the objective is decided independently by the evaluator or team and is based more on the availability of measurable indicators than on the relevance of the question being asked. For obvious reasons, the perceptions of the key issues are very different when viewed by the evaluating team, the program director, the administrator of the institution, the granting agency (if any), and the general public (see Table 6-2).

An evaluation that discloses deficiencies or defective elements in any program constitutes a threat to the position of active participants, either by the evaluation process or in subsequent decisions. In the specification of objectives, it is frequently preferable to phrase the question "How can this program be improved and what are the criteria for success?" The elements of the program that are most crucial for such a study should be listed and given priorities. The operational indicators can be identified and developed, if possible. In general, a program evaluation that is undertaken in the presence of conflict or controversy is likely to end up with questionable results. Important ingredients at the outset are mutual agreements on definitions of objectives and general consensus regarding their applications. In complex systems, a single concise target is rarely identified, since there exist a multiplicity of components with complex interactions. For this reason, it is necessary to distinguish carefully between the overall aims, long range goals, and the immediate objectives. For each of the components of a system under study, care must be taken to identify indicators most suitable for judging the performance or outcome of the process. Finally, there is an implied responsibility to carefully consider undesired or unintended consequences from any change that might be recommended or introduced. It is often useful to ask "What is the worst possible thing that could go wrong with this program?" Such queries can profitably be addressed to people who honestly believe the program will not succeed or to those in corresponding institutions with similar problems (6).

OPERATIONAL INDICATORS

The end result of the objective-setting process usually takes the form of action-oriented statements, each associated with operational indicators, preferably variables which are subject to quantitative measurement. Hypertension is a convenient example, because blood pressure represents a quantitative measurement that is commonly used and generally trusted as an objective operational indicator for an evaluation. Unfortunately, such a generally accepted outcome measurement is the exception rather than the rule in most program evaluations. To the greatest extent possible, the indicators used should be chosen on the basis of as wide a consensus as possible among those who are involved in (1) evaluating and (2) using the acquired data.

Categories of Evaluations. Among the many types of evaluations, a few deserve mention. The magnitude of an *effort* is frequently measured in terms of time spent at various activities and use of resources and services. The evaluation of *performance* requires operational indicators that provide insight into the effectiveness of the activities. *Relative performance* refers to a comparison between groups and individuals engaged in comparable activities or in accordance with standards. *Efficiency* is commonly regarded as an assessment of performance in relation to cost. The question may be oriented toward the possibility of maintaining or increasing output at lower cost. *Process* evaluation is intended to explore the underlying factors or features that cause a program to either function well or poorly by examining the procedures being used. *Cost/benefit* relationships are most difficult to assess in health delivery processes, since the values assigned to the benefits are almost always intangible, conjectural, or controversial.

Components of Program Evaluation (An example). Programs never exist in isolation. It is therefore important to consider and evaluate the preexisting conditions which affect the program in critical ways before the evaluation is initiated. Factors which must be considered are more readily visualized by means of a schematic diagram. Program evaluation is best regarded as a cyclical effort which begins with the identification of the objectives of the effort, by far the most important step. Planning of the evaluation program is followed by the mobilization of the resources required to collect the necessary information and to analyze it. The performance of the program under study is evaluated and compared to the original objectives of the study. Critical reviews of performance generally lead to mechanisms for improvement which lead to new objectives and, ideally, the process begins anew (Table 6-1).

More specifically, a quality assurance program might begin with consideration of the preexisting conditions in a hospital as they are affected by the medical staff organization and the relations to other activities within the institution. The principal program elements could be inputs in the form of program objectives, personnel, available resources, and the specific activities required to undertake such an evaluation. Interventions that can affect functioning of the organization might include reorganizations within the institution and also external factors. Impact could be expressed in terms of disease-specific morbidity or mortality, duration of illness, or other measurable indicators. Additional consequences might include greater patient satisfaction and other favorable results, as well as undesirable consequences such as increased unit costs in the laboratory or discontent from altered staffing patterns (Table 6-1).

Experimental Design. Methodology used in program evaluation stems largely . from disciplines outside the traditional medical boundaries, such as sociology,

208 Assessment of Health Technologies and Services

TABLE 6-1. Components of a Program Evaluation Process

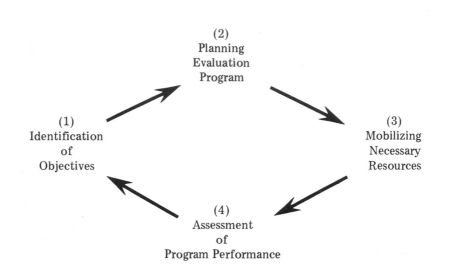

Essential Elements in an Evaluation Process

Program Status (Initial)	Program Components	Interventions Imposed on Program	Effects of Interventions (Impact)	Consequences (Ultimate Outcome)
Organization of program	Objectives	Evaluation design	Data processing	Interpretation
Function of program	Personnel	Modifications	Analytical assessment	Evaluation
Relation to other programs	Facilities	Perturbations	Validity appraisal	Projection
Overall environment	Support Activities Records	Additions Measurements	Indicators of significance	Implementation

See also Shortell and Richardson (6).

anthropology, statistics, and behavioral sciences. Until relatively recently, health professionals were quite content to accept as evidence of successful procedures the statements of satisfaction by their patients or their own subjective impression of the consequences of their ministrations. Such impressions are not adequate for purposes of arriving at rational decisions. For near-term or long-range planning, valid data are essential for reasonable conclusions about whether an intervention actually has an effect, whether the intervention is the cause or the effect, what other factors are significant, and whether or not the results can be extrapolated to other situations. Many factors must be considered in assuring valid results, such as methods of randomization, establishing control groups, avoiding bias induced by the testing process, or artifacts resulting from the selection process or attrition of participants. Extensive discussions of such issues are to be found in many standard sources (12, 13, 14).

A cornerstone of experimental evaluation is the random allocation of subjects to treatment and control groups in an effort to avoid some of the complications mentioned above. When the sizes of samples are necessarily restricted, improved design can often be achieved by matching or pairing of equivalent individuals in the experimental and control groups. Lacking opportunities to engage in more structured research, it is sometimes possible to obtain valuable information from quasi-experimental designs, such as *time series* experiments. For this purpose, multiple measures are obtained, both before and after the introduction of a particular program. This process is particularly useful in situations where programs are not likely to vary significantly during the period of study.

Cost/Benefit Analysis. There are many instances in which a program produces results of unquestioned value. For example, the mass immunization against poliomyelitis produced dramatic effects such as reducing the number of cases from 20,000 in 1950-1954 to only 61 cases in the entire country in 1965. Cost/benefit analysis is undertaken more commonly in instances where the results are more difficult to discern, or where the allocation of resources becomes crucial (see also Fig. 6-2a).

Benefits derived from programs focused on specific diseases are frequently expressed in economic terms, such as the estimated cost of premature death and disability, the costs of labor lost, or reduced expenses from moribidity or debility. The estimated return from public investment in biomedical research or health manpower training have quite consistently suggested that the benefits outweigh the cost, whether couched in terms of a rate of return, cost/benefit ratio, or estimated value (15). There are strong incentives to make assumptions that are likely to bias results toward such desirable conclusions.

Cost/Effectiveness. *Cost/effectiveness* is a term applied to the analysis of the relative merits of different mechanisms for providing similar health services. The most common outcomes from cost/effectiveness analyses have been recommendations to: (1) start new health programs or (2) expand existing ones in order to achieve the potential benefits. Despite the obvious advantages of rendering such decisions on the basis of valid and rigorous data, opportunities for doing so have been relatively infrequent. The process is extremely complicated, the issues tend to be poorly defined, and the values are intangible and difficult to assess in any quantitative terms. The nature and extent of these problems are considered in more detail below (see the section on conceptual consideration in health services research). An additional impediment is the great diversity of attitudes and motives which are represented among the many necessary participants in the process of health program evaluation (see Table 6-1).

Diverse Perceptions by the Participants. New knowledge is almost universally regarded as a worthy objective and a useful product deserving support. In contrast, critical evaluation of programs necessarily evokes many types of

TABLE 6-2. Perspectives and Motivations of Participants in Program Evaluation

Components of Program Evaluation	Evaluation Team	Health Care Team	Responsible Administrator(s)	Funding Agencies	Patients and Public
Objective	Improvement in services	Patient satisfaction	Efficiency	Protecting public	Personal safety and well-being
Target	Current practice	Current practice	Cash flow	Tangible results	Improved service
Type of evaluation	Critical analysis	Subjective impressions	Cost-effectiveness	Curtailing costs	Maximize benefits
Experimental Design	Valid data requirements	Unaltered routines	No added costs	Convincing data	Lack of concern
Measurements	Reliable, relevant data	Minimal disruption	Minimal load on staff	Familiar	Painless, without hazard
Analyses	Statistically significant	Individual patient	Relevant to administration	Far-reaching	Applicable to individual
Interpretations	Supported by data	Upsetting to traditions	Improvements at lower cost	Potential regulations	Effects on confidence
Applications	Powerless to effect	Resistant to change	Limited power	Possible legislation	Uncertainty

responses from the various participants in the scenario (Table 6-2). The motivation of the evaluating team is very frequently viewed with suspicion or even alarm by the people engaged in providing the service under scrutiny. A favorable review would be nice and reassuring, but the prospects of criticism, backed by data, can threaten the position, professional prestige, or even the livelihood of the "targets." Similarly, the responsible administrators may gain valuable information for setting priorities but at the possible expense of revealing past mistakes in judgment. Program evaluation always carries the prospects of changes with the accompanying uncertainties that this implies. Agencies that support critical program evaluation desire valid information but prefer to avoid inciting powerful opposition.

The general public is often upset by revelations indicating that processes and procedures in which they have had great confidence may not be as effective as they had been led to believe (Table 6-2). The health professions have always been extremely dependent upon the confidence and faith of their patients as an essential ingredient for their successful ministrations. Anything that undermines the patient's confidence in the effectiveness of the procedures prescribed or used by physicians tends to depress the effectiveness of medical management, particularly for ailments lacking definitive therapy (see the section on the value of doing something: the placebo effect, below). Wide diversity of perceptions among the participants and beneficiaries of program evaluation is suggested by the examples presented in Table 6-2. The implications of these differences in perceptions by the evaluation team, health care team, administrators, funding agencies, and the public can best be visualized by trying to imagine the impact and obstacles that could arise from proposals to critically evaluate any one of the following: coronary bypass surgery, CAT scanners, automated chemical laboratory procedures, and so forth.

CONCEPTUAL CONSIDERATIONS IN HEALTH SERVICES RESEARCH

The principal participants in program evaluation (Table 6-2) exhibit differences in both perceptions and priorities resulting from very different points of view. The patients, the physicians, the health teams, the health evaluation teams, and the "third parties" have different motivations which are justifiable, rational, and considered in the "best interests of the general public." However, these differences represent "divergent problems," which are characterized by significant discrepancies between the best interests of the person and the best interests of society. For example, the detection of a disabling disease in one person by extensive and expensive screening of 10,000 nonsymptomatic adults is an extreme example of such a discrepancy. It might seem valuable to the one individual and a less appropriate use of public money to the remainder. Less obvious is the fact that the allocation of limited resources to one category of diagnosis or treatment also implies that the same funds are not available for other options. Similarly, the process of establishing facilities for health services tends to be somewhat irreversible, limiting future choices. Once a method of diagnosis or treatment has become established, it tends to become entrenched despite impressive evidence or wisespread doubts regarding efficacy. All these issues are made more complex by ambiguity regarding the definition of health and the scope of health care. This issue is considered in more detail in the next chapter (see Figs. 7-6 and 7-7). The operational relationship between the "demand" for health services and the "need" for health services was mentioned in previous sections.

USAGE, DEMANDS, AND NEEDS FOR HEALTH SERVICES

The demands for health services are readily recognized by tabulating the numbers of requests for particular types of encounters or procedures by people or professionals acting for the benefit of their patients. The "usage" can be regarded as the actual delivery of health services and therefore represents approximate equality of desires of the patients and prescriptions by the health professionals. The needs of the public for health care may be represented by an iceberg (Fig. 6-1), the exposed tip representing the clearly defined requirements that have been well established by both performance and tradition (16). Unmet needs represent a discrepancy between the available resources and demands for their availability. These commonly become expressed as waiting lists or underserved populations. Progressing below the level of clearly recognized need is a huge volume of ill-defined or poorly documented "needs," which extend out of sight and have no natural limits. These include methods of doubtful value that persist in common practice. The scope of "health and health care" has been progressively extended to encompass symptoms and stresses in a growing array of nonmedical problems (see Chapter 7). The symptoms and functional disturbances resulting from domestic friction, cultural stresses, psychological aberrations, and many other factors of modern living have become defined increasingly as "health hazards."

Appropriate allocation of resources, through health services research, ultimately involves some elements of cost/benefit analysis in attempting to establish perspectives and priorities among myriad options. It is difficult enough to estimate the costs of health services. The problem of arriving at an economic equivalent of health benefits is a challenge that still defies our most conscientious efforts.

COST/BENEFIT BALANCE

The health professions are suddenly confronted with new requirements to consider the relationship between the cost of services and the benefits they provide. The value of human life and health must now be more seriously considered due to an uncontrolled upward spiral of medical costs.

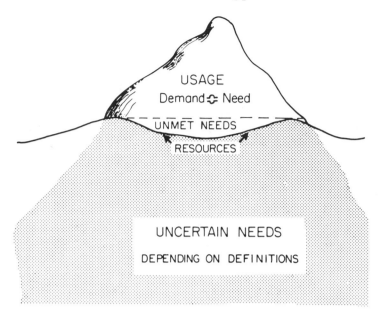

Figure 6-1. Utilization of health services is the visible part of an "iceberg" where the *demands* of the patients are approximately equal to the needs perceived by the health professionals. A vast and invisible volume of uncertain needs for health services lies under the surface, including services which "might be useful." Areas of responsibility extend beyond disease or disability into realms of psycho-social, behavioral, and cultural problems impinging upon health. Planning and assigning priorities to health services do not normally encompass vast invisible or intangible needs and tend to focus on more sharply defined requirements of current practice (After J.R. Ashford [16]).

Many health providers and decision makers disclaim the ability to place a value on life, despite the fact that policy decisions on highway design, auto safety, traffic control measures, mining hazards, and safeguards against health hazards all imply an economic evaluation of the value of life. Our failure to arrive at a broader and more realistic spectrum of values has left the health professions with a remarkably limited array of measurable variables on which most of the policy decisions have been made in the past.

The actual costs of health care are generally difficult to estimate with accuracy, because most hospital facilities have originated as nonprofit organizations with correspondingly loose accounting procedures. Estimating expenditures for drugs, personnel, facilities, and materials may be difficult enough but it appears impossible to assign monetary value to intangible items such as reassurance, prognosis, symptomatic relief, improved health, or life expectancy (Fig. 6-2a). A large number of the ailments suffered by humans are due to unknown causes and/or resist treatment of the suspected mechanisms, as indicated in Chapter 4.

214

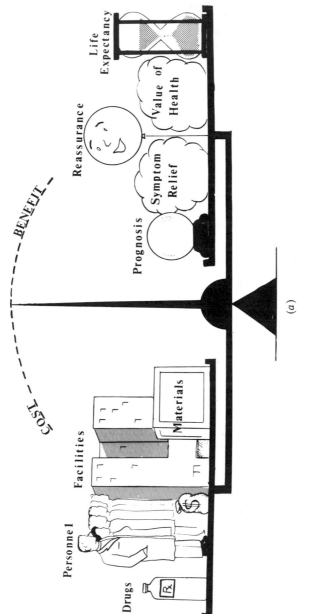

Figure 6-2. (a). Cost/benefit analysis is extremely complicated because health care involves many complex components that are not readily assessed. The benefits of health services include intangible factors such as relief of pain, reassurance, diminished disability, or the value of life and health. (b) The balance between cost and benefit can be considered in certain general categories. Benefits of health services are perceived as worthwhile when they are rendered apparently free by third party payments even if the outcome is little affected. Effective methods of either cure or prevention are unquestionably of great value. Conditions lacking effective therapy or definite diagnosis are not likely to be greatly improved by medical management. Extremely costly techniques and technologies for conditions with poor prognosis are inherently less beneficial than for conditions with more definitive diagnosis and therapy (From Rushmer RF: *Humanizing Health Care* [17] reproduced with permission of MIT Press, Cambridge, Mass.).

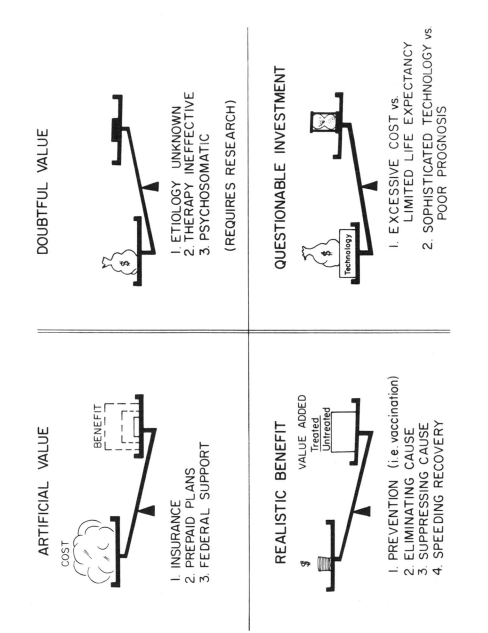

Figure 6-2. (b)

215

Prognosis, symptomatic relief, and reassurance constitute a very large proportion of medical practice, impelling both physicians and patients toward physical examinations and "routine" laboratory tests without specific indications. The perceived value of these procedures is as difficult to estimate as the value of health or of life itself (17). Traditional scales for judging the balance between the costs and the benefits have been the self regulatory mechanism of supply and demand. The amount of money a consumer was willing to pay for a service nominally established a value in a free market. Modern mechanisms cushion the costs of care and obscure the relationship between price and perceived benefit (Fig. 6-2a).

Artificially Cheap—Apparently Free. Modern societies tend to equalize wealth by providing essential services apparently free or at a reduced cost through subsidies. Economists have generally failed to make the important distinction between goods and services obtained for a price or offered "free." "Free" goods or services generally fall into two classes, namely collective public services, such as defense, police, and fire protection, or public health, and individual goods and services, such as education, health services, school lunches, free transportation, and so forth. "Free" does not mean costless, it simply refers to goods and services for which the consumer does not *pay more* if he *uses more*. Subsidized freeways, utilities, or services all tend to remove economic restraints. Such public support stimulates excessive utilization, soaring costs, uncontrolled demand, and threatened breakdown. Every country attempting to provide easy and equal access to personal services has found that it can never meet the essentially unlimited demand, inevitably leading to congestion and waiting lines.

Health insurance renders health care an "apparently" free or cheap service, because a consumer can obtain more services without increased costs. When access to health care is greatly increased through insurance and federally supported health programs, people demand service even when benefits are limited or doubtful. When the requirement to pay for service has been removed, any benefit or improvement can appear to be "well worth it," even if it were only a drug, a massage, or free meals in a hospital bed (Fig. 6-2b). Experience in other countries indicates that the single most pressing problem stemming from artificially "cheap or free" medical care is the universal tendency to clog the system through expanded demands (see Chapter 9). Patients generally derive little improvement in self-limited ailments from expensive encounters with physicians or with hospital staffs, when therapy is solely symptomatic. The health professions should be more candid in recognizing and acknowledging such inadequacies, actively pursuing more effective mechanisms either within the health care system or by innovations. This problem is particularly acute in problems for which medicine shares responsibility with other segments of society, such as drug abuse, aging, or mental illness.

Since there is no prospect of meeting the expanding demands for health care, we must face the painful prospect of establishing criteria that will channel patients toward the most effective use of the available resources and provide the maximum benefit to the largest number of persons. This prospect inevitably arouses the specter of using some form of triage to allocate health services in favor of those patients whose prospects are best for deriving maximum benefit from services rendered. The denial or reduction in treatment for some patients in favor of others is barely acceptable in the exigencies of military campaigns when demand by wounded or sick greatly exceeds supply near the battlefields. The American people have preferred to blindly retain the delusion that this rich country of ours can afford to provide all the health care that all the people think they need or desire. Estimates of the relationship between the magnitude of expenditures and the consequences of care for patients with many types of illness remain vague and clouded by uncertainty (Fig. 6-3).

OUTCOME ASSESSMENT: VALUE ADDED

The "effectiveness" of medical care might be gauged by the relationship between the specificity of diagnosis and nature of the therapeutic result (Fig. 6-3). Prevention of illness or direct treatment of the cause can best be assessed in those conditions in which specific diagnosis can be established by quantitative tests. When the nature and severity of an illness can be reliably indicated by quantitative measurement, the extent to which the physician has successfully suppressed or eliminated the cause can be most accurately assayed. Medical management provides unquestioned benefits to patients having conditions that have a high level of diagnostic specificity coupled with an effective therapeutic attack on the disease. Diagnosis of a condition, lacking effective therapy, can provide reassurance and prognosis but little change in course of illness or health status. Quacks can be recognized by promises or assurance of "cures" for illnesses of unknown cause or indeterminate diagnosis.

Virtually any ailment could be assigned an appropriate position on the matrix in Figure 6-3 with a reasonable degree of consensus among health professionals, based solely on diagnostic specificity and therapeutic effectiveness. Using such criteria, health care resources might be preferentially allocated for medical management of those conditions which provide greatest benefits. Greater candor is needed in advice to patients about conditions with unknown cause or cure. Resources for medical *research* need to be appropriated for conditions lacking either effective diagnostic or therapeutic methods (see Chapters 3 and 4). Theoretically, a systematic approach could facilitate evaluations based on more specific and realistic criteria than are now in use.

THE CONCEPT OF "VALUE ADDED"

The single greatest deficiency in our ability to evaluate health services is the general lack of means for gauging the outcome. Criteria or weighting factors have never been widely accepted for use in assigning economic

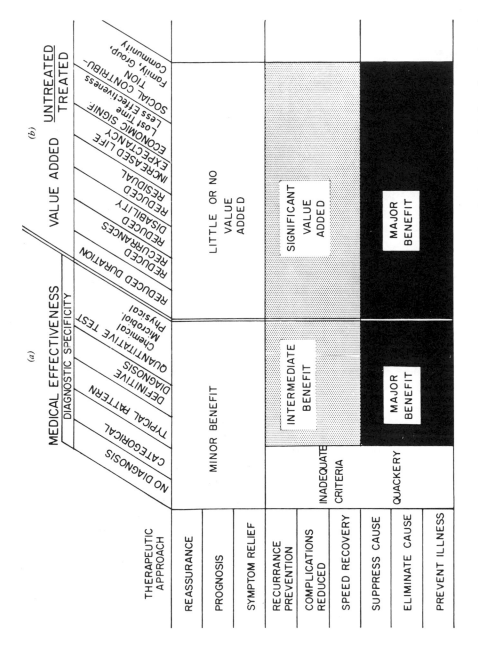

Figure 6-3. (*a*) Benefits of highest order are achieved for conditions in which the diagnosis is based on relevant quantitative measurements. Minor benefits can be provided for conditions in which the cause(s) is unknown and/or the diagnosis is uncertain and the therapy is manifestly ineffective. (*b*) The "value-added" by health services could be assessed by the relation between the effectiveness of the available therapy and the extent to which the medical management favorably altered the duration or course of "typical illness." (From Rushmer RF: *Humanizing Health Care,* Ref. 17, reproduced with permission of MIT Press, Cambridge, Mass.).

equivalents (i.e., dollars) to intangible properties such as life, health, relief of pain, or improved quality of life. Economists have increasingly engaged in estimating the value that is added to raw materials during each stage of manufacture and distribution of a product. This is the conceptual basis for the "value-added" tax widely assessed in European countries. If the desired product of health services is healthy patients, then the concept of value-added might be applied to the differences in conditions before and after therapy. A number of authorities have proposed this approach. The difficulties of assigning relative values to such intangibles as discomfort or restriction of activity etc., have been emphasized by Sir Richard Doll (18). In those conditions where the existence and severity of an illness can be objectively estimated or quantitatively measured by diagnostic technologies, it should be possible to estimate the extent to which therapy has shortened the course or avoided complications as compared with untreated individuals following a "typical course." Unfortunately, such definitive monitoring is available for an extremely small proportion of ailments and "typical courses" are not generally accepted by medical authorities.

Some measureable criteria that might be employed for such assessments would include changes in the duration of ailments, reduced incidence of recurrence, shortened duration of disability, and reduced residual impairment. Increased life expectancy would be more difficult to assess but has been attempted in the case of cancer, heart disease, and other major categories of illness. The economic significance of the time lost from work and the reduced effectiveness in employment are components considered in the "burden of illness" (see Fig. 3–5).

A more attractive alternative would be to assess the "value added" in accordance with the nature of the diagnostic and therapeutic methods employed. There are certain large categories of ailments for which the nature and extent of improvement that could be expected from therapy can be quite clearly specified at the outset. For this purpose, the effectiveness of management methods needs to be more completely and consistently assayed by methods described near the end of this chapter. Pending such developments, it should be possible to provide rough categories that would be useful to decision-makers in prioritizing programs or allocation of resources.

VALUE ADDED BY PREVENTION OF DISEASES

Preventable diseases are prone to disappear as illustrated schematically in Figure 4–1. Although the costs involved in the control of contagious and epidemic diseases have been very large (i.e., sanitation, water supplies, immunization programs, and vitamin supplements), the inherent values have always been so apparent that there have been very few who question the wisdom of making these expenditures. There has been no "tax revolt" against the costly measures that have been responsible for virtual elimination of the scourges of the past. Indeed, the mild objections expressed regarding such methods as fluoride treatment of water supplies have been based largely on philosophical grounds rather than economic consideration. On this basis, the highest level of "value added" is attained in the case of primary prevention. In general, the greatest cost/effectiveness, cost/benefit and value-added can be attained by preventing the development of disease or disability as opposed to managing the consequences.

VALUE ADDED BY DEFINITIVE THERAPY

When physicians can couple definitive diagnosis with definitive therapy, the value added is too great for argument. For example, the antibiotics were quickly shown to be effective in suppressing certain infectious diseases but were very costly at first. However, the "value added" was so obvious that few hesitated to prescribe them for even an instant on the basis of cost or consequence. Through the years, surgery has always provided dramatic and definitive therapy by incision or excision of diseased elements, repair of injury, or reconstruction of defective structures. The preeminent professional and financial position of surgeons appears to derive from the fact that their skills provided definitive therapy during eras when medical management was largely palliative.

Application of sound and scientific evaluations has produced some surprising results. Controlled clinical trials and program evaluations have elicited data and doubts about the outcome benefits and cost/effectiveness of indiscriminate use of many treatments mentioned above (i.e., tonsillectomies, coronary care units, coronary bypass operations and insulin in adult diabetes). There is obviously need for critical evaluation of many more therapeutic modalities.

VALUE ADDED BY SUPPORTIVE AND SYMPTOMATIC MANAGEMENT

The natural recuperative powers of the patient may be favorably influenced by supportive measures such as nutritional, environmental, and physical factors, without directly affecting the course of illness. Similarly, symptomatic relief may be all that a physician can provide in the absence of more directly effective treatments. These measures are obviously useful and highly valued by patients and physicians alike. However, the value-added by these management mechanisms is of a different order of magnitude when contrasted with more definitive therapies (see also Fig. 5-4). Health professionals have little to offer beyond symptomatic management for a very large proportion of many mild and serious illnesses (i.e., colds, "flu," arthritis, hepatitis, etc.). Such ailments greatly outnumber the more significant and serious ailments.

VALUE ADDED BY DIAGNOSIS WITHOUT EFFECTIVE THERAPY

The impact of technology on medicine has provided diagnostic capability far in excess of the therapeutic accomplishments, as indicated in Chapter 5. For this reason, diagnostic efforts are commonly exerted at great expense for the detailed identification and definition of conditions for which effective therapy has not yet been developed. It is a long medical tradition that diagnosis is a part of therapy. The advent of more "scientific" medicine has added impetus toward the liberal utilization of diagnostic technologies for untreatable ailments. A vivid example is presented by the computerized axial tomography (CAT scanners), which can provide impressive and interesting cross-sectional views of the brain, thorax, or abdomen. These devices have not displaced traditional diagnostic tests, and their contribution to the outcome of therapy remains controversial and largely unexplored. Similarly, physicians are prone to order extensive testing repeatedly under conditions in which there is no anticipated therapeutic result (i.e., infectious hepatitis). The "value added" by such relatively fruitless pursuits has rarely been considered. Similarly, the "value added" by periodic health appraisals on patients without signs or symptoms is increasingly being questioned on scientific grounds, even while it is being widely recommended by many in the health professions.

VALUE ADDED BY "DOING SOMETHING": THE PLACEBO EFFECT

The benefits derived from the actions of physicians when caring for patients extends beyond the direct effects of their attentions because of the well-known "placebo" effect. Patients from earliest times have "felt better" as a result of even the simplest ministration of physicians such as the "laying on of hands." Symptomatic relief is often obtained from prescriptions known to be without pharmacological effect. In recent times, more scientific evaluation has demonstrated that completely inert substances administered with assurance that they will reduce pain have demonstrated reduction in susceptibility to organic pain, including that from conditions like cancer (19,20). The positive effects of placebos are now recognized despite the recognition of their psychological origins. The placebo effect has greatly enhanced the effectiveness of physicians' treatments but has greatly complicated the problem of scientifically assessing the "value-added" of various forms of therapy. This single factor has undoubtedly been responsible for the persistent use of manifestly useless treatments—typified by the peculiar sequence of surgical approaches to coronary insufficiency described in Chapter 4.

The inexplicable power of placebos exceeds any rational explanation in common practice. Only recently has the effectiveness of these quasi-medications been demonstrated convincingly by controlled experiments. Beecher (19) was intrigued with the remarkable effectiveness of placebos in treating postoperative wound pain, and was impelled to explore reports from other investigators. Included were well-conceived studies demonstrating relief of discomfort from angina pectoris, headaches, seasickness, anxiety, and tension. More specifically, severe pain after surgery was relieved by morphine in 52% of the cases, while placebos were found to be effective in 40% of the cases. "Less easily open to challenge, however, are the following data: The average effectiveness of placebos in relieving pathological pain is

35%, whereas the average effectiveness of placebos with experimentally contrived pain is only 3.2%. In other words, the placebo is *ten times* more effective in relieving pain of pathological origin than it is in relieving pain of experimentally contrived origin" (19).

A sensitive discussion of the doctor's dilemma in dealing with the use of placebos was presented by Norman Cousins (20). Virtually all physicians use placebo action for a wide assortment of conditions, including Parkinsonism, mental depression, allergies, arthritis, morphine addiction, and many others. They necessarily are faced with a fundamental dilemma of medical ethics. A placebo has little or no effect if the patient is aware that it is not pharmacologically active. Therefore, the physician must either deceive his patient or withhold a potential source of relief. Cousins (20) recounted a fascinating anecdote about a visit to the African Hospital of Dr. Albert Schweitzer, who said: "Some of my steadiest customers are referred to me by witch doctors. Don't expect me to be too critical of them. . . . The witch doctor succeeds for the same reason that all the rest of us succeed. Each patient carries his own doctor inside him. We are at our best when we give the doctor who resides within each patient a chance to go to work."

Now that the effectiveness of prescriptions as placebos is generally recognized, it is even more obvious that the drama and mysteries surrounding the surgical operation can serve as extremely potent placebos, leading to a very large proportion of people undergoing operations for relief of pain to report favorable responses and significant relief. A notable example was Preston's (21) assessment of the potential contribution of the placebo effect among persons having coronary bypass operations for angina pectoris (see also Chapter 5). Favorable results from coronary bypass surgery are known to persist in patients in whom the bypass channel can be demonstrated to have closed.

The need for carefully designed and judiciously analyzed experiments in the evaluation of outcome from therapy is due in large measure to the fact that virtually anything a physician does for the benefit of patients elicits varying degrees of satisfaction and relief, even when there is no scientific basis for it. Thus, extreme care must be utilized to randomize both control and experimental groups of subjects, administer placebos as needed, and take precautions to avoid spurious positive results which have no basis in pathophysiological terms. For this reason, double blind studies have become recognized as essential for most types of clinical program evaluation.

EVALUATING EFFECTIVENESS: CLINICAL TRIALS

The need for large-scale multicenter clinical trials has been recognized in NIH for many years as an indispensable method for assessing the efficacy and applicability of innovations stemming from the research and development effort. The National Heart, Lung, Blood Institute has mounted an extensive program of clinical trials, beginning in 1972 (see also Chapter 2).

The quality of these assessments has been gradually improved through past failures, careful accumulation, and critical analysis of data, taking into account the various obstacles to successful program evaluations. The magnitude and scope of evaluation efforts are indicated by allocation of about one-eighth of the total research budget of the NHLBI to clinical trials (22). This investment is even greater than that figure suggests, since a large proportion of research funds are committed to ongoing programs. The targets for evaluations and the relative funding for some of them is indicated in Table 6-3 as of the year 1976.

Coronary artery surgery is a dramatic technology that has swept the nation without adequate evaluation as to its efficacy. Alleviation of the pain of angina pectoris occurs in a very large proportion of patients, but controversy persists regarding the placebo effect mentioned in the preceding section. The extent to which the function of the heart is affected by the operation remains conjectural. A large-scale study has been organized with cooperation of 16 selected clinical centers beginning in 1973 with funding totaling over $5 million as of 1976 (23). The results of this study have not been fully analyzed and released at this writing.

Other large-scale clinical trials have been directed at such diverse therapeutic interventions as the use of aspirin in patients who have had at least one antecedent myocardial infarction. A $40 million study is directed at consequences of a hypertension detection, therapy, and followup program. The effectiveness of risk reduction is being explored by monitoring mortality and morbidity as affected by avoidance of smoking and fatty diets, or lowering of blood pressure (Table 6-3).

The administration of steroids before delivery is being studied as a means of avoiding respiratory distress syndrome in newborn infants beginning in 1976. Two clinical trials have been conducted on blood diseases, namely hemophilia and sickle cell anemia. A list of additional clinical trial topics that are being introduced includes the effectiveness of devices (such as membrane oxygenators and intermittent pressure breathing equipment), therapeutic administrations (oxygen and propanalol), and further studies on control of hypertension.

This list represents a huge commitment of funds but does not reveal any inherent rationale or consistent criteria which have been utilized to select the targets for these massive clinical efforts. It is not selfevident that hypertension is such an overwhelming and overriding consideration that it warrants three huge evaluations—particularly when the last one is directed toward the treatment of "mild" hypertension. Selection of the target topics appears to be based more on available measures than on rational priorities.

CHOOSING TARGETS FOR PROGRAM EVALUATION

Program evaluation is an exceedingly complex issue that defies simplistic solutions. The process appears more appropriate for use on medical interventions directed toward acute conditions that produce predictable sequences,

TABLE 6-3. Clinical Trials Supported by the National Heart Lung Blood Institute[a]

Title	No. of Centers	Initiated	Funding to 1976	Objectives
Coronary artery surgery trial	16	1975	$ 5,050,040	Efficacy of bypass surgery
Aspirin-myocardial infarction study	30	1975	7,529,658	Effect of aspirin on subsequent MI
Hypertension detection and follow-up program	14	1971	40,605,227	Effectiveness of anti-hypertension therapy on mortality and morbidity
Multiple risk factor intervention trial	20	1972	52,750,854	Effectiveness of risk-reduction (i.e., blood pressure, smoking, lipids)
Prevention of neonatal respiratory distress	5	1976	134,355	Antenatal administration steroids
Hemophilia and its relation to Factor VIII inhibitors	11	1975	1,274,397	Relation of inhibitor to course of disease
Sickle cell screening clinics	22	1972	13,967,693	Clinics for testing methods of service.

Additional Clinical Trial Topics[b]

Extracorporeal Membrane Oxygenator Study. To examination, indications, use, and efficacy in patients with respiratory failures

NHLBI Veterans Administration Clinical Trial in Mild Hypertension. To determine if treatment of mild hypertension reduces the incidence of heart attack

Nocturnal Oxygen Therapy Trial. A six-center study of efficacy of nocturnal low flow oxygen therapy in patients with chronic lung diseases

Effects of antiarrhythmic drug (propranolol) on sudden cardiac death and total mortality in patients recovering from acute myocardial infarction

Techniques designed to protect ischemic myocardium associated with acute myocardial infarction

Effects of long term, intermittent positive pressure breathing (IPPB) as an adjunct to overall care of chronic obstructive lung disease.

[a]Fact Book for Fiscal year 1976. National Heart Lung Blood Institute DHEW Publ. No. (NIH)77–1172.

[b]Fourth Report of the Director of National Heart Lung and Blood Institute March 1, 1977. DHEW Pub. No. (NIH) 77–1170.

because the effects of treatment and overall outcome could be more directly discerned. The greatest single deterrent to unequivocal evaluations is the general lack of outcome criteria for so many of the diagnostic and therapeutic methods in practice. The total number of techniques and technologies that clearly deserve critical analysis of efficacy is truly enormous, since it could include a large proportion of all of the procedures in current practice. It would seem presumptuous to recommend specific criteria for setting priority for the vast spectrum of health technologies. However, there are some considerations that appear to deserve more attention than has been awarded in the past.

FIRST, DO NO HARM!

A pervasive attitude among physicians is to always suspect illness and to proceed on the basis that it is "better to be safe than sorry." Another common tendency is to "do something," as indicated above. Both of these impelling forces need to be tempered by the time honored injunction that the prime responsibility is to *avoid doing harm* (24). When confronted by patients with either symptoms or concerns about health, physicians have powerful incentives to apply all diagnostic or therapeutic modalities that seem appropriate. The possibility that such steps involve varying degrees of risk to the patient is undoubtedly considered as one of the factors in making choices. However, past experience has clearly demonstrated what devastating results can accrue from conscientious efforts of physicians to provide the best and most modern methods for the benefit of their patients. A few examples will suffice to illustrate the point.

Retrolental Fibroplasia. It is generally recognized that virtually any substance found in nature can be deleterious to health if taken in excess. This general rule applies to food, water, and even the air we breathe. In the early 1940s, a form of blindness arose abruptly among infants, particularly among those born prematurely. The loss of vision was due to opacities developing just behind the lens (25), and so the condition became known as retrolental fibroplasia. The disease was found to be widespread as soon as the initial descriptions and name became familiar to physicians. It was widely believed that the condition was congenital, despite some observations that it occurred in babies whose eyes were normal at birth. The proliferation of scar tissue was ascribed to more than 50 separate causes. About half of them were investigated; only four were tested by prospective experimental clinical trials. One of the treatments widely employed was ACTH, but with mixed and confusing results. A clinical trial was conducted, and about 30% of the infants became blind after receiving ACTH and only 20% of the infants in the control group developed the condition.

After 10 years and observations on hundreds of tragic cases, attention became focused on the oxygen-enriched atmosphere routinely provided for premature babies. A hotly contested debate evolved regarding whether the cause of blindness was too much oxygen or too little. Early in 1953, the oxygen issue was discussed at NIH and a majority of participants urged the development of a controlled study. A minority argued that there was sufficient data to indict oxygen and that a clinical trial would be unethical. A study was conducted on 800 premature infants (each weighing less than 1.5 kilograms). The results were conclusive in that 23% of infants in the routine-oxygen group developed retrolental fibroplasia in contrast to only 7% of the group receiving oxygen in lower concentrations (<50%). Now, more than 20 years later, crucial questions persist. There is evidence that infants receiving oxygen have lower incidence of both hyaline membrane disease and spastic diplegia (paralysis of the lower limbs) (25). Estimates suggest that the curtailing of oxygen to avoid retrolental fibroplasia may be responsible for increasing the death rate in infants by about 700 per year. Such a vivid and frustrating experience serves to emphasize the hidden and enigmatic risks that are taken daily by the prescription of drugs and other substances on the basis of incomplete knowledge with best intentions of contributing to the health of patients.

Adverse Drug Reactions. Among the most serious problems associated with the increasing numbers of drugs in contemporary medical practice is the problem of adverse drug reactions (26). The word Thalidomide immediately calls to mind the dreadful deformities in babies born after this apparently innocuous sedative was employed in early stages of pregnancy. Thirty years ago diethystilbesterol (DES) was commonly prescribed as a means of reducing the tendency toward spontaneous abortions. Years later, the drug was found to be associated with the production of precancerous transformations in cervical cells of the offspring. The National Library of Medicine prepared a bibliography of 80 citations from the years 1970 to 1974 on this subject. Some other examples include the development of thromboembolic diseases in peripheral blood vessels from the administration of estrogen, serum hepatitis from vaccines made from human sera, and scores of others (26).

Patient sensitivity to different drugs is difficult enough to predict or detect, but growing numbers of people are simultaneously consuming many pharmaceutical preparations. Self-medication is also extremely common, with a choice of over 100,000 nonprescription drug products available over the counter. The overwhelming magnitude of the risks of "therapeutic" drugs was summarized by Rabin and Bush (27) to the effect that as many as 20% of patients in five university medical services experienced iatrogenic complications of which over 50% were classified as drug reactions. Many of these were relatively mild, but some can be fatal. Engaging in multiple-drug therapy can place some 7 or 8% of recipients at risk. There is urgent need for much more definitive knowledge regarding the magnitude and extent of risk from various individual and combinations of drugs. As a threat to life and health in this country, the much publicized risk from smoking and fatty diets seems out of proportion to the rampant dangers of drug overuse (both prescription and nonprescription). An important example is the widespread use of tranquilizers and mood-altering drugs to which many individuals have been habituated and dependent. They may interfere with ability to cope with the very problems for which the medication was originally administered. There is clear and certain need for improved surveillance of drug usage by a wide variety of approaches including spontaneous or required reporting by physicians, case-control studies, multipurpose data systems, and specially mounted ad hoc clinical trials. The dangers of drug reactions can be diminished by routine computer checks of possible drug interactions by means of computer terminals in pharmacies. A successful prototype of such a mechanism is being used routinely in Group Health Cooperative of Puget Sound, which serves 250,000 members. There is need for two data sets at least (1) information on drug use (i.e., through pharmacy records) and (2) data on incidents of significant drug reactions attributable to pharmaceutical agents. This area of concern seems appropriate as an addition to the present programs of the various departments of health at state, county, and city levels (see the section on departments of health, below).

Dangers from Diagnosis. It is commonly assumed that the diagnostic process is innocuous. While most diagnostic procedures are designed to be without risk to the patient, some carry the potential of having complications. A notable example is the recent flurry of concern about roentgenographic screening for breast cancer. A critical evaluation of mammography led to the conclusion: "There seems to be a possibility that the routine use of mammography in screening asymptomatic women may eventually take almost as many lives as it saves." (28). The radiation exposure could theoretically induce about as many breast cancers as would be discovered through the screening process.

Recognition of the radiation hazard of mammography led to a major technology assessment of the sort indicated as needed in the preceding chapter (29). The data collected in four studies initiated by the Cancer Institute were reviewed by a multidimensional panel along with the opinions of dozens of witnesses. The technical "consensus" pointed to the advantages of continuing mammography among high risk women (i.e., over 55) and discontinuing the practice in favor of other alternatives (i.e., self-examination, etc.) among younger women. Although most other forms of diagnostic tests impose little hazard, there is need to weigh the potential value against even slight risk in such procedures as cardiac catheterization, angiocardiography, and other situations calling for invasion of the body or rapid injection of test materials.

There are fundamental issues at stake in evaluating exposure to diagnostic radiation. There is general agreement that the ionizing radiation has cumulative effects with respect to both the recipient and genetic effects on future generations. Furthermore, there are many potential sources of radiation in addition to diagnostic x-ray studies. Measurable quantities of radiation can be emitted by television sets, nuclear power plants, and cosmic rays (30). A balance is badly needed between overreaction and complacency in arriving at rational approaches to these potential health hazards. There is appreciable danger that the nation might enter an era of irrational phobias. The massive propaganda in the multi-media regarding cancer, heart disease, stroke, hypertension, diabetes, and a host of other diseases cannot help but adversely affect the perceived health status of otherwise healthy citizens. Very little consideration has been given to the deleterious effects of "cancer-phobia" on both the psychological stability of people and the economic health of the country as a growing number of substances are being pronounced as carcinogenic and forcibly withdrawn from products on the basis of data that sometimes appear flimsy.

"Doing something" diagnostically may provide substantial relief for patients from placebo effect, but "saying something" thoughtlessly can have the reverse effect of inducing or accentuating problems or symptoms. The discovery of an "innocent heart murmur" can produce varying degrees of cardiac crippling. When patients become aware that diagnostic test results are beyond the limits of normal, undesirable psychological effects may occur.

Surplus Surgery. Although no one doubts the enormous contributions that have been made by surgeons in removing, repairing, reconstructing, and replacing diseased or deficient organs, unnecessary surgery must be regarded, by definition, as an unwarranted assault, even if the patient "feels better" as a result. There are few effective mechanisms for assaying the extent to which unnecessary surgery is being conducted. Comparisons of surgery in different geographic regions or different populations have disclosed disturbing variability. In general, surgery is used more frequently when surgeons are numerous, in fee-for-service practice (rather than prepaid), and with ample beds available (31). Monitoring the quality of surgical care by retrospective examination of charts or by panels of specialists can be accomplished, but bias seems inescapable. An alternative approach has involved the assessment of need for operations by having second opinions by board-certified specialists (32). This step revealed surprisingly large proportions of surgical procedures *not* recommended, in the following specialty categories:

General surgery	16.4%	Ear, Nose, Throat	16.3%
Gynecology	31.4%	Ophthalmology	28.2%
Orthopedics	40.3%	Urology	35.8%

These data lend credence to the concept that "a second opinion," particularly before elective surgery, could be a most significant addition to present procedures.

Among the clinical trials being conducted by the National Heart, Lung, Blood Institute (Table 6-3) is a critical evaluation of the coronary artery bypass operation. The variation in the extent to which this type of operation is performed in different geographical locations is indeed startling. In areas in which the physicians' income is not based on fee-for-service, the frequency is only a small fraction of that occurring in an area served by exceedingly enthusiastic surgical teams.

Rates of Coronary Bypass Operations

Sweden, Finland, England	2/100,000 population
Prepaid Plans in U.S. (i.e., Kaiser)	4/100,000
Total U.S.A. Rates	28/100,000

Western Washington State*	45/100,000
Eastern Washington State*	90/100,000
Spokane (a city in Eastern Washington)*	116/100,000

*From Guidelines for Heart Surgery Programs, Washington State Medical Association, May 1977.

The 50-fold difference in these rates clearly indicates a major discrepancy in the criteria for recommending surgery and a need for developing more definitive and effective mechanisms for modulating overly-enthusiastic adoption of surgical practices prior to critical assessment. The number of coronary bypass operations increased from about 2,000 in 1971 to 49,000 in 1975, and probably mor ͻ than 70,000 in 1978. An estimated average cost of $13,000 brings the total cost to more than $1 billion. Clinical evaluation revealed some patients return to work after the operation, but there appears to be inadequate data comparing patients treated medically with those receiving surgery. The greatest benefit from the operation appears to decline five years after surgery, with relation to both symptomatic relief and survival rates. A growing number of patients are undergoing surgery a second time. The most significant aspect of the problem is the need to recognize that coronary bypass surgery is essentially a palliative pseudosolution (see Chapter 5), and is no substitute for ultimately developing definitive therapy for the underlying disease process.

Variations in Postoperative Mortality. Postoperative mortality varies rather widely among different hospitals, as might be expected on the basis of differences in size, specialization, support services, and other factors. A particularly interesting set of data emerged as a byproduct of a study on the possible complications from Halothane anesthesia. These data disclosed rather large (seven-fold) differences in postoperative mortality among the various participating hospitals, which had been selected for this cooperative study. Subsequent evaluation indicated that differences in age and other factors in the "patient mix" might account for much of the difference (34). However, two overlapping studies disclosed residual differences of significant magnitude among the hospitals examined. If gross differences in mortality and morbidity occur from the same procedure in different hospitals, corrective action seems warranted. For this purpose there is unquestioned need for a substantial increase in the quantity and quality of information obtained routinely from the many readily available sources in terms of the outcome of therapy. If physicians can be required to report contagious diseases, routine institutional reporting and monitoring could also be required to discover substandard quality of care so that remedial actions might be taken more promptly and effectively.

Early Warning Systems. A guidance system has been proposed by Rutstein (35), based on early warning signals that the system was not functioning up to standard. Even individual instances of readily preventable diseases (i.e., diphtheria, plague, etc.) could serve as indicators that available mechanisms have not been adequately utilized. "The disability rate from paralytic poliomyelitis, bone rickets, or from occupational diseases such as silicosis should be zero" (35).

Sentinel Health Events. The occurrence of preventable or unnecessary disease, disability, or untimely death can serve as indexes of the quality of health care. There are certain ailments which should never occur so that the appearance of a single instance is sufficient to warrant a probe or inquiry. Rutstein and a working group on preventable diseases (36) assembled such a list containing some 100 specific ailments that could serve such a role (Table 6-4). Alternatively, an observed increase in the prevalence of some other diseases or disabilities could be used to stimulate a controlled scientific search for remediable underlying causes. A similar approach was successful in illuminating and correcting causes of the maternal mortality elicited by studies by the New York Academy of Medicine in the 1930s. The general principle is similar to the comprehensive examinations of the sites of aircraft accidents by highly qualified teams to find, and thereby avoid, preventable causes. Some selected samples from such a list are presented in Table 6-4 to indicate the kinds of conditions that might be used for the purpose. Such an approach may be regarded as negative (i.e., looking for medical failures or deficiencies). The advantage lies in the fact that the signal events are quite rare and therefore avoid the need for widespread and comprehensive evaluations of a very large number of highly successful cases to find an occasional defect in the quality of health services. Mechanisms for monitoring health care performance already exist. For example, the role of departments of health across the country could be expanded to include collection, analysis, and channeling of data selected as guidelines and early warning indicators to provide an ongoing weathervane of the health care delivery services being rendered in various localities.

Dangers of Immunization. Immunization against contagious diseases represents the most cost/effective and desirable method of preventing diseases. Every effort is exerted to determine that the vaccines employed are both safe and effective. The need for such caution is implicit in the basic concept of developing immunity in large populations by administering microorganisms believed incapable of producing the typical disease. Despite conscientious efforts to avoid undesirable complications, tragic consequences can occur. An extreme example was the massive immunization against a phantom epidemic of swine flu. The development of a rare and unexpected form of paralysis has resulted in more than 1,000 claims, totaling $1.5 billion, against the government and more are expected. Even if the government were to win every case and pay no reparations, the cost of litigation alone would mount to some $25 million. The ultimate consequences of this ill-conceived program are even greater, because it undermined the public confidence in mass immunization programs which have a long history of great efficacy and safety. As a result, it is safe to predict that thousands of children will be susceptible to preventable infections because they have not been fully immunized against poliomyelitis, diphtheria, tetanus, and a variety of other important and preventable diseases.

TABLE 6-4.

Single Case Indexes[a]		Indexes Based on Rates[b]
Cholera	Neoplasms of Lip,	Dysentary, bacillary
Typhoid fever	mouth, skin, cervix,	Food poisoning, bacterial
Salmonella inf.	eye, bladder, thyroid	Hepatitis, infectious
Botulism	Goitre	Hepatitis, serum
Tuberculosis	Cretinism	Malaria
Silicotuberculosis	Myxedema	Malignant neoplasms of colon, rectum, and vagina
Plague	Avitaminosis	Hodgkin disease
Tularemia	Nutritional deficiences	Leukemia, lymphatic
Anthrax	Gout	Diabetes
Rat-bite fever	Hypervitaminosis	Hemophilia
Diphtheria	Anemias	Epilepsy
Whooping cough	Blindness, glaucoma	Hypertensive disease
Strep throat	Otitis media	Cerebral Vascular disease
Scarlet fever	Pneumoconioses	Dental caries
Poliomyelitis	Osteomyelitis	Ulcer, stomach, or duodenum
Smallpox	Rh Complications	Congenital anomalies of heart and great vessels
Measles	Maternal deaths	Mental Retardation associated with cerebral palsy
Rubella	Mental retardation	metabolic disorders such as phenyl-
Yellow fever	nutritional	ketonuria and aminoacidurias
	rubella	neonatal sepsis
Psittacosis	Rh	toxoplasmosis
Typhus	Tay Sachs disease	
Spotted Fevers	Environmental and occupational hazards	Accidental poisoning
Congenital syphilis		Surgical complications
Acquired syphilis		Medical complications
Gonorrhea		Nosocomial infections
Yaws		Iatrogenic disease
Trichinosis	Surgical operation rates	Surgical operate rates
Hookworm		Tonsillectomy
		Appendectomy
Ascariasis		Hysterectomy

[a] Examples of unnecessary Disease, Disability, or Untimely Death.
[b] Examples of unnecessary Disease, Disability, or Untimely Death.

APPROPRIATE UTILIZATION OF
AVAILABLE TECHNOLOGIES

The enormous progress in preventing epidemics of contagious diseases is being increasingly threatened by growing apathy on the part of the general public. In many areas of the country, large proportions of children are not receiving adequate immunization against important and potentially devastating diseases. At least three explanations can be proposed: (1) Many of the diseases have become quite rare in the experience of the individual and no longer seem so threatening. (2) "If other children are immunized, then mine will not be exposed." (3) Growing concerns about the hazards of immunization (i.e., from the swine flu experience). These trends persist despite powerful arguments in favor of intensive immunization on the basis of humanitarian, social, and even economic grounds.

There is little excuse for the impending poliomyelitis epidemic that is almost sure to occur if present trends continue. The tragedies that will result could be prevented and the costs of the program are trivial in relation to the losses avoided by preventing this dread disease.

Estimated Financial Gains from Polio Immunization (37)

Estimates	*Millions of Dollars*
Loss avoided	$ 326.8
Medical care costs	6,389.7
Gross lifetime income lost	$6,716.5
Costs of avoidance	
Vaccine purchase	$ 128.9
Physician fees	468.6
Vaccine administration costs	13.3
Government funded research and trials	41.3
	$ 653.0

These estimates indicate that a net return of more than $6 billion on investment has been attained by preventing paralytic poliomyelitis during the period 1955–1961 in the United States alone. Similar evaluations would provide equally convincing evidence of the cost/effectiveness and cost/benefit derived from the eradication or control of smallpox, cholera, bubonic plague, and so forth. However, there is disturbing evidence of an increasing incidence of mumps, measles, and even diphtheria, for which effective immunization is widely available. Furthermore, the unnecessary tragedies of congenitally deficient or deformed infants from measles occurring in pregnant mothers defy computation or economic equivalents. The epidemic of gonorrhea which is rampant among the youth of the nation may be a reflection of altered moral values. However, the growing evidence of organisms resistant to effective antibiotics is an overt example of irresponsible overuse by physicians of some of the most effective remedies available. Future generations are likely to suffer from the reckless and unrestrained prescription of antibiotics for conditions which do not respond to these drugs or do not warrant such a profligate use of them.

EMERGENCY CARE OF THE INJURED

Accidental injuries and trauma from violence represent the most common cause of death and disability between the ages 1 and 35 years. We have failed to fully utilize our most highly developed technologies (communication and transportation). In general, emergency clinics, ambulances, communication networks, facilities, and services are notably deficient among the various components of health care delivery mechanisms. Despite the diversity and intensity of the problems encountered in emergency rooms, there are very few physicians trained and certified in this unique type of general practice. Significant strides have been made in the past few years in the training of emergency technicians rendered highly mobile by emergency vehicles. However, few communities in the nation even remotely approach the effectiveness with which injuries have been successfully managed at or near battlefronts. The mortality from battle casualties have declined since the Crimean War (16.7%), World War I (8.2%), World War II (4.5%), and Viet Nam War (1%), reflecting the availability of improved methods for rapid evacuation and emergency care (38). In one operational experiment, helicopters were reserved and hospital units maintained in state of readiness for immediate care of the wounded. The mortality was reduced to 0.368 or 5 deaths from 1,368 casualties. The average time interval between injury and arrival at the operating table was between 15 and 20 minutes with minimal times of 7.5 to 10 minutes for the most seriously wounded. This kind of system is extremely expensive and probably not economically feasible on a universal scale. However, remarkably little effort has been expended toward approaching such capabilities as nearly as possible on the home front.

ASSURANCE OF EFFICACY

A major discrepancy between the soaring costs of health care and tangible benefits in terms of health of the public (see Fig. 5-8) has elicited questions regarding the efficacy of the increasingly sophisticated technologies being widely used across the country.

Coronary Care Units. Coronary care units have been installed in hospitals, large and small, to meet demands by patients, physicians, and community pride. In this country, a patient with an acute myocardial infarction who was unable to gain admittance to a well equipped coronary care unit could feel deprived and threatened. As a result, coronary care units have multiplied rapidly all over the country. Specifically, a carefully considered health plan for Massachusetts determined that the people would be better served by 39 coronary care units with 336 beds as contrasted with the 94 units—446 beds—actually in use. This smaller number could still provide 95% chance of having a bed within a traveling distance of 30 minutes. It was anticipated that the fewer units would provide a higher quality of care by reducing the number with patient flows below the number required to maintain proficiency (39).

A randomized clinical trial to test coronary care using a control group would require considerable courage and conviction. However, such tests have been conducted in Britain with unexpected results (40). A cooperative study of 1,203 episodes of acute myocardial infarction was conducted to compare the outcome of treatment at home as compared with intensive care in a hospital of a randomly selected group. There was some bias introduced by the fact that a slightly larger number of patients with low blood pressure was sent to hospital. Cochrane (11) felt impelled to make a few significant points. First, he was convinced that effective randomization had been achieved in the study. He proposed the simple hypothesis that some people become so intensely frightened in the CCU that their susceptibility to cardiac arrest is increased over the more familiar and reassuring environment at home. Even more important, the results of this evaluation of "accepted" therapy illustrate the importance and value of continuing such carefully designed explorations in this and other important areas.

AVOIDING UNNECESSARY EXTRAVAGANCE

The expanded arrays of clinical laboratory equipment have greatly increased the sources of diagnostic data available to the average physician (see Figs. 5-2 and 5-3). The number of different biochemical determinations in typical laboratories in large hospitals doubled every five years from 1946 and now reach levels of several hundred different options (41). Automation of chemical determinations provides multiple test results from single small samples at significantly reduced unit costs. However, the greatly increased utilization of these tests has substantially escalated the cost per patient per day. The ideal clinical test would unequivocally identify a certain disease and indicate its severity from a single quantitative determination. Very few disease states can be recognized with this degree of specificity. Instead, most conditions are recognized on the basis of patterns of signs, symptoms, and laboratory data. "For many illnesses, indirect tests are performed because we simply have not discovered what to measure." (42). As a consequence of this and other factors, most laboratory services are grossly overutilized in this country and in many others. Some of the reasons for such excesses can be readily appreciated.

Unnecessary Use or Repetition of Tests. Clinicians may fail to ask themselves whether each of the tests they are ordering will contribute to the management of that particular patient. Multiple tests are often used when one would do, or a more pertinent one is needed. Retesting is a very standard practice, and often becomes almost automatic. If clinicians were occasionally asked what the second and third repetitions have contributed, they might find it difficult to justify their actions. The origins of such profligate usage are not hard to find. Impressionable young medical students are exposed to exorbitant uses of laboratory tests during their medical training (see also Chapter 7). One study of a teaching hospital disclosed patterns of laboratory tests bearing little relation to the needs of the patients for optimal care. The data suggest that followup laboratory studies are excessive. From an average 14-day hospitalization, the average patient received 69 tests at a cost of $469, roughly one quarter of the hospital bill (43). A 17-fold difference was found in the use of laboratory testing among faculty internists caring for a homogeneous population at a university clinic (44). Disclosing the results of this audit to the physicians was followed by a 29.2% decrease in laboratory expenditures.

Diagnostic Radiology. Physicians naturally place high reliance on the roentgenographic images containing information about the size, shape, position, and character of internal organs. Approximately 125 million medical x-ray examinations were made on the United States population in 1970. Obtaining x-ray pictures is rapid, painless, and apparently free of hazard (if one ignores exposure to radiation). Unfortunately, x-ray films are used in such excess as to assume a form of "radiological overkill." (45). For example, a study of 1,500 head examinations in patients who had had some degree of head trauma disclosed 93 skull fractures. However, further study revealed that the detection of fractures failed to influence treatment in most instances. Of the total, 510 examinations were apparently for medicolegal reasons, and revealed only five fractures. To detect fractures by films taken for medicolegal reasons alone would require an investment of $7,500 in films alone. Furthermore, therapy for most patients with skull fractures is limited in both its versatility and effectiveness.

Radiography for screening purposes is expensive. For example, mammography has an expected yield of one to two unsuspected breast cancers per thousand women in the high risk age group. This could amount to $18,000 to $20,000 per detected lesion. Such examinations are not without hazard (see Mammography above).

LABORATORY SCREENING: THE LIMITING FACTORS

The concept of preventive medicine is strong in this country. Many recall the successful use of the chest x-ray film for case finding of tuberculosis in large segments of the population, and its important role in the virtual elimination of this disease. As a consequence of such experiences, the idea of early diagnosis through mass screening retains a high level of popularity. The routine admission testing in hospitals is an example of mass screening which is widely accepted throughout the country. In addition, there is a strong movement toward extending this concept to the screening of large numbers of people in hopes of disclosing previously undetected disease so that early treatment could be instituted. Economic and practical considerations implied by large-scale screening programs are rarely considered in detail. The tests must be simple, precise, relevant, sensitive, specific, and have predictive value.

It is equally important that these tests accomplish the purposes for which they are used. Criteria for assessing the potential value of screening were considered by Sackett (46), who proposed that efforts at early diagnosis should lead to an improvement in end results, as defined in terms of mortality and physical, social, and emotional function.

In addition, health services of sufficient quantity must be available to insure diagnostic confirmation. The long-term beneficial effects must outweigh the long-term detrimental effects of the therapeutic regimen used or the labeling of a person as diseased and/or at high risk (46). Few of the screening procedures which are currently in widespread use can conform to these clearly stated criteria. The progressive increase in the availability of highly sophisticated technologies have encouraged screening of individuals under conditions where the costs are great and the most optimistic estimates of the rewards are meagre at best. A prime example is the periodic health examination.

Periodic Health Appraisal. Regular inspections of machines are a useful process by which the components of mechanical devices can be inspected and defective parts replaced. These advantages are not so applicable to preventive maintenance of the human body because direct inspection and replacement of parts is rarely easy or even possible. The public has been encouraged to see their physician at least once a year for a periodic checkup. This widespread recommendation apparently stems from the successful endeavor by dentists to get their patients to see them twice a year on a similar basis. It is worth noting that both complete examination and direct repairs of carious teeth are generally possible. According to Lewis Thomas:

> Most conspicuous and costly of all are the benefits presumed to derive from 'seeing the doctor.' The regular complete checkup, once a year or more often, has become a cultural habit, and it is only recently that some investigators have suggested cautiously that it probably doesn't do much good. There are very few diseases in which early detection can lead to a significant alteration in the outcome: glaucoma, cervical cancer, and possibly breast cancer are the usually cited examples, but in any event, these do not require the full expensive array of the complete periodic checkup, EKG and all. Nevertheless, the habit has become fixed in our society, and it is a significant item in the total bill for health care (47).

Spitzer and Brown (48) have posed penetrating questions regarding the utility of periodic health examinations and concluded that the list of conditions which conform to reasonable criteria is extremely short (see Table 6-5).

SOURCES OF STANDARDS FOR EVALUATION OF HEALTH CARE

Until fairly recently, the prime sources of information regarding the health of the public have been based on vital statistics, particularly mortality. A sudden surge of interest has been manifest in developing more

TABLE 6-5. Targets for "Appropriate" Pre-Clinical Detection of Disease

Stage in Life	Targets for Selective Screening
The fetus and first year of life	Rh incompatibility Phenylketonurea Congenital dislocation of hip Some congenital heart defects
Preschool age	Hearing abnormalities Amblyopia
Childhood and adolescence	Smoking Congenital heart defects
Adulthood	Smoking Breast cancer Cancer of the cervix Cancer of the colon and rectum Hypertension Bacteriuria in pregnancy
The aged	Hypertension Conditions and states amenable to rehabilitative intervention where the goal is not cure or extension of life but improvement of quality of life

Spitzer, Walter O., and Brown, Bruce P., Unanswered questions about the Periodic Health Exam, Ref. 48, pp. 257-263.

specific and useful information regarding the incidence and prevalence of death, disease, disability, and other health factors among various segments of the population according to age, sex, economic conditions, etc. (see Fig. 3-5). A deluge of data is now flowing from a wide variety of sources into the National Center for Health Statistics for accumulation, analysis, and dissemination.

SOURCES OF HEALTH STATISTICS

The most obvious of the countable criteria available for health statistics is the total number in the population, as derived from census profiles. In the United States, census has been taken every 10 years since 1790. The counting of the citizens extends beyond merely enumerating their numbers, but also includes gathering of information useful for projecting the needs for facilities and services. The profile of populations based on the 1970 census included demographic characteristics, such as age, race, sex, marital status, household composition, and the like. In addition, housing characteristics were explored, and socioeconomic characteristics of the target populations were included with measures such as income, poverty status, educational attainment, participation in the labor force, family stability. In addition to the federal census bureau, many state, regional, and local areas have initiated their own population estimation and projection programs. In fact, some states have a state demographer, usually in the state health department, who can supply population estimates. All these data tend to provide the necessary denominator in the fractions used to describe the prevalence and incidence of diseases as they are encountered in the general population, either locally or on a national scale.

Vital Statistics. Vital statistics are data provided on the records obtained in relation to birth, death, fetal death, marriage, and divorce. Uniformity of vital statistics data throughout the United States has been achieved through the development of standard certificates, the content of which is closely followed by most states. The data collected on the local level are transmitted to the National Center for Health Statistics, either on tapes or microfilm and published in annual volumes entitled *Vital Statistics of the United States* (49). Despite some variability in the procedures in different states, the coding rules and procedures for most items of information are sufficiently uniform to insure relatively comparable data on these issues.

Mortality Data. Analyses of mortality statistics have been an essential source of vital information for disease control for centuries (see Fig. 1-1). Mortality data have served as the most prominent bases for action needed to improve public health in local areas. Death rates are generally regarded as being more reliable than other reportable items, because of several distinct advantages.

· Completeness
· Universality
· Economy
· Availability
· Diversity

Virtually all deaths are reported in this country—to a level of approximately 99%. These data are readily available and economical to use since they are already collected, coded, and tabulated. The simplest measure of mortality is the crude death rate, namely the number of deaths per unit of population in a particular area. However, this information lacks the necessary specificity to suggest needed action. For this reason, specific death rates are computed to render these data more useful. For example, age-specific death rates indicate the number of deaths for each designated age group. In addition, there are sex-specific death rates and cause-specific death rates. Death rates can be rendered even more specific by combinations of such characteristics. However, the more specific the death rate, the more difficult it is to obtain the necessary numbers of cases in the numerator to make the statistics valid. When the data are not adequate in numbers for the various ages and so on, an indirect method of standardization may be used for estimation purposes (50).

Cause-Specific Death Data. Probably the most common vital statistic in use today is the specification of death rates by cause of death (51). For this purpose, an international classification of diseases has been adopted in the United States. Examples of disease-specific death rates are illustrated in other chapters (see Table 4-1). Such data are commonly used for justifying appropriations.

SOURCES OF STATISTICS ON MORBIDITY

Morbidity is defined by the National Center for Health Statistics as a "departure from a state of physical and mental wellbeing, resulting from disease or injury, of which the affected individual is aware" (52).

Disease Registries. The most obvious sources of morbidity data are compilations of reportable diseases available from the various state health departments. These differ from state to state and are usually maintained for communicable epidemic diseases for which reporting is required. The registries are generally detailed and have traditionally focused on such conditions as tuberculosis, venereal disease, and other communicable diseases. They reflect primarily the local health department concerns and may not be useful on a broader scale. Thus, only certain categories of sickness are regularly reported, particularly the infectious diseases. Among the 36 diseases included in morbidity and mortality weekly reports, only 12 can be considered significant in the United States (chicken pox, hepatitis A and B, measles, mumps, German measles, salmonella infections, shigella infections, tuberculosis, syphilis, and gonorrhea). Some 50 additional categories of disease are reported to various state health departments. These include hepatitis, diarrheal disease, rheumatic fever, influenza, strep throat, and measles. There may be other state registries such as those pertaining to diabetes, hypertension, phenylketonurea, sickle cell anemia, and the like. Since reporting of these diseases is not generally mandatory, such registries tend to understate actual prevalence. Clearly, many categories of diseases which are of extreme importance in the United States are not reported. Indeed, there is substantial evidence of extreme under-reporting of significant diseases, particularly those which might be regarded socially sensitive (i.e., venereal disease).

Specific Disease Registries. Certain states, localities, or individual hospitals have developed registries for specific disease categories. Perhaps the most common examples are the cancer registries maintained by some 800 hospitals under an approved cancer control program of the American College of Surgeons. Recent emphasis on local or regional cancer data and subsequent epidemiological analysis has found additional support in the development of 17 cancer centers funded by the National Cancer Institute.

SURVEYS BY THE NATIONAL CENTER FOR HEALTH STATISTICS

The sources of information regarding diseases which do not necessarily terminate fatally have long been recognized as inadequate. Over the past several years, the National Center for Health Statistics has developed important and rich new sources of information regarding the magnitude and distribution of health problems on a nationwide scale.

HEALTH INTERVIEW SURVEY

The National Center for Health Statistics is undergoing a continuous sampling and interviewing of samples of civilian, noninstitutionalized populations in the United States for information on health-related areas (52). The individuals are selected and interviewed according to a carefully designed protocol to render the collected information representative of the nation as a whole. The interviewer obtains descriptive information about members of the household, and then asks questions eliciting data about the occurrences of illnesses, injuries, or physician visits in three time-frames. Current illnesses are explored during the period of two weeks before the interview. A three-month period is probed to identify more chronic conditions. The preceding year is queried to stimulate recall of notable events such as periods of hospitalization, the first occurrence of chronic condition, and the number of bed-days. For each condition, a nonmedical description is obtained. If the condition has resulted in restriction of activities or days of disability, these are tallied. Those conditions which result from an accident or injury are explored as to the nature of the injury and the attending conditions which led to it. The reliability of a respondent's statements and the accuracy of recall have been explored in several studies. The findings indicated that respondents in a health interview tend to report conditions that are important to them— conditions which are costly, severe, or require treatment. The results of these studies are published in Series 10 of *Vital and Health Statistics.* The listing and topical index to the *Vital and Health Statistics* series (1962–1976) encompasses 112 reports presenting a wide variety of information derived from these interviews and analyzed for the purpose of eliciting information of a widely varied sort (53).

National Health Examination Survey. Another source of morbidity data is the Health Examination Survey, which was carried out by the National Center for Health Statistics. For this survey, individuals selected in the sample were examined and tested to provide information unobtainable through an interview. The first cycle of examinations (6,300 adult civilians, 18–79 years of age) was conducted between 1959 and 1962. A second cycle was performed on persons 6–11 years of age between 1963 and 1965, and cycle three was conducted on persons 12–17 years of age between 1966 and 1970. The voluminous data produced by this health examination survey are published in Series 11 of *Vital and Health Statistics* (53). At least 160 reports have evolved from these three cycles of examinations.

Hospital Discharge Survey Report. The records accumulated in hospitals provide far more extensive and comprehensive information about illness but are necessarily restricted to those disabilities severe enough to require hospitalization. Thus, the morbidity profile of the population as a whole does not match that seen in hsopitals. The result of an extensive hospital discharge survey has been reported through 1971 in *Vital and Health Statistics*, series 13. The hospital discharge survey was carried out on a sampling basis on non-federal, short-stay hospitals. About 70% of hospital discharges from these hospitals are accounted for by 6 diagnostic groups:

1. Diseases of the circulatory system—13%
2. Diseases of the digestive system—13%
3. Complications of pregnancy and childbirth—13%
4. Diseases of the respiratory system—11%
5. Diseases of the genito-urinary system—11%
6. Accidents, poisonings, and violence—11%

The National Ambulatory Medical Care Survey. A recent component of the National Health Survey is concentrating on private physicians' offices, which in 1972 accounted for about 82% of all physician visits. The data are collected on a sampling basis from a stratified random sample of office-based physicians in the United States. Morbidity data were collected from two perspectives: (*1*) patients' chief complaints or present problems and (*2*) physicians' diagnosis. Major discrepancies between the prevalence of problems presented to physicians by ambulatory patients have been discussed with relation to the distribution of research resources (Chapter 3), targeted research (Chapter 4), and health technologies (Chapter 5). The implications of common presenting problems are discussed in relation to medical education in the next chapter (Chapter 7).

NEEDS FOR NEW MECHANISMS FOR CLINICAL ASSESSMENT

The foregoing discussion was directed primarily at data acquisition for two distinct purposes: (*1*) for discrete program evaluation and (*2*) for large-scale assessment of health status of populations and their utilization of health services. These are necessary and commendable objectives and deserve continuation and expansion. However, neither approach can be expected to provide crucial answers to the pressing questions that permeate the fields of health.

Clinical trials designed to evaluate the efficacy of coronary bypass operations deserve the high priority prescribed by the NHLBI (see Table 6-3). The costs of such large-scale clinical trials (approximately $1,000 per patient per year) are so large that only a slender selection can be addressed. The targets for such assessments must be identified with great care according to clear and consistent criteria.

The costs of clinical trials are high in part because they tend to be conducted by experts in some of the most prestigious institutions in the country whose participation is obtained by rather generous appropriations of funds. In many instances, the grant or contract pays for elements of the patient care that would normally be covered by the patients' insurance coverage or other sources. The common tendency toward recruiting the most eminent clinicians for such clinical trials gives added weight to the results. They skew the results toward the best that could be expected under idealized conditions and cannot be extrapolated with confidence to the services rendered in all other settings in the country. Clearly, there is also a need for developing techniques of assessing the performance, outcome, and quality of health care as provided by physicians in widely representative conditions. New and innovative approaches are essential, with attention directed toward two considerations:

1. Targets for evaluation must be carefully and consistently given priority by means of rational and consistent criteria to assure most effective return on the large investments.
2. A wide variety of new mechanisms must be developed for conducting program evaluations and technology assessments on the wide variety of targets and situations in which they are employed.

In the limited space available in a publication of this sort, only a few representative examples can be discussed. These must be regarded as specific indications that other alternatives are worth exploration rather than as specific recommendations.

NEW PRODUCTS AND PROCEDURES: NEED FOR ORDERLY INTRODUCTION

Mechanisms for orderly introduction of new products have been developed as an expanded responsibility of the Food and Drug Administration (FDA). A great deal of impatience and criticism of this restraining influence has surfaced. The evident advantages of care and control in evaluating new procedures as well as new products can be suggested by past experience (54). It is enlightening to compare surgical operations for portal hypertension with the more deliberate introduction of artifical hip prostheses (55). The over-enthusiastic introduction of shunts to relieve hypertension in the portal circulation was finally exposed to careful randomized clinical trials (RCTs) only after decades of unbridled use. They disclosed no difference in survival between patients selected at random for medical and for surgical therapy. The incidence of hemorrhages was reduced in the surgical group, but the end result was not significantly different. "As one reviews the disorderly history of the innovation of shunting procedures, it is obvious that decades were wasted by the failure to introduce, standardize, and carry out RCT's from the beginning" (56).

The recent introduction of total hip joint replacements followed a much different course, partly because of peculiar circumstances (55). The basic technique was originally described by Charnley in Manchester in 1961, but failures resulted from excessive wear of a plastic joint surface. Methylmethacrylate was substituted and corrected the deficiency. However, the FDA ruled that this plastic fell under the regulations covering a new drug, including the requirements to present protocols before orthopedic surgeons were permitted to proceed with the new operation. The provision of complete and updated information was regarded as a great nuisance by the surgeons, but provided a continuous flow of very useful data as the procedure became more widely used. The safety and efficacy of the operation were considered to have been established by late 1971 and the total hip replacement was then released by the FDA for general use. From that time onward, national experience with this procedure is unknown for the most part. Despite the natural opposition of physicians to such surveillance and regulation, a case can be constructed for the development of mechanisms by which new procedures and devices can be brought on line in a sequence that protects the patients, physicians, and the general public from complications during spontaneous spread of untested treatments. In the early stages of development, the new procedure should be explored in "feasibility studies" for which independent review would indicate when development had reached a level warranting careful collaborative trials on patients in accordance with rigorous criteria.

The costs of acquiring data for clinical evaluations in current clinical trials are extremely great (i.e., $1,000 per patient per year). Huge amounts of clinical data are routinely collected in the course of regular practice by highly competent physicians which could be rendered much more useful by careful preparation of protocols. These could be rapidly and conveniently filled out by groups of physicians recruited specifically to take advantage of their practice settings and approaches to management of patients. For example, a comparison of the outcome from two different operations or between medical and surgical therapy can be approached without ethical or status problems engaging the cooperation of groups of physicians who have elected to approach specific clinical problems by different methods. A much more comprehensive approach to objective evaluation of the myriad clinical procedures can be obtained by innovative methods of utilizing more of the mountains of patient data being collected every day.

An Institute of Health Care Assessment was proposed by Bunker et al. (55) with a mandate and funding to provide independent evaluation of new and selected older procedures where sufficient uncertainty persists. The function might be delegated to a private agency such as the Institute of Medicine or to a federal agency such as the National Center for Health Services Research. Evaluations could be pursued by designated groups of physician investigators in approved institutions utilizing protocols developed under supervision of such a center to provide valid and relevant data for analysis on a national scale.

Attractive Alternatives as Sites for Evaluations. Special clinical centers were once established by NIH Institutes in medical schools and hospitals for the purpose of engaging in research and development and introducing innovations into practice. Such multidisciplinary groups could engage more actively in the process of evaluation of new and traditional modes of diagnosis and therapy if that responsibility is not now adequately incorporated into the program. Many such groups are not adequately endowed with individuals thoroughly trained in the difficult task of devising protocols and analyzing the resulting data. In such instances the addition of an experienced epidemiologist might increase the validity and relevance of the data being collected in the normal course of studies. Such groups might also be encouraged to make use of protocols and experimental designs which could be developed by NCHSR or NCHS for projects of corresponding nature.

Schools of Public Health. Health services research is most commonly a designated field of teaching and research within Schools of Public Health. The communication and collaboration of such departments with Schools of Medicine (even when geographically nearby) leave much to be desired. Efforts should be directed to devise and to use incentives that would encourage closer cooperation between the faculties engaged in health program evaluation and medical faculties who are daily conducting examinations on a wide spectrum of patients in an environment conducive to critical examination of such issues.

Medical Schools. Although each physician is assumed to be using critical judgment in the selection of procedures and the interpretation of his results, there is very little effort to provide the necessary background as part of the medical school curriculum. A closer relationship between the Schools of Public Health and Medicine in planning of curricula could provide a means of inserting material and experience in health services research into both the basic science and clinical years of study. The clinical faculties of most medical schools are steeped in a traditional attitude that their judgment of the effectiveness of therapy is not only adequate but maybe superior to randomized clinical trials. One justification of the attitude is the fact that physicians normally deal with individual patients, and each successive instance of the same disease or disability has unique characteristics known best by the attending physician. Awareness of physicians regarding the importance of random clinical trials deserves greater emphasis. Perhaps the best place to initiate the process is during the years of medical education.

Prepaid Clinical Settings. Resistance to engagement in critical evaluations of clinical processes is a natural reaction among people who derive both professional and financial benefits from them. For this reason, the average physician practicing in fee-for-service settings might not be able to preserve a completely unbiased point of view during health services assessments. Physicians who are practicing in situations where income is divorced from the procedures they employ should experience less bias from this origin. In recent years, the Veterans Administration hospitals have served as important sources of such evaluations. By the same reasoning, highly qualified physicians practicing in prepaid plans or HMOs might be a particularly appropriate means for engagement in such critical evaluations. The administrators of prepaid plans and government funded hospitals have greater inherent incentives to provide highest quality care at most reasonable costs. The need to exercise care and consideration that none of the patients be deprived of necessary therapy must be exercised by all such institutions. Nevertheless, there is ample evidence that physicians in prepaid plans are less likely to refer patients to hospitals than are physicians functioning in fee-for-service. There is little or no incontrovertible evidence that the outcomes are inferior in either one of the two types of institutions. Such differences in style and emphasis in practices appear to provide opportunities to engage in evaluations without violating the ethical problems implied by typical randomized studies. If patients would not receive a certain type of treatment in one setting anyway, a comparison of outcome with another group of patients regularly receiving the treatment might provide valid data by suitable protocols and experimental designs. Under these conditions, the cost of conducting a program evaluation or a technical assessment could be greatly reduced compared to the massive clinical trials currently being conducted. These are undoubtedly issues that require very large and comprehensive evaluations. Useful data can be obtained at much lower costs by applying appropriate protocols to carefully selected situations.

Selected Physicians in Private Practice. During the past decade, widespread experience with randomized clinical trials in this country and abroad has amassed considerable background of experience. A large and growing array of proven approaches can now be identified for application in a variety of clinical settings (56,57). It should be possible to recruit well-trained and dedicated physicians to meticulously follow established protocols of data collection on their patients (58). Selection for such participation could be established as recognition of clinical proficiency and awarded as an honor. In addition, such physicians could be reimbursed for services as consultants and the *added* costs of treating of their patients involved where necessary. With such an approach, numbers and diversity of clinical trials could be greatly expanded at lower unit cost and with the prospects of more rational extrapolation to the rest of the medical community. Such a process would appear to be particularly appropriate for assessing new drugs or procedures before they became established in common practice.

Departments of Health: Expanded Roles. The country is studded with departments of health of various dimensions and scope at state, county, and city levels. The original objectives of these departments was the monitoring of threats to life and health, mainly from communicable diseases and occupational hazards. Most communicable diseases have been brought under control, except for persistent problems such as venereal diseases and resistant organisms. The occupational and environmental hazards have become the responsibility of other agencies as well. Departments of health are generally deployed and prepared for collection of large amounts of health-related data and their personnel is generally trained for that purpose. These organizations appear entirely suitable for a substantial expansion of roles for the purpose of engaging more actively in the process of program evaluation and technology assessment conducted by selected individuals and groups of physicians in accordance with tested protocols and accepted experimental designs of proven utility during the past several years.

SUMMARY

1. The National Center for Health Services Research is a response to recognized need for critically evaluating many and varied procedures, processes, and outcome encountered in health care delivery. The techniques for evaluating the processes and programs and for assessing outcome are a new requirement in the fields of health and are being adapted from approaches employed in other disciplines such as biostatistics, and behavioral and social sciences.

2. The components of program evaluation include cost/benefit and cost/effectiveness assessment, both of which are complicated by third party payments rendering health services "artifically cheap" or apparently free. The benefits derived from health services are difficult to appraise in terms of economic equivalents. However, the potential improvement in health of patients can be considered in terms of the "value added" by (1) prevention, (2) definitive therapy, (3) supportive and symptomatic management, (4) diagnosis without effective therapy, and (5) "doing something" —the placebo effect.

3. Large-scale clinical trials are being conducted as a major new element in the programs of the NIH, particularly the National Heart, Lung, Blood Institute. The techniques and technologies presently undergoing clinical evaluation do not appear to have been selected on the basis of consistent criteria. Among the factors that need to be considered in the selection of targets for critical appraisal are the following: (1) "first, do no harm," (2) appropriate utilization of available technologies, (3) assurance of efficacy, and (4) avoiding unnecessary extravagance.

4. The National Center for Health Statistics is an important resource for the collection, analysis, and interpretation of data collected on a nationwide basis according to sound design and tested protocols to provide information regarding the health status of the public, the utilization of resources, and ultimately to assess the influence of health services on the health and welfare of the American public.

5. Among the sources of important health statistics are (1) national census, (2) mortality data, (3) cause specific mortality and morbidity data, (4) various registries at state and local levels, and (5) extensive surveys conducted by trained field workers of the National Center for Health Statistics.

6. In addition to the wealth of new information being collected through the various agencies of government, there is a pressing need for a wide variety of new and innovative methods for gathering relevant data regarding the various forms of clinical diagnosis and therapy. The number and diversity of processes and procedures used in health care are so vast that there is no prospect of keeping up with the rapid pace of development without devising effective, routine reporting by large numbers of practicing physicians utilizing protocols and incentive systems. Such information could become valuable supplements to the information gathered by the professionals in

the governmental agencies for improved planning and development of health facilities and services.

REFERENCES

1. The Program in Health Services Research. Health Resources Administration, DHEW, Pub No (HRA) 78-3136, October 1976.
2. NCHSR Research Funding Priorities, FY 1979-80, National Center for Health Services Research, 1978.
3. Quality of Medical Care Assessment Using Outcome Measures, National Center for Health Services Research, DHEW Pub No (HRA) 77-3176, August, 1977.
4. Controlling Cost of Health Care. National Center for Health Services Research, DHEW Pub No (HRA) 77-3182, May 1977.
5. Recent Studies in Health Services Research, Vol II, National Center for Health Services Research, DHEW Pub No (HRA) 78-3183, December 1977.
6. Shortell S, Richardson WC: *Health Program Evaluation.* St. Louis, The CV Mosby Company, 1978.
7. Assessing Quality in Health Care: An Evaluation. Report of a Study, Institute of Medicine Publ. No 76-04, Washington, D.C., National Academy of Sciences, November, 1976.
8. Clearinghouse on Health Indexes, Accumulated Annotations, 1976, National Center for Health Statistics, DHEW Pub No (PHS) 78-1225, September 1978.
9. Holland WW. The epidemiologist, in McLachlan G (ed): *Positions, Movements, and Directions in Health Services Research.* Published for the Nuffield Provincial Hospital Trust by Oxford University Press, 1974.
10. Goldman L: *When Doctors Disagree; Controversies in Medicine.* London, Hamish Hamilton, 1973.
11. Cochrane AL: *Effectiveness and Efficiency; Random Reflections on Health Services,* London, The Nuffield Provincial Hospital Trust, 1971.
12. Campbell DT, Stanley JC: *Experimental and Quasi-experimental Designs for Research.* Skokie, Ill, Rand McNally & Co, 1966.
13. Deniston OL: The validity of non-experimental designs for evaluating health services. *Health Serv Rep* 88:153-164, 1973.
14. DeCosta A, Sechrist L: Program evaluation concepts for health administrators, Washington DC, DHEW Bureau of Health Manpower, 1976.
15. Dunlop DW: Benefit-cost analysis; a review of its applicability in policy analysis for delivering health services. *Soc Sci Med* 9:133-139, 1976.
16. Ashford JR: Planning local health services, in McLachlan G (ed): *Framework and Design for Planning; Uses of Information in NHS.* Published for the Nuffield Provincial Hospital Trust by Oxford University Press, 1977.
17. Rushmer RF: *Humanizing Health Care; Alternative Futures for Medicine.* Cambridge, Mass, and London, The MIT Press, 1976.
18. Doll R: Surveillance and monitoring, approaches to epidemiology of health. *Internatl J of Epid* 3:305-314, 1974.
19. Beecher HK: Quantitative effects of drugs on the mind, in Talalay P (ed): *Drugs in Our Society.* Baltimore, the Johns Hopkins Press, 1964.

20. Cousins N: The mysterious placebo; how mind helps medicine work. *Saturday Rev* 5:8-17, October 1, 1977.
21. Preston TA: *Coronary Artery Surgery: A Critical Review.* New York, Raven Press, 1977.
22. Report of the Director, National Heart Lung Blood Institute, DHEW Pub No (NIH) 77-1170, March 1, 1977.
23. Fact Book for Fiscal Year 1976. The National Heart Lung and Blood Institute, DHEW Pub No (NIH) 77-1172, October 1976.
24. Haney CA: *Psychological Factors Involved in Medical Decision-making in Psychological Aspects of Medical Training.* Springfield, Ill, Charles C Thomas, 1971.
25. Silverman WA: The lesson of retrolental fibroplasia. *Scientific American* 236:100-107, 1977.
26. Sartwell PE: Iatrogenic disease; an epidemiologic perspective. *Internatl J of Health Services* 4:8994, 1974.
27. Rabin DL, Bush P: The use of medicines; historical trends and international comparisons. *Internatl J of Health Services* 4:61-87, 1974.
28. Bailar JC: Mammography; a contrary view. *Ann Intern Med* 84:77-84, 1976.
29. Culliton B: Mammography controversy; NIH's entree into evaluating technology. *Science* 198:171-173, 1977.
30. Morgan KZ: Never do harm, in Haven B (ed): *Man, Health, and Environment.* Minneapolis, Burgess Publishing Company, 1972.
31. Bunker J: Surgical manpower, a comparison of operations and surgeons in the United States and in England and Wales. *N Engl J Med* 282:135-144, 1970.
32. McCarthy EG, Widmer GW: Effects of screening by consultants on recommended elective surgical procedures. *N Engl J Med*, 291:1331-1335, 1974.
33. Miller DW: The economics of bypass surgery, in: *The Practice of Coronary Artery Surgery.* New York, Plenum Press, 1977.
34. Staff of the Stanford Center for Health Care Research: Comparison of hospitals with regard to outcomes of surgery. Health Services Research, pp. 10-27, Summer 1976.
35. Rutstein DD: *Blueprint for Medical Care.* Cambridge and London, The MIT Press, 1974.
36. Rutstein DD et al.: Measuring the quality of medical care; a clinical method. *N Engl J Med* 294:582-588, 1976.
37. Melnick V, Melnick D, Fudenberg HH: Participation of biologists in the formulation of national science policy. *Fed Proc* 35:1957-1962, 1976.
38. Weil MH, Shubin H, Boycks EC, et al: A crisis in the delivery of care to the critically ill and injured. *Chest* 62:616-620, 1972.
39. Blood BS, Peterson OL: Patient needs and medical care planning. The coronary care unit as a model. *N Engl J Med* 290:1171-1177, 1974.
40. Mather HG, Peargon NG, Read KQ, et al: Acute myocardial infarction; home and hospital treatment. *Brit Med J* 3:334-338, 1971.
41. Brown JHU, Dickson JF: Instrumentation and the delivery of health services. *Science* 66:334-338, 1969.
42. Kinney TD, Melville RS: Mechanization, automation, and increased effectiveness of the clinical laboratory. Medical Laboratory Sciences Review Committee of the National Institute of General Medical Sciences, DHEW Pub No (NIH) 77-145, 1976 edition.
43. Griner PF, Liptzin B: Use of the laboratory in a teaching hospital; implications for patient care, education, and hospital costs. *Ann Intern Med* 75:157-163, 1971.
44. Schrodder SA, Kenders K, Cooper JK, et al.: Use of laboratory tests and pharmaceuticals; variation among physicians and effect of cost audit on subsequent use. *JAMA* 225:969-973, 1973.

45. McClellan JL: Wasted x-rays. *Penn Med* 72:107-108, 1969.
46. Sackett DL: Laboratory screening; a critique. *Fed Proc* 34:2157-2161, 1975.
47. Thomas L: On the science and technology of medicine, in Knowles J (ed): *Doing Better and Feeling Worse*. New York, WW Norton and Company, 1977.
48. Spitzer WO, Brown BT: Unanswered questions about the periodic health examination. *Ann Intern Med* 83:257-263, 1975.
49. Vital Statistics of the United States, Vols I, II, III, US Department of Health, Education, and Welfare. National Center for Health Statistics, Rockville MD, 1970.
50. Hill AB: *Principles of Medical Statistics*. New York, Oxford University Press, 1966.
51. Mortality Trends for Leading Causes of Deaths; US 1950-69. National Center for Health Statistics DHEW Pub No (HRA) 74-1853, 1974.
52. Health Survey Procedure; concepts, questionnaire development, and definitions in the Health Interview Survey (National Center for Health Statistics, Rockville MD, 1964.)
53. Current Listing and Topical Index to the Vital and Health Statistics Series, 1962-1976, DHEW Pub No (HRA) 77-1301, May 1977.
54. Tukey JW: Some thoughts on clinical trials, especially problems of multiplicity. *Science* 198:679-684, 1977.
55. Bunker JP, Hinkley D, McDermott WV: Surgical innovation and its evaluation. *Science* 200:937-941, 1978.
56. Byar DP, Simon RM, Friedewald WT, et al.: Randomized clinical trials; perspectives on some recent ideas. *N Engl J Med* 295:74, 1976.
57. Peto P, Pike MC, Armitage P, et al: Design and analysis of randomized clinical trials requiring prolonged observation of each patient. Introduction and design. *Brit J Cancer* 34:585, 1977.
58. Frazier HS, Hiatt IIH: Evaluation of medical practices. *Science* 200:875-878, 1978.

Part Four

Attractive Alternatives for the Future

The final three chapters are devoted to ways in which health in the future might be enhanced through improved training of a new mix of health professionals (Chapter 7), increased involvement of the public through increased self-reliance (Chapter 8), and prototypes developed in foreign countries that might be adopted or modified for use in this country (Chapter 9).

Medical education has been greatly affected by the overriding influence of research as a priority goal of medical faculties. A time of transition is approaching which provides a valuable opportunity to consider mechanisms for improving quality and distribution of the major unmet need in this country, namely primary care. The overabundance of certain specialists, defiencies in general practitioners, and deficient preparation of biomedical scientists could be improved by establishing parallel pathways in medical schools with curricula more discretely tailored to the ultimate professional careers of the students. The qualifications of health professionals have been greatly upgraded by more extensive and comprehensive curricula (i.e., for nurses, dentists, pharmacists, optometrists, and many others). The competence of many recent graduates greatly exceeds the level of responsibility generally delegated to them. Many exciting examples across the country bear witness to their competence in providing primary care to patients, particularly in situations where physicians do not choose to practice (remote, rural, and central city areas). Opportunities to introduce medical students to cooperative team functions with other health professionals would also be worth consideration for inclusion in health science education.

A precipitous plunge into a national health insurance program seems ever more imminent. Many countries in Western Europe and elsewhere have approached these problems by a wide variety of mechanisms, tried and modified over many years. Unfortunately, the vast experience and knowledge gained through these extremely costly "feasibility" studies is being largely neglected in America. We could never afford to undertake corresponding investigations here so we would be wise to take maximum benefit from the experiences of others, including both the successes and complications. To this end, certain interesting aspects of biomedical programs in Britain, Sweden, and Canada have been selected for description to give some sense of the potential value of more detailed exploration and evaluation of such programs in search of methods that might prove valuable in the United States.

CHAPTER 7

Professional Pathways:
Evaluation of Education

From earliest times, the training of physicians has been based in large measure on apprenticeship, and vestiges of this orientation are clearly visible today in the clinics and on the wards of teaching hospitals. The clinical faculties of medical schools are predominantly specialists highly trained and focused on discrete topical research areas and clinical responsibilities. The multiplication and dominance of specialties is a natural consequence of accelerated progress in research, rapidly accumulating new knowledge, and increasingly sophisticated technologies (see Chapter 5).

The preeminent position of specialists is visible in medical school curricula, in the administration of medical schools, in the mix of physicians in practice, and in advisory roles in governmental agencies and other institutions. In the United States, the educational processes leading to the M.D. degree are clinically oriented with relatively limited training in experimental methods. Intensive research training is generally attained in pursuit of the Ph.D. degree in basic medical sciences or other academic disciplines. This tradition is at variance with the academic traditions of other countries where intensive training in research is typically superimposed on the medical degree in preparation for academic careers in either basic medical sciences or clinical disciplines. For this reason, clinical specialists in academic and advisory positions in other countries generally have more extensive experience with research concepts, practices, and procedures than obtained on balance in this country. Some implications of these differences are discussed in relation to foreign prototypes (see Chapter 9).

The overwhelming clinical influence of specialists in medical schools is also reflected in the medical community where they outnumber general practitioners by about four to one. Until very recently, many deficiencies of health care delivery had been attributed to a doctor "shortage." As a consequence, medical schools were strongly encouraged to increase enrollment. The output of physicians has approximately doubled in the last 10 years, with correspondingly large proportions of graduates entering the specialties in practice, in academic positions, research, or administrative roles. The fundamental shortage of family practitioners has not been alleviated significantly, but the costs of health care have been soaring.

METAMORPHOSIS OF MEDICAL SCHOOLS

In 1906, the AMA Council on Medical Education reported that, in their view, only half of the 160 medical schools were prepared to teach modern medicine, that 30% were doing a poor job, and the other 20% were unworthy of recognition. Important changes occurred in consequence of the efforts of Flexner, aided by the influence of the Association for American Medical Colleges and the American Medical Association. By 1930, the number of medical schools in America had dropped from 148 to 66 (1) (see also Chapter 1). The gradual improvement in education and the beginning emphasis on medical research during the first half of this century set the stage for the dramatic expansion that followed World War II (2).

The Flexnerian format decreed that medical schools should be organized around certain disciplines (i.e., anatomy, physiology, biochemistry, pathology, medicine, surgery, etc.). These organizational components are readily recognized today. After World War II, research funds became available for support of individual research projects. At first, the medical school faculties were suspicious of these funds, because of justifiable concern that it might lead to federal regulation of an undesirable sort in the long run. However, the attractiveness of having available research funding overcame this reluctance. Research-oriented members of the medical school faculties responded to the obvious advantages of becoming independent entrepreneurs. The NIH policy of leaving the initiative and selection of research topics in the hands of the individual faculty members proved very successful in recruiting a wide diversity of investigators in the various biomedical disciplines. The availability of research grants permitted the purchase of essential equipment, the hiring of laboratory technicians, and the collaboration of colleagues to engage in more and more sophisticated research. In many departments, active members of the faculty became the key figures in empires of diverse size and scope.

Energetic and perceptive faculty members identified their own research interests with the programs of the several granting agencies which had overlapping areas of responsibility (see Chapter 2). Gradually, each medical school department branched into divisions and subdivisions (Fig. 7-1). These branches were generally organ-oriented or disease-oriented, reflecting to varying degrees opportunities provided by federal and voluntary agencies supporting medical research. Through such a process, neurological, cardiovascular, gastrointestinal, genitourinary, metabolic, infectious disease, and

GREENING OF MEDICAL SCHOOLS

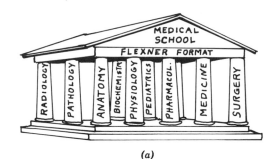

(a)

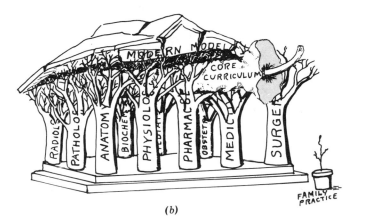

(b)

Figure 7-1. (a) The Flexner report identified specific
academic disciplines that emerged as the traditional departments in an organizational format for medical teaching
and research. (b) Rapid expansion of research, specialization, and empire building by individual faculty members
stimulated growth of many specialties in each department,
represented by intertwining branches. The interdisciplinary
borders became blurred and "core" curricula were developed as means of providing cohesive, organ-oriented approaches to medical school teaching.

cancer components could be readily identified in basic science and clinical
departments in virtually all medical schools. As a result, the areas of interest
within each medical school department became broadly overlapping with
other departments, obscuring the previously distinctive interdisciplinary
borders.

Research grants and programs were obviously attractive to most faculties, since they provided a very high level of autonomy and independence,
enhanced their professional prestige, provided means of going to professional meetings, and engaging competent technical support and colleagues to
enhance their research productivity. The incentives become increasingly

powerful as the criteria for professional advancement and salary increments became progressively oriented toward research productivity. The internal relationships within medical schools became increasingly complex and unmanageable. Medical administration was strained even further by development of large program projects, centers, and institutes sponsored by granting agencies.

DISPERSION OF POWER

Before World War II, the deans and departmental chairmen had substantial influence over their faculties by control of both funding and space. When individual faculty members could develop substantial external support, they became more independent and autonomous. The prospects of bringing substantial sums of money into the departmental activities often prompted the allocation of additional space, which further eroded the control and planning function normally exerted by chairmen and deans. For these reasons, the administrators of medical schools had a very high level of responsibility but greatly diluted authority.

THE INCENTIVE STRUCTURE

Medical schools have always been dedicated to teaching, research, and community service. The prestige endowed by scholarly pursuits of research rapidly supplanted teaching ability as the primary basis for professional advancement. The reward system carried little incentive to engage in teaching, other than the inherent desire on the part of most faculty toward replication of graduates in their own images. Those faculty members whose abilities and interests inclined toward teaching, rather than research, frequently had difficulty getting promoted. Thus, the basic medical scientists tended to be drawn strongly toward research with some tendency to avoid heavy teaching involvement. For most clinical faculty, the priorities were research, clinical service, and teaching, in that order.

COMMON CONCEPTS OF MEDICAL EDUCATION

The teaching functions of medical schools are generally based on a few assumptions, the validity of which are subject to debate.

- Patient care can be regarded as a form of scientific investigation (see Flexner quotation, page 11, Chapter 1).
- Active research is a necessary prerequisite for a scholarly job of teaching.
- Research productivity is the key criterion for academic performance meriting professional advancement.

· Faculty with primary interest in teaching to the neglect of experimental research are not truly scholars in the academic sense.

These perceptions have widespread acceptance to the point that teaching has commonly been relegated to lower level of priority. The rewards for teaching are far less tangible than the fruits of active research. Under these conditions it is a tribute to the dedication of medical faculty that the teaching efforts are as intensive and effective as they appear to be.

Research Training of Physicians. The educational processes of medical schools are strongly oriented toward creating highly competent physicians capable of dealing with the myriad diseases and disabilities by applications of growing spectra of new knowledge and arrays of new and complicated technologies. Despite deep interest and desire to also inculcate concepts of the scientific method, the medical curriculum is too congested to provide much training or experience in rigorous research, even during the prolonged residency periods leading to board certification in the various specialties. Some graduates of these educational programs gravitate into the medical school faculties where they are expected to engage in independent laboratory investigation of the highest quality. (See also the section on Competence and Creativity.)

CORE CURRICULA

As the areas of involvement in the medical school departments became overlapped and intertwined, the boundaries between various disciplines became increasingly obscured. Faculty members often developed bonds of mutual interest with investigators with common interests in organ systems or diseases in other departments. Duplication of teaching efforts became unavoidable. During recent years many different institutions have developed innovative curricula, by which faculty from different departments collaborate in formal courses covering the functions of organ systems or other special areas. Core curricula (see Fig. 7–1) melded the overlapping interests in the branching disciplines for a more effective integration of material for instructional purposes.

The generous support of research by federal government coupled with the financial constraints of medical school budgets, has led to increasing dependence on the federal government for both teaching and research activities. The federal support of teaching functions has been justified on the premise that it is impossible to distinguish between research and teaching. The predictable dependence on outside agencies for funding is now leading to a degree of federal control and interference with the inner workings of medical schools that were feared when NIH first appeared on the horizon. Despite all these factors, the medical schools of this country are universally regarded as being among the finest in the world and in many cases, models for those in other countries.

CAREER OPTIONS FROM COMMON CURRICULA

The roles of physicians in our society have extended far beyond the care of the sick, to encompass a wide variety of career opportunities. The educational processes leading to the M.D. degree opens the door to a remarkable diversity of careers. Although the basic orientation is toward the training of physicians to engage in family practice or medical and surgical specialties, the M.D. degree is also the key to careers in basic medical research, research administration, hospital administration, health planning, and many other opportunities. Until recently, the medical school curriculum was so congested and tightly knit that it resembled a rigid lock-step with very little opportunity for elective options. However, in recent years the development of core curricula has been accompanied by a greatly expanded opportunity for the students to take courses of their choice, more appropriately preparing them for this wide diversity in ultimate careers.

Medical students are entering medicine from a wider variety of university disciplines, including biology, chemistry, and engineering. Furthermore, there is a growing tendency to encourage students to strengthen their premedical experience by including the humanities and social sciences. However, the competition for entrance into medical school is so keen, that many students are reluctant to engage in these perimedical subjects if it appears to threaten their opportunity to compete for places through the admission process (3).

Modern medical schools have been organized to provide the basic background for entering students with diverse educational experiences in preparation for a wide spectrum of professional careers (Fig. 7-2). For example, physicians are engaged in health planning, public health activities, administration of hospitals, and research institutions. Research careers have emerged and expanded in many areas such as basic medical sciences, clinical medicine, laboratory medicine, health services evaluation, and others. All these options have tended to syphon off graduates from schools of medicine whose principal products remain the medical and surgical specialties and general practitioners engaging in family practice.

The information explosion since World War II has been a major factor in the proliferation of specialties of many different types. The deluge of new data coupled with increasingly complex technologies challenges the ability of health professionals to keep fully informed of progress even in relatively restricted areas of medicine or surgery. As a consequence, the clinical faculties of medicine have successively formed into many different specialty groups which have subdivided even further as subspecialties indicated in Figure 7-1. The natural tendency of teachers to proselytize students virtually assures that many graduates will elect specialties. The attractive aspects of specialization include professional prestige, economic advantages, extensive support by personnel, facilities, and technologies, and conditions of practice that are convenient, pleasant, and satisfying.

The organ-oriented medical and surgical specialties focus attention on the structural systems of the body (nervous, cardiovascular, reproductive,

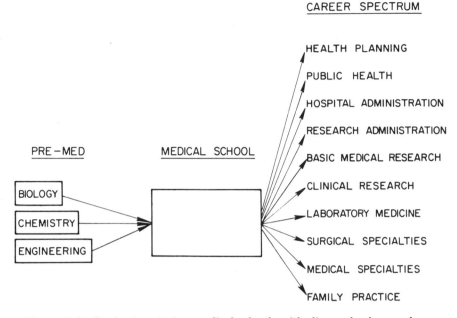

Figure 7-2. Students entering medical schools with diverse backgrounds are nominally prepared to enter a very large selection of professional careers. Clearly, no single curriculum can provide optimal training for such diversity, even with a wide selection of electives. The success of medical school graduates in the many different lines of endeavor is a reflection more of the students' innate ability than the relevance of the educational process.

urinary, musculoskeletal, etc.). There are also disease-oriented divisions or disciplines (infectious, allergic, and neoplastic), as well as age-oriented components (pediatrics, gerontology). In short, the internal components of medical schools display the same kinds of overlapping areas of responsibilities that emerged in NIH (see Table 2-2 and Fig. 2-5).

CLINICAL CURRICULA

Clinical faculties in medical schools are composed almost exclusively of highly specialized physicians whose research interests tend to converge attention on unusual ailments, of particular interest for research and teaching. As a consequence, clinical experience and exposure of virtually all medical students is heavily oriented toward specialties and subspecialties of medicine, surgery, or laboratory medicine. A very large proportion of student time is spent in the specialty wards and specialty clinics of teaching hospitals or their affiliated institutions. The residents, training to be specialists, usually serve as surrogate faculty for both interns and medical students. This complex process requires access to "good teaching material."

In order to get a concentration of good teaching material, the teaching hospitals must be able to attract referral of special types of cases from the local physicians. The practicing physicians in a region are loath to refer patients that they can handle themselves, so referred patients tend to be those which are sufficiently difficult that the average practitioner is willing or pleased to refer them to a teaching hospital or medical school faculty. To be successful, the medical school faculty must remain recognized authorities in the most difficult and complex types of cases which are represented by their particular clinical specialty. Furthermore, the diagnosis and management of these complex cases requires the most modern equipment which can be used as lavishly "as necessary." As a consequence of this process, the wards and clinics of teaching hospitals tend to be populated with exceptional or exotic patients. The typical patient population is grossly different from the spectrum of patients usually seen by any physician in general practice.

Benevolent Extravagance: Education by Example. In addition to exposure to rare and exotic types of patients, the medical students and interns are also exposed to extreme examples of benevolent extravagance by their instructors. In a teaching situation, the student observes the residents and faculty ordering extremely large numbers of tests on their patients, partly because the patients are complicated, and partly because this is a means by which teaching benefits of each case can be maximized. The profligate use of hospital resources is not a very sound object lesson for physicians who enter private practice and treat large numbers of much less complicated disease processes. Not only is the number and diversity of tests exorbitant but the frequency with which they are repeated is also in excess of that needed by the patient's care. The extent to which such practices lead to waste have been analyzed by Griner and Lippzen (4), using data pertaining to laboratory studies for 855 adult patients over a three-month period at the University of Rochester Medical Center (see also Chapter 6). The clinical implications of the individual tests were analyzed and their potential contribution to the care of the patient evaluated. The volume of laboratory data bore little relationship to the needs of the patient. The data also suggested that the followup studies were excessive. It is a common observation that students, interns, and residents are rarely, if ever, subject to criticism for ordering too many tests, but failure to obtain a test, later deemed desirable, is commonly a cause for vitriolic comment. Current concerns about malpractice allegations provide additional incentives to err on the side of caution to rule out the possibility that any patient could be suffering from an unsuspected or complicated disease. The medical school instructors should serve as examples of discrimination and judgment to train medical students to use those tests and treatments that are really necessary for the proper management of illness.

The International Brain-Drain. It was estimated in 1970 that there were approximately 48,000 foreign graduates in the United States, and the number entering the country was estimated to range from 8,000 to 10,000 a year (see also Fig. 7–3b).

This drain on the world supply of physicians adds to an oversupply in the United States and depletes areas that are seriously deficient. A substantial portion of these physicians is attracted by the glitter of American medicine. Even worse, some of these physicians have been trained at the expense of the governments of developing nations. This diversion of an essential resource from countries that need it worse than we is reprehensible and is being corrected much too slowly.

GENERAL PRACTITIONERS: AN ENDANGERED SPECIES?

The many obvious attractions of general practice have not proved adequate to prevent progressive decline in both numbers and percentages of family physicians. Medical progress is extremely rapid in both information and methodologies, so that even specialists have trouble keeping abreast of new developments in relatively restricted areas of medical, surgical, or laboratory specialties. General practitioners are responsible for keeping sufficiently conversant with all branches of health care that they can judiciously treat most and refer many patients to appropriate consultants. General practice in small cities or rural areas remote from the metropolitan and medical centers presents added problems in keeping up with progress. Family physicians in solo practice also have unremitting responsibilities, many being subject to call day or night the year around, leaving little time or opportunity for either intellectual or family life. The need for general practitioners in cities and centers of population is just as urgent as the demand in remote or rural areas. Metropolitan areas provide somewhat greater opportunity to attend meetings, refresher courses, and engage in group practice to ease the incessant load.

The net result of all these factors has been a progressive decline in the numbers of general practitioners as the total number of physicians has increased from 220,000 in 1950 to 324,000 in 1973 (Fig. 7-3a). Less than 20% of practicing physicians are in general practice in the United States in contrast with conditions abroad where general practitioners represent about 50% of the practicing physician population.

Patients in need of primary care but unable to locate a general practitioner are relying to an increasing degree on various kinds of specialists. The specialties of internal medicine and pediatrics have long provided primary care for adults and children respectively. The newly developing specialty of family practice is adding significantly to the supply. In many metropolitan areas, excess numbers of specialists are also providing primary care. For example, orthopedic surgeons report that patients previously treated for injuries may return to them for diverse problems unrelated to their particular specialty. Many women return to "their" obstetricians for relief of symptoms having no obvious relation to pregnancy. Cardiologists are commonly called on to provide remedies for problems unrelated to the heart. These are all expressions of distorted roles by both patient and physician. Such patients are tacitly assumed to be able to arrive at a provisional diagnosis in deciding which specialist to consult. Under these conditions the specialists often function in areas outside their fields of special training. As a con-

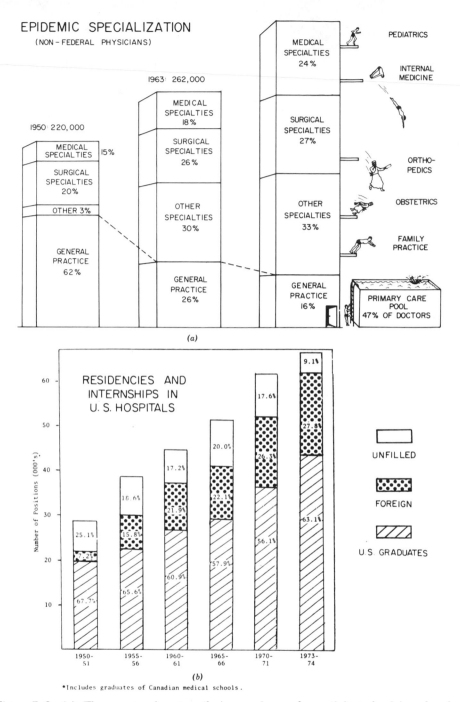

Figure 7-3. (*a*) The progressive growth in numbers of practicing physicians has been characterized by enormous expansion in numbers of specialists of many types with a dwindling supply of general practitioners. Many requirements for primary care are being met by an expanded "primary care pool" comprised of general practitioners supplemented by various specialists who make up some deficiencies at great cost. (*b*) Increasing numbers of residency positions have been utilized to train the growing numbers of specialists. Many of these available positions are unfilled and even more are being occupied by "foreign" doctors, a serious "brain drain" on many underdeveloped countries (From Crowley A [ed]: Medical Education in the United States: 1973-74. *JAMA*, suppl, January 1975, p 49. Permission requested from A.M.A.).

262

sequence of all these factors, the primary care pool is believed to represent some 47% of doctors. This might be regarded as a very desirable trend to make up for the deficiencies in numbers and distribution of family doctors. However, the coverage of common complaints by highly trained specialists is an extremely expensive way to solve simple problems.

The general public perceives an unmet need for the services of general practitioners or family doctors in virtually all portions of the country except the more affluent sections of metropolitan areas. The public has been encouraged to seek medical consultation for signs or symptoms of virtually any sort for early detection of ailments. The increasing complexity of both diagnosis and therapy have rendered patients increasingly dependent upon health professionals—even for self-limited ailments that formerly were managed equally well by grandmothers or maiden aunts. In addition, the public is admonished to have a periodic health appraisal at regular intervals even when no signs or symptoms are present. These calls for professional services are overloading the family physicians without contributing very much to the health status of their patients.

FAMILY MEDICINE AND PRIMARY CARE

The patients seen by students in a teaching hospital differ from general practice experience. An illuminating example of this discrepancy was documented by Keith Hodgkin, a general practitioner in Yorkshire, England. Dr. Hodgkin (5) kept careful records of patients encountered as a student over 3½ years and incidence of illness encountered in hospitals as an intern on surgical, medical, pediatric, obstetric, and neurosurgical services. He also kept records of every patient encountered over a period of 10 years, as a National Health Service physician responsible for a "list" of 2,500 people. The results of this tabulation computed as an annual exposure to patients, is presented in Figure 7-4. These data have been reorganized according to organ systems to make clearer the pathophysiological relationships. Horizontal bars extending toward the left represented the accumulated experiences as student and intern computed on an annualized basis. On the right is the corresponding annual exposure to patients as a general practitioner in the National Health Service. Corresponding information comparing teaching encounters with general practice encounters are lacking for American physicians but there are good reasons to believe that the situations are roughly comparable. Such figures make it abundantly clear that the exposure to patients in a teaching hospital or clinic is not comparable to the experience of a general practitioner in private practice. This discrepancy is not surprising, considering the manner in which medical schools are organized and their patient load is filtered. Current efforts are directed toward corrections in many medical schools by providing students opportunities to serve as clinical clerks to general practitioners for several weeks, often accompanying them during visits to hospitals or homes in addition to observing office practice. Such experience still remains a relatively small proportion of the total medical curriculum.

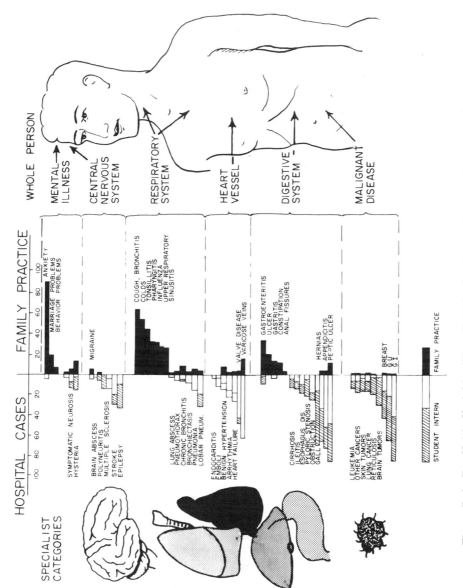

Figure 7–4. Dr. Keith Hodgkin (5), a British physican, tabulated the types of patients encountered during medical school and internship in teaching hospitals. They bore little relationship to the patients seen during several years of active family practice. A corresponding disparity is probably experienced by general practitioners graduating from American medical schools.

264

There is growing recognition that a very large proportion of encounters with physicians are for trivial problems that do not really require the unique competence provided by highly trained physicians. The nature, numbers, and distribution of the problems presented by patients to their family physicians has not been systematically evaluated until very recently.

PRESENTING PROBLEMS IN FAMILY PRACTICE

The problems presented to family practitioners have been compiled in a comprehensive tabulation by David Masland and his colleagues (6). Some 526,196 problems were presented by patients to 82 family practice residents and 36 family practitioners in the state of Virginia. Some 567 categories of problems were employed for the purposes of the analysis. More than half of these problems were encompassed within the top 23 categories (Table 7-1). According to these data, the highest incidence was found to be physical examinations or annual checkups under the general heading of prophylaxis or preventive medicine. Intensive screening programs to detect individuals with elevated blood pressure ranked second. (Other preventive measures— Pap tests and inoculations—occurred much less frequently.) Pharyngitis, which includes febrile sore throat and tonsillitis, was fourth in frequency, followed by acute bronchitis. By grouping the various presenting problems in this extensive tabulation into some simple categories, a more intelligible picture emerges as indicated in Figure 7-5. The leading impetus for visiting family physicians is seen to be prophylactic (i.e., health appraisals or screening for preclinical conditions). There is growing awareness that such screening elioits a very small percentage and total number of treatable ailments—that it should be carried out much more selectively on patients in high risk categories. The very common diseases of the respiratory system are also a dominant factor. The frequent occurrence of injuries, particularly lacerations, abrasions, sprains, and strains, usually require relatively simple first aid measures. Mental illness, as characterized most frequently by neuroses and functional ailments, also ranks high. A relatively small proportion of the commonest problems presented to family physicians actually require or respond to their intervention.

FAMILY PRACTICE: AN
EXPANDING SPECIALTY

It is not surprising that only some 20% of medical students elect to go into general practice. As students, many have very little exposure to general practice in contrast to the direct contact with attractive specialties. The current efforts to induce greater numbers of medical students to enter family medicine has led to the development of an increasing number of departments of family practice in medical schools.

TABLE 7-1. Presenting Problems Ranked by Frequency*

Rank	%	Cumulative %
1. Medical examinations for preventive and pre-symptomatic purposes	8.4%	8.4%
2. Hypertension—benign or unspecified with or without heart disease	5.6	14.0
3. Trauma—lacerations, amputations, abrasions	4.1	18.1
4. Pharyngitis, including tonsillitis and febrile sore throat	3.8	21.9
5. Bronchitis, acute	2.6	24.5
6. Sprains and strains	2.4	26.9
7. Diabetes mellitus	2.4	29.3
8. Coryza—nonfebrile common colds	2.1	31.4
9. Obesity	2.0	33.4
10. Colds and influenza-like ailments—febrile	1.8	35.2
11. Otitis media—acute	1.7	36.9
12. Neurosis—depressive	1.5	38.4
13. Cervical smears	1.5	39.9
14. Pregnancy and prenatal care	1.3	41.2
15. Neurosis—anxiety	1.3	42.5
16. Arteriosclerosis—including cardiovascular disease	1.2	43.7
17. Vaginitis, vulvulitis, cervicitis—nonvenereal	1.2	44.9
18. Abdominal pain—excluding colic	1.1	46.0
19. Congestive heart failure	1.0	47.0
20. Urinary infections	.9	47.9
21. Sinusitis—acute	.9	48.8
22. Signs or symptoms unaccompanied by diagnosis (Category 8)	.8	49.6
23. Arthritis, rheumatism	.8	50.4
24. Other signs or symptoms or incomplete diagnoses (Category 16)	.8	51.2
25. Pneumonia and pneumonitis	.8	52.0
26. Physical ailments—presumably psychogenic	.7	52.7
27. Headache	.7	53.4
28. Dermatitis, contact	.6	54.0
29. Anemia—iron deficiency	.6	54.6
30. Asthma	.6	55.2

*Data from Masland, Wood, and Mayo, (6).

266

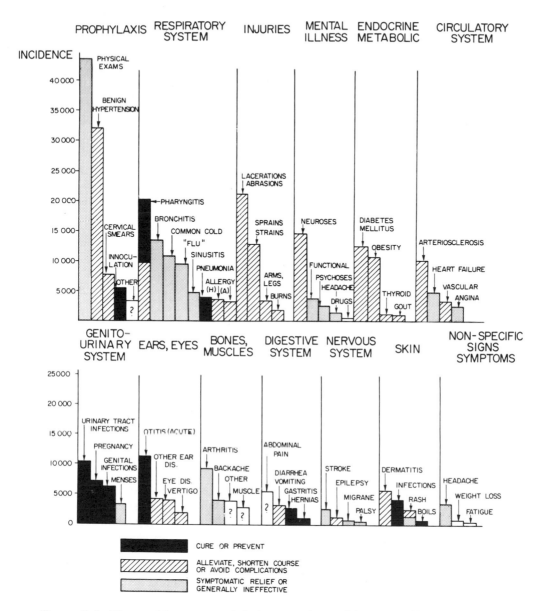

Figure 7-5. The problems presented to general practitioners in Virginia during 526,196 patient encounters have been compiled in accordance with various common categories (6). The distribution of patient problems is indicated by the heights of the vertical colums. A rough estimate of the most probable resolution or outcome is indicated as cure or prevention (black bars), alleviation with shortened course or complications avoided (cross hatched sections), and symptomatic relief or ineffectual therapy (stippled areas).

Family physicians have become widely acknowledged as an under-developed resource. To fill the void, medical schools have encouraged students to go into family practice and some 310 family practice residency training programs have been established since 1969 with approximately 4,500 students currently enrolled. The responsibility to be thoroughly grounded in the basic aspects of all components of medical practice is so demanding that family practice is now regarded as a specialty. The family practice faculty may encounter obstacles to professional advancement in medical schools whose clinical departments are dominated by specialists. By nature of their specialty, the faculties in family practice are not strongly oriented toward engaging in the kind of academic research that normally leads to professional advancement. As a consequence, they do not rank high in the pecking order of a medical school (Fig. 7-1). For such reasons, departments of family practice are not likely to accomplish the task of supplying family physicians in the numbers that the country requires.

EXPANDING DEMAND FOR PRIMARY CARE

The areas of responsibility of health professionals have been extended far beyond care of the sick to encompass many problems of modern society. The American people are living much longer and most chronic diseases do not succumb readily to available methods of management. Major interest and concern is now directed at ways in which individuals can remain healthier by changes in their living conditions, lifestyle, and health habits. There is growing belief that avoidance of risks and excesses may be the most important way of sustaining the health of the average American citizen. Most Americans engage in activities which are known to be hazardous to health, particularly excesses in eating, smoking, drinking. Reckless driving and failure to use seat belts greatly increase the hazards of the highways. The home is the most common location for injuries, due most commonly to unnecessary risks. Hazardous sports account for a large proportion of bodily injuries. The health problems that stem from behavioral and psychosocial origins are increasingly encompassed within the mandate of the health care delivery system. Examples include nonconventional, criminal, or even "sinful" behavior or actions which are characterized by such phenomena as drug addiction, alcoholism, certain forms of sexual aberration, criminal tendencies, and violence. This broadened definition of health would challenge the ability of psychiatrists, psychologists, social workers, criminalogists, and a host of other highly trained and specialized professionals. Yet there is an increasing tendency for most or all these conditions to be laid at the door of physicians. Neither training nor experience of physicians prepares them to cope with this diversity of responsibilities (7). The time seems ripe to identify the categories of malfunction which are to be included under health, to define and to characterize them specifically and to delegate responsibility for the various components in terms of the education, training, and experience required to manage them appropriately (7).

MEDICAL ENVELOPMENT OF PSYCHOSOCIAL PROBLEMS

The expanding horizons of health appear as a double envelopment by which the core of medical care is extending ever further beyond the traditional care of the sick (8). Justification for these trends are reasonably based on the fact that there are medical implications easily distinguishable in each instance. For example, the health professionals have obvious roles in the management of patients with physical handicaps that pose pressing psychological, social, and economic problems. The proper position of physicians is somewhat more obscure in their contributions to patients with either emotional problems or mental retardation (Fig. 7-6a). Aging is obviously accompanied by increasing tendencies for medical malfunction. However, senility and the impact of retirement cause psychosocial problems for which physicians are rather poorly prepared. Current cultural stresses may result in activities which could be injurious or dangerous to health. Occupational hazards and psychosocial problems associated with employment are recognized as factors which may interfere with good health.

One consequence of such "medicalization" of psychosocial issues is the tendency to funnel patients with behavioral problems into costly facilities equipped with technologies for diagnosing physical ailments. Judged by current trends, the process of incorporating behavioral and social sciences into the biomedical research enterprise appears to be progressing inexorably. It seems timely to develop a more appropriate model of the relationship between the behavioral and biomedical communities (8).

The interfaces between behavioral sciences, social sciences, and health sciences appears to be more appropriately represented by a series of salients, as illustrated in Figure 7-6b. The extension of the medical and surgical core can be envisioned as finger-like projections, or salients, extending into the domains of other segments of society represented by other academic disciplines. For example, persons with handicaps (emotional, physical, or mental) may have medical implications, but the problems they face are predominantly social and psychological. Similarly, there are important elements of health care among the aging population, as represented by the malfunctions which are characteristic of older people. There are medical implications of senility and consequences of retirement affecting health, but the major problems require social and personal services. Cultural stresses are manifested by domestic problems, occupational hazards, and unhealthy habits, which obviously threaten health but fall only partly in the province of the health professionals. By the same token, environmental threats produced by urban blight, inadequate living conditions, or contamination of the atmosphere are problems which are shared between the medical profession, the sociologists, behavioral scientists, politicians, and others.

Thus far, there has been very little effort devoted to delineation of these boundaries or to establish reasonable distribution of activities and responsibilities among the various groups involved. So long as these boundaries remain obscure, long-range planning and rationalizing of research and development will be complicated and retarded by conflict over turf and duplica-

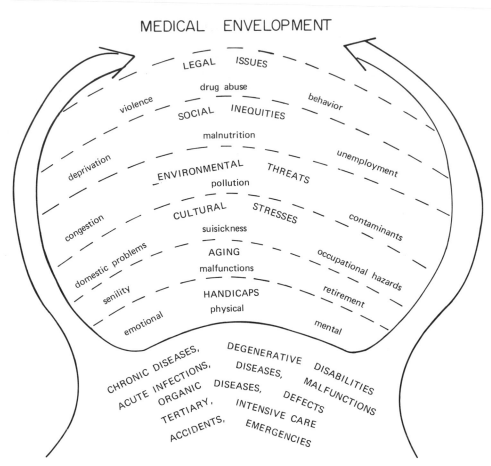

Figure 7-6. (*a*) During recent years, the medical professions have increasingly encompassed an expanding array of behavioral and social influences on health, extending far beyond the more traditional problems of disease and disability.

tion of efforts. The greatest need is for effective cooperation and collaboration in approaching these complex problems. They are far more amenable to teamwork than to the sum of many individual and unrelated efforts. The present wide-scale interest in developing forward plans provides a unique opportunity to actively engage in the essential steps of clarifying the goals, objectives, policies, and priorities and developing organizational and operational mechanisms that more accurately reflect the scientific relationships among the various components of our society.

ROLES AND RESPONSIBILITIES OF PHYSICIANS

Modern medicine imposes on the practicing physician a large number of varied responsibilities and roles beyond those which were characteristic of his predecessors of earlier times. Not only is he expected to serve as a healer

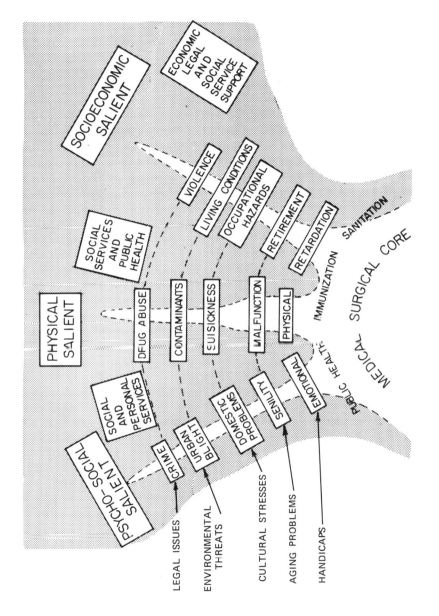

Figure 7-6. (*b*) The medical implications of behavioral, social, and economic problems can be more realistically represented by salients extending into the psychosocial and socioeconomic fields. There is pressing need to explore the interface between the health professions and other related disciplines to more clearly define and delegate the appropriate nature and extent of responsibility that each should bear.

271

for his patients, but he is expected to be a qualified nutritionist, psychological counselor, and scientist. His scholarship is expected to keep him at the forefront of biomedical advances. He often serves as the manager of an entrepreneurial business. A most important and extensive role is rarely mentioned. Modern physicians serve as professional purchasing agents for their patients (9).

PROFESSIONAL PURCHASING AGENT

The physician acts on the authority delegated to him by his patients to determine how the patient's money, or the money of his insurance company, will be spent for the various components of medical care. At the same time, the physician bears no financial responsibility for these decisions. This role is schematically illustrated in Figure 7-7, indicating a functional relationship between a physician and the very large number of facilities and services represented by hospitals, laboratories, drugstores, and manufacturing companies. These institutions employ the 4.5 million people tabulated in Figure 5-5. Physicians' fees are relatively small proportions of the total expenditures for health, yet doctors are deciding factors in determining the kinds and amounts of diagnostic and therapeutic resources which are brought to bear on the individual patient's problems. The following types of decisions are reflected in patients' medical bills and affect the way society's resources are allocated.

1. The decision to hospitalize rather than to treat the patient on an outpatient basis.
2. The techniques chosen for diagnosis, the number and types required.
3. Decisions regarding the choice of alternative methods of treatment.
4. The selection of drugs, devices, and services to be utilized.
5. Referral for consultation or specialized technologies.

Physicians as Primary Filters. The physician's role of professional purchasing agent involves not only selecting tests and treatments but also referring patients to other physicians and health professionals. The medical profession has retained its commanding position as the interface between the general public and the other elements of the enormous health enterprise. Each physician is positioned at the small end of a huge funnel, through which patients are channeled to many other facilities and services, as illustrated in Figure 7-7. For example, patients gain access to the huge number of nursing services or laboratory technicians mainly through the intervention of a physician. Dental care is ordinarily obtained by direct access to dentists without intervention of physicians. Patients gain access to other health professionals such as pharmacists, optometrists, psychologists, podiatrists, and others primarily through the physician, although the individual citizen may elect to go to these professionals directly, as illustrated in Figure 7-7.

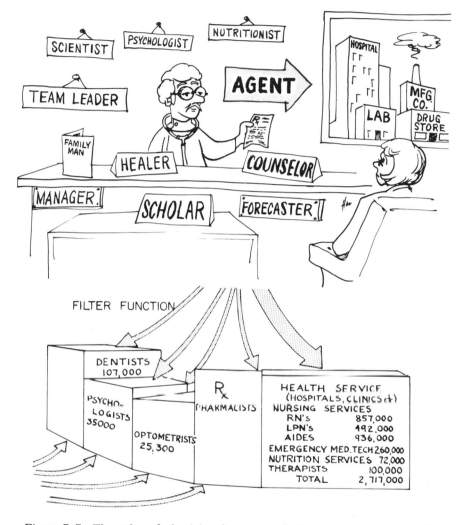

Figure 7-7. The roles of physicians have expanded in recent years to include a variety of responsibilities as scientists, team leaders, managers, counselors, psychologists, nutritionists, and in other advisory capactities. The predominant role of most practicing physicians is to serve as purchasing agents for patients in selecting from the vast array of health services and products the ones most suited to the presenting problem. Physicians also serve as a primary filter directing their patients to a varied assortment of health services.

DEFICIENCIES OF MODERN MEDICAL EDUCATION

Modern medical schools are richly endowed with highly trained faculty superbly qualified to teach and practice their individual specialties at the forefront of both knowledge and technology.

However, medical schools are singularly deficient in training opportunities with relation to many other key functions of modern medicine. Some notable examples warrant specific mention.

1. *Purchasing Agent:* Professors and preceptors provide rather poor examples of the discrimination and judgment required to select programs of diagnostic testing and therapeutic regimens that balance the needs of the patients against the rising costs of care.

2. *Proficiency in Primary Care:* The typical medical school curriculum is so dominated by specialties and specialists that the average graduate is ill prepared to respond effectively to the wide diversity of problems encompassed by the common concept of holistic medicine. The deficiencies in first contact or primary care on a national scale cannot be overcome solely by the limited number of general practitioners, or primary care specialists, but necessarily involves collaborative teams composed of a variety of relevant health professionals (see also Chapter 9).

3. *Management Methods:* Medical students receive remarkably little exposure to the principles and practices of developing and maintaining efficient practices. Long waiting periods and relatively high overhead costs are common signs of inadequate attention to organizational relations and operational procedures.

4. *Medical Economics:* The peculiar properties of medical economics are not well covered in medical schools with the result that physicians have little inclination to exhibit reasonable restraint and little motivation to consider such important factors as cost/benefit in their ministrations to patients.

5. *Nutrition:* The average physician is expected to provide authoritative advice and guidance regarding nutrition, despite manifestly insufficient background or training in the subject. The courses in biochemistry and superficial contact with diets on the wards are totally inadequate for this particular role.

6. *Psychological Counseling:* A very large proportion of encounters with physicians involve the need for personal counseling or management of signs or symptoms stemming from stresses of socioeconomic, cultural, or domestic origins. Most physicians are ill-prepared to deal with such problems on the basis of their medical school education or postdoctoral experience (7).

7. *Technical Training:* Most medical students have backgrounds in biological or chemical disciplines; few have significant educational exposure to mathematics, physics, or engineering sufficient to afford the necessary insight into the inner workings of modern medical technologies. Decisions regarding the appropriate use of diagnostic technologies and prescriptions for therapy need to be based on an understanding of at least the basic principles of the devices involved.

8. *Preparation for Research Careers:* The medical curriculum is not designed to develop the necessary background, skills, and technological base for careers in medical research. The provision of postdoctoral training enhances the research potential of clinicians but is a rather poor substitute

for the training and experience required for technical competence, experimental design experience, analytical capabilities, and the rigor necessary for conversion of biomedical research into a quantitative science.

UNDERUTILIZED PROFESSIONAL PERSONNEL

Joseph Califano, former Secretary of the DHEW, urged the medical colleges to cut down on the class size, a proposal that was warmly received by the representatives of American medical colleges. Curtailing the size of medical school classes would provide a valuable opportunity to modulate the curricula to provide a mix of graduates that conforms more closely to the recognized national needs. While continuing to provide educational experiences for the types and numbers of specialists that are in short supply (i.e., anesthesiologists), the basic science and clinical faculties and facilities could be adjusted to accommodate two additional pathways; namely, a) primary care and b) biomedical research careers. The gross differences in educational requirements for specialties, for primary care, and for research clearly warrant the provision of curricula more attuned to these special requirements as indicated schematically in Figure 7-8.

PROVISIONS FOR PRIMARY CARE

Any service that brings clients directly into first contact with the most highly trained and costly member of the organization is inherently inefficient. Surely the country would be in chaos if citizens were directed to bank presidents, mayors, or senators to gain access to necessary services. The medical profession has successfully retained a unique position as the ultimate authority on all matters of health to the point that the average citizen is commonly unsatisfied with health care that did not include a direct encounter with a physician. In most instances, physicians serve as the entry point or first contact in gaining access to the health care system. It is commonly assumed that only a physician has sufficient insight into medical problems to refer patients to the various elements in this complex and confusing system. The numbers of general practitioners and family physicians are grossly inadequate to afford the luxury of initial contact with physicians as the standard procedure. This problem is compounded in those areas where shortages of health services exist such as remote areas, rural areas, many small communities, and central cities. When physicians do not elect to practice in such areas, a void is left that can be filled by other categories of health professionals. Fortunately, the standards and educational requirements for many of the other health professions have been progressively increased.

Education of Other Health Professionals. Pharmacists undoubtedly have a sounder education in the details of dosage and distinctions among pharmaceutical agents than do physicians. Similarly, optometrists have a more extensive exposure to the basic principles of physiological optics than do physicians. In 1974, the annual meeting of the Association for Academic Health Centers was attended by most of the presidents of the nation's health educational associations, including nursing, pharmacy, dentistry, optometry, podiatry, and so on. As a consequence of this meeting, an educational synopsis was developed for the 11 health-related professions. The characteristics of their programs of education were assembled to provide improved perspectives of these health professions (10). From this synopsis some interesting information was extracted regarding 5 of the 11 health-related professions in Table 7-2. Here the general characteristics of education for nursing, pharmacy, optometry, and podiatry are compared with medical school training. It can be noted that each of these has state board requirements and four of the five have national boards. All these educational institutions require accreditation at regular intervals. The admission requirements for medicine are less specific or demanding than in some other categories. Each of these educational processes involves some years of basic sciences, preclinical education, and clinical experience. The postgraduate education is clearly more extensive for physicians entering specialties but not greatly different from the experience of many general practitioners. In general, the basic educational experience of these five professions are remarkably similar and cannot account for consistent underutilization of "nonmedical" health professionals.

NEW NURSING FUNCTIONS

During its long history since Florence Nightingale, the nursing profession accepted a role which was supportive and largely subservient to the medical profession. To a large extent, nurses were prohibited from engaging in active diagnostic or therapeutic actions without the specific orders of a supervisory physician. As a consequence, nurses were generally overtrained for the roles they were permitted to play. The past two decades have witnessed a major expansion in nursing roles, accompanied by a diversification of nursing curricula. It is now possible to engage in nursing careers through programs having duration of two years, three years, four years, or graduate study. Between 1950 and 1975, the number of registered nurses increased by nearly 2½ times to a level of 906,000. (There are approximately 300,000 registered nurses who are not employed in nursing but maintain their licenses.) The number of practical nurses ranges around 500,000, and the nursing aides, orderlies, and attendants number nearly 1,000,000.

More important than the change in numbers is the diversification of training and of professional scope. Nursing is practiced in many types of health care institutions and community agencies, as well as in schools, industry, and homes. Nurses are specifically trained to perform the following functions (10):

· Give direct physical and emotional care as well as continuing assistance to persons with a variety of health-illness problems, in order to promote, maintain, and restore health.

TABLE 7-2. Education of Selected Health Professionals

	Medicine	Nursing	Pharmacy	Optometry	Podiatry
Practitioners					
Total number	330,000	778,000 (1972)	130,000	19,271	7,120
General Practice %	32%	?	95%	95%	83%
Schools	114	311	72	13	6
Public	65	162	52	7	1
Private	49	149	20	6	5
Accredited every:	1–7 yrs.	8 yrs.	6 yrs.	5 yrs.	5 yrs.
Total admissions	15,295	32,672	8,750	1,024	654
Graduates/yr.	11,613	17,049	6,712	865	350
State Boards	+	+	+	+	+
National Boards	+	+	0	+	+
Aptitude tests required?	+	0	0	+	+
Admission Requirements	88%–4 yrs. (variable)	2 yrs.	1–3 yrs.	2–3 yrs.	95% 4 yrs.
Biology	+	–	+	+	+
Inorganic Chemistry	+	–	+	+	+
Organic Chemistry	+	–	+	+	+
Physics	+	+	+	+	+
Microbiology		+		+	
Psychology		+		+	
Anatomy-Physiology		+		+	
Math, Statistics		+	+	+	
Sociology		+			+
Economics			+		

277

TABLE 7-2. (continued)

Curriculum (years)	Medicine	Nursing	Pharmacy	Optometry	Podiatry
Basic Sciences					
1st	80-100%	90%	60%	85%	80%
2nd	40-60%	60%	30%	60%	60%
3rd		10%		40%	
4th				5%	
Pre-Clinical					
1st	0-20%	5%	10%	5%	19%
2nd	40-60%	20%	50%	20%	30%
3rd		15%	60%	10%	16%
4th			40%	5%	7%
Clinical					
1st	10-20%	10%		5%	
2nd	60-100%	60%	20%	10%	8%
3rd	60-100%	90%	40%	40%	78%
4th				80%	

- Engage in health education of patients, family, and community, help understand the directives from other health team members, and cope with psychosocial stresses related to health problems or impending death.
- Provide direct care and assistance in the following areas:
  - Assessment of health status and lifestyle
  - Promotion and maintenance of health
  - Prevention of illness and reduction of functional losses
  - Promotion of comfort
  - Participation in the curative process
  - Adaptation to physical limitations

The emphasis in both nursing training and in nursing practice on health education and on dealing with psychosocial stresses as well as providing the "tender loving care" all represent areas which are too often neglected by physicians. In this sense, the expanding roles of the nurse are fulfilling important, unmet needs to large segments of the population, which are supplemental rather than competitive with the roles of the medical profession. Some are areas in which medical curricula are recognizably deficient (see the section on doctors' deficiencies, above).

Inventory of Nursing Innovations. During the past few years a number of health agencies and educational institutions have conducted a variety of programs to improve distribution of nursing skills and services. An inventory of innovations in nursing (11) was published in November 1976, summarizing 159 programs and prototypes of community health services, home health care agencies, school health programs, independent nursing practices, hospital and nursing care functions, and educational programs in various parts of the country. Some notable examples of these exploratory programs were located in the state of Washington, for an interesting reason. The town of Darrington, Washington, an isolated, remote logging community of about 4,000 people, has a high incidence of severe traumatic accidents and other health problems. Efforts had been unsuccessful in obtaining a physician over many years. To fill this gap, two registered nurses developed a primary care clinic under the nominal supervision of a physician in Arlington, some 70 miles away. These nurses provided primary health care to this isolated community for several years, partly supported by the National Health Service Corps, until July 1976, when it became independent of all outside funding. Critical evaluation by both the National Health Service Corps and the Washington-Alaska Regional Health Program revealed that the clinic is a self-supporting primary health care center staffed by nurse practitioners and delivering high quality primary care in all its facets. This effort was so successful in meeting a crucial medical deficiency, that within a brief period (about two years), the state legislature passed specific legislation authorizing nurses and nurse practitioners to carry increased responsibility for primary care.

Ghetto areas and poverty-stricken central cities are generally medically underserved because physicians gravitate to more lucrative and satisfying practice in other parts of metropolitan areas. The skid row of Seattle and its international district are served effectively by the Pioneer Square Neighborhood Health Station. In this case, the original staff consisted of two nurses and a physician, with the nurses learning primary care skills on the job. (This was before nurse practitioner training had developed in this state.) Over the years, the nurses' practice has expanded in scope and today they engage in full evaluation and treatment, consulting the physician only if they are in doubt.

By virtue of the very heavy concentration of physicians in metropolitan and suburban areas, there are many remote and rural areas which are unable to support or attract physicians. For example, Champlain Islands off Vermont had depended upon a visiting nurse program for its health care until a health center was established in the town of Grand Isle in May of 1974. This center is now staffed daily by a nurse practitioner who performs preventative maintenance examinations on infants, children, and adults, and treats acute and chronic illness, using protocol guidelines and telephone consultation as needed. During the first year the average cost per visit was $11.55, after deducting developmental expenses. There are many other examples of nurse practitioners providing primary care in remote areas. For example, the Checkerboard Health system operates several health clinics in a distressed rural area serving 10,000 low income people in northwestern New Mexico.

Triage Incorporated is conducting a pilot project to coordinate a system of care for elderly residents living in their own home environment in Plainville, Connecticut. A rural nursing service (Circuit Rider) is serving a six-county area of Montana, in which the distance to medical facilities and physicians is often 100 miles. The service includes care for 14,000, many aged 60 or over, spread over this large area. The total responsibility is carried out by 13 registered and two licensed practical nurses. This service helps maintain 288 persons in their own homes, who otherwise would have been institutionalized.

Nursing specialists are being trained to care for the seriously ill and dying patients. One example is a program at Harrisburg Hospital at Harrisburg, Pennsylvania. The Cancer Center in Cleveland, Ohio, has a program called SERENE, to provide families with assistance needed to remain productive and comfortable during the advanced illness of a patient. It also serves as a specialized facility for handling the unique problems encountered in the terminally ill. Satisfaction with nurse practitioners has been high among both the patients and the professional personnel (12). The quality of care has been assessed and found to be equivalent to that provided by qualified family practitioners in terms of diagnostic accuracy, therapeutic effectiveness, and outcome. In addition to the roles enumerated above, nurse practitioners have proved extremely effective in pediatrics, as womens' health care specialists, and as effective members of teams sharing an increasingly extended scope of responsibilities. Public health nurses also work with a high degree of autonomy under diverse conditions from the management of widely dispersed people out of Ketchikan, Alaska, to the indigent population in Cleveland.

PHARMACISTS: UNTAPPED TALENT

The curricula of schools of pharmacy have been greatly extended and improved in recent years. Pharmacists rarely mix or concoct prescriptions themselves. The convenience of prepackaged pills, capsules, and solutions relieves responsibility for concocting prescriptions, but the consumption of huge quantities of drugs of wide variety greatly increases the incidence of adverse drug reactions (ADR). The majority of adverse drug reactions consist of minor gastrointestinal disorders, rash, itching, drowsiness, weakness, headache, fever, and other common complaints. There exist reports that as many as 15 to 20% of hospital patients have had drug reactions—some severe and a few fatal. The true magnitude of the problem is difficult to assess because the data tend to be incomplete and difficult to analyze with confidence (13). Adverse drug reactions in 6 to 15% of hospital patients (average 10%) might be a more reasonable figure (14). Part of the difficulty may stem from a lack of emphasis on pharmacology in the medical schools, leading to injudicious selections of drugs by practicing physicians. It is widely acknowledged that too many medical students receive too little instruction in pharmacology. In some institutions it is an elective course. In contrast, the educational programs in schools of pharmacy have responded with a substantial upgrading of the curricula. This is evident by a comparison of admission requirements and course content with those of other health professionals (Table 7-2).

Two professional degrees are now awarded in pharmacy—the B.S. in Pharmacy and the Doctor in Pharmacy. The bachelor level program requires a minimum of five academic years of collegiate study, at least three years of which must be spent in a school of pharmacy. The Doctor of Pharmacy requires at least one additional year of study. During the past six to eight years, emphasis in schools of pharmacy has shifted from information about various drugs and products toward application of this knowledge to the direct care of the patient. Pharmacy students are receiving training in health care settings such as hospitals, clinics, nursing homes, and community pharmacies. Unfortunately, all this education is largely wasted on those pharmacists who dispense drugs which are already prepared and packaged by major drug houses. They must faithfully fill prescriptions that are prescribed by physicians with far less training in details of the drug interactions and the options for achieving the desired results. Recent graduates of schools of pharmacy study anatomy, pathology, physiology, and microbiology, with coverage quite similar to that of physicians. Many have clinical clerkship courses, by which the students observe the effects of drugs in clinical situations. The current curricula in pharmacy prepares graduates to serve as sources of information, not only to physicians but also to the general public. If adequate provisions were made for them to dispense this information, the pharmacists could play an important role in primary care and patient education. Many studies have demonstrated that therapeutic failures are most commonly the result of the failure of patients to follow the course of therapy directed by the physician. Many patients fail to take medications as directed, and a substantial portion of them use medications in a manner that could threaten their welfare. A greatly increased degree of compliance resulted when pharmacists took more active roles in consulting with patients as to the action of the drugs, the intent of the physician, and the manner in which best results could be obtained. Finally, well-trained pharmacists can play an extremely important role for self-care in providing the necessary counseling regarding the most appropriate medications that can be prescribed over the counter for functional disabilities or self-limited illness (see Chapter 8). Pharmacists can enhance the quality and safety of self care. They are also in a position to greatly reduce the cost of drugs by substituting generic drugs for proprietary drugs which are equivalent but very costly. If the medical profession were willing to rely more heavily on pharmacists to select the drug with the appropriate action, they could reduce costs and minimize the likelihood of drug interaction.

PARAPROFESSIONAL POTENTIAL

The medical school experience is extremely comprehensive in scope and therefore has unavoidable limitations in depth of many elements of health care for which physicians naturally assume responsibility (15). For example, physicians generally assume the role of ultimate authorities in the field of nutrition and unhesitatingly provide detailed advice regarding all manner of dietary problems. In point of fact, the course content devoted to nutrition during four years of medical school is miniscule.

Clinical Psychology. A very large proportion of encounters with physicians revolve around emotional or psychological problems as the underlying issue. Physicians have some exposure to psychiatric issues in didactic lectures and exposure to psychiatric and psychosocial problems in their clinical experience. For many of these problems the training and experience of clinical psychologists may well be more extensive and appropriate than the rather meager training of general practitioners. The resolution of psychosocial problems seems more likely to be advanced by an hour-long appointment with a clinical psychologist than with a brief encounter with a busy practicing physician.

Social Work. The role of social work in the delivery of health care is becoming increasingly apparent and important as the mechanisms for access and payment for medical services become progressively more complicated. Its place is well established in institutional settings, such as hospitals. However, the potential contribution of social workers in ambulatory settings has not been effectively exploited in this country as it has in others (i.e., in Great Britain—see Chapter 9).

Optometry. Physicians in general are legally entitled to test eyes and prescribe glasses. Ophthalmologists are fully trained to recognize diseases of the eyes and to prescribe appropriate treatments, including glasses. However, the upgraded curricula of optometry schools generally provide more extensive basic knowledge, training, and experience in correcting refractive errors than most opthalmologists receive. Training and clinic experience in detection of eye pathology now renders recent graduates of optometry schools capable of filling an extremely important role in this specialized area of health care. The persistent opposition of the medical profession has retarded but only partially impeded optometrists from providing ever expanding service in the care of the eyes.

These few examples are representative of a much longer list which could include podiatrists, physical therapists, and a variety of allied health professionals.

NEW HEALTH PROFESSIONALS

The pressures for expanding the coverage and improving the quality of health care delivery has stimulated the creation of whole new categories of health care personnel. In recognition of the need for personnel qualified to assume newly developing responsibilities, a wide variety of "physician's assistants" has emerged in recent years. One potent stimulus for this trend was the recognition that thousands of medically trained and experienced medical corpsmen were unable to identify slots in the health care delivery system or to derive advantage from their unique experience and abilities (16).

In 1965 Dr. Eugene Stead (17) initiated the training at Duke University for men from a large pool of medical corpsmen (8-10,000) discharged from military service each year. Intensive training was provided to fill gaps and assure competence in areas which might not have been encountered by the individual in the military service. Military corpsmen in the Army, Navy, Air Force, and Coast Guard provide primary medical care, often with substantial amounts of autonomy under stress. They are prepared for such service by training. For example, some Navy corpsmen received 1,400 hours of formal medical training, which often included several weeks of clerkships. Corresponding training has been provided for Army corpsmen. Many have 3-20 years of experience, including independent duty on battlefields, aboard ship, or other isolated stations. In an effort to create an identifiable professional category, the MEDEX program was established by Richard Smith (18) at the University of Washington. A group of general practitioners, overworked by an increasing patient load and unable to find time for continuing education or relief from the continuous load, were mobilized for the purpose of providing clinical experience as the final stage of training of these highly selected corpsmen. In most instances, the preceptor hired the MEDEX immediately after graduation, at a time when an effective working relationship had been established. While most of these cooperative efforts proved very rewarding, it was discovered that the physician's assistants increased the volume of the practice by 15 to 25% and relieved the load mainly among the simpler kinds of medical problems. Fees for the services of physician's assistants were not reimbursed by Medicare or Medicaid, unless performed directly in the presence of the supervising M.D., a requirement which greatly reduced either the efficiency of the assistant, or impaired the efficiency of their operation.

A special panel was created by the Board on Medicine of the National Academy of Sciences to explore the needs and establish categories of physician's assistants (16).

It was recognized that these new health careers should be open to members of either sex, and that they should function as members of a health team, under general supervision and authority of a physician or a group of physicians.

The past 10 years have seen an explosive growth of a wide variety of new health practitioners graduating from 50 or 60 training programs across the country.

Approximately 7,000 new health practitioners of various types have been trained, and most of them have jobs, but the demand is not swelling. Physicians in solo practice see physician's assistants as requiring a substantial income, increasing their malpractice liability, and somewhat lowering their productivity because of required supervision. Patient volume increases, and produces a heavier daily load. Two principal problems prevented the complete realization of the potential of adding new health practitioners as members of the health team. First, some policies have precluded appropriate reimbursement for the services of physician's assistants. These militate against the most effective utilization. In addition, most physicians are very reluctant to delegate responsibility to anyone else. Although more than half of physicians polled in a large survey (19) believe that physician's assistants are needed, and 42% said they would use such an assistant in their practice, there are many traditional, legal, and emotional impediments to the delegation of the types and degrees of responsibility that would be required to fully implement this potential. One consequence of this attitude is that many counties and communities are functioning without access to any readily available medical care that might otherwise be provided by new health practitioners with demonstrated ability to perform extremely valuable, albeit restricted, professional services. Many of the natural concerns regarding the consequences of such a program should be allayed by the success of an innovative approach to providing care for remote villages in Alaska.

Village Health Aides in Alaska. The Bureau of Indian Affairs has established a very practical prototype designed to provide medical care for the remote, isolated native villages (75–175 people) in the huge expanse of Alaska. A program has been established by which the people of each native village select from its numbers an individual to serve as a village health aide (alternatively identified by the term community health aide). This individual is then intensively trained by the Alaska Native Medical Service over a period of several months in the techniques of gathering specific data, performing simple tests, and introducing specific kinds of therapy, using a very comprehensive and well-illustrated textbook for the purpose. After this intensive training, the village health aide returns to the home village equipped with powerful radio. The village health aides provide essentially all primary care. They dispense drugs, including narcotics, administer drugs intramuscularly, and give intravenous fluids. They suture minor lacerations and are capable of such medical procedures as washing out the stomach and catheterizing the bladder. At predetermined times, the village health aide makes direct radio contact with a specific physician in the closest regional hospital for needed advice or guidance regarding any problems that have arisen. In the course of such contacts, the physician can ask the health aide questions about the specifics of the patient problems and can advise regarding appropriate therapeutic action that should be taken.

Another experimental prototype was developed for providing health care to larger communities (450–800 population), through an agreement with the National Health Service Corps. Three communities were selected, ranging 200–800 miles from the nearest medical facility. The most distant was on Unalaska—an island far out on the Aleutian chain. Such a community is too small to support a physician, so a physician "extender" or physician's "assistant" was selected for each village. Support was provided by radio-telephone communication, chart reviews three times a week, patient management protocols, and standing orders for medications. Through community efforts, new clinics were developed to provide a wide range of outpatient services, including blood counts, x-ray examination, electrocardiography, and bacteriology. The staff consisted of a physician's assistant or nurse practitioner, and a health aide. A part-time visiting nurse conducted house calls and provided services not only for the immediate village, but for miles around.

The logistics of providing health care at the large distances under adverse weather conditions are impressive. If such mechanisms can provide highly satisfying health care where temperatures drop as low as -80° in winter and physicians are unavailable it seems clear that the many possible modifications of this kind of program should be applicable in the continental United States.

With the development of effective communication and transportation capabilities within the continental United States, this type of program, coupled with the prospects of training new health professionals specifically for the purpose, should make it possible to greatly enhance the health care provided in the medically deprived remote and rural areas. The opportunities and needs to provide such service in the medically indigent areas of central cities is even more pressing, and yet more readily solved by the proximity of many surplus physicians and facilities.

Emergency Medical Technicians. Many large metropolitan areas are now served by a cadre of emergency medical technicians trained and equipped to answer promptly to medical emergencies anywhere within their area of responsibility. A large proportion of the calls relate to unexpected heart attacks or other kinds of medical emergencies. Through a combination of news media and melodramas, the roles of these remarkable young men are becoming widely recognized by the entire population. By virtue of extensive and intensive experience, utilizing the best of modern technologies, these technicians have proved themselves to be more effective than the average physician in the management of such emergencies and possibly equal to the best of the medical specialists in these restricted areas. Such experience lends credence to the idea that a great responsibility could safely be allocated by physicians to other health professionals, particularly for common and self-limited kinds of ailments, which represent the huge majority of problems confronting the population as a whole (see Fig. 7–5).

Current efforts at long-range planning for health have generally focused on minor modification of the present organizational relationships when far more fundamental changes in both organizational and operational mechanisms are needed. Physicians are naturally reluctant to encourage expanded training or utilization of paraprofessionals providing services over which they have no supervisory control. With the spread of private insurance plans and government reimbursement procedures, physicians are under far greater nonmedical pressure and control.

ORGANIZATIONAL AND OPERATIONAL MECHANISMS

The penetration of the health fields by growing numbers and diversity of qualified health professionals has the net effect of diluting the influence of the medical profession (Fig. 7–7). It is no longer rational to assume that physicians are the ultimate authority and sole font of knowledge in fields of health for which their training is manifestly less comprehensive than others. It is no longer completely clear that the primary filter function (Fig. 7–7) should be uniquely reserved for physicians when there are abundant examples of primary care being delivered with success and satisfaction by qualified nurses and others with different backgrounds and experience. In geographical areas or environmental situations where physicians choose not to practice (i.e., remote and rural areas or central cities), other health professionals can help fill the voids. Many prototypes have appeared to demonstrate the effectiveness of these alternatives. The techniques of program evaluation discussed in the preceding chapter have not yet been adequately applied to these situations. There is urgent need for more definitive data regarding the favorable and unfavorable consequences of various types of primary care provided by the various available mechanisms so that more rational judgments could be made for future planning.

RATIONALIZING ROLES: TEAM TRAINING

The provision of primary care by persons other than physicians has proved eminently successful in a wide variety of settings. So long as the various categories of health professionals are educated by separate faculties with individual curricula, there is little or no opportunity for them to become knowledgeable regarding the capabilities of their colleagues in other disciplines. The development of a primary care pathway to expand the training of family physicians could provide an opportunity for development of health care teams during the process (see Fig. 7–8). Students of medicine, nursing, dentistry, pharmacy, optometry, psychology, and social work could have the experience of working collaboratively with shared responsibilities during appropriate phases of their training. By this means, the potential contributions of each category of health professionals to the overall effort could be more accurately gauged and utilized in preparation for a balanced delegation of responsibilities after graduation. The increasing complexity of health care inevitably leads to a growing interdependence, since no single curriculum can hope to provide the necessary competence to take full advantage of the vast arrays of health technologies that are currently available. The present period of transition could provide an opportunity to reorient the curricula and educational experiences to improve the interaction and cooperation of the many and diverse professionals and support personnel involved in modern medicine. Important prototypes can be found in other countries (see Chapter 9).

PREPARATION FOR DIVERSE PROFESSIONAL CAREERS

Parallel Pathways for Health Practitioners. A single medical curriculum, accomodating students with widely different backgrounds (i.e., biology, chemistry, physics, etc.), has been used to turn out graduates prepared to engage in even greater diversity of professional careers (see Fig. 7–2). This approach has not been responsive to changed needs for either research or practice.

The deficiencies in numbers of general practitioners and family physicians have not been reduced very much by the expansion of medical school enrollment during the past decade.

The recently proposed retraction in the numbers of medical graduates will not solve the problem either. Neither incentives nor regulations by government or other mechanisms show sufficient promise of shifting the current educational output from specialties toward family practice to meet the pressing needs of the American people. It seems timely to consider the development of preferential pathways with expanded provisions for training general practitioners and opportunities for family practice residencies for a substantial proportion of them (Fig. 7–8). Alterations should include more educational experience in management of patient populations likely to be encountered in family practice, avoiding discrepancies illustrated in Figure 7–4. In addition, the training should include teamwork among the various professionals on which family physicians are dependent, including nurses, pharmacists, optometrists, and clinical psychologists and social workers, to name a few. The clinical training of these and other professionals might be organized to provide a higher level of personal interaction to enhance recognition of the various contributions that each is prepared to make to the management of patients.

Pathways leading toward the individual specialties could be maintained

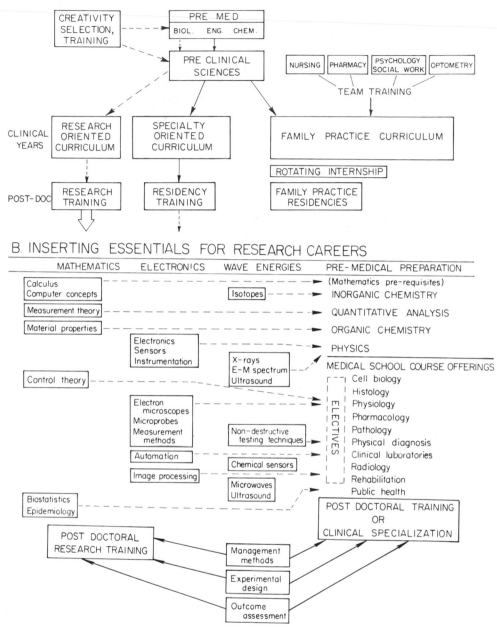

Figure 7-8. Deficiencies in numbers of family physicians and in thoroughly qualified academic investigators might be diminished by providing three separate pathways in medical schools. A family practice pathway that included opportunities for team training would provide opportunities for various health professionals to realize more fully the extent to which they could be mutually supportive. The numbers of specialists in training could be limited by the number of positions for that pathway. Investigators could be selected for either competence or creativity and then provided training that was tailored to provide the necessary backgrounds in basic sciences, clinical medicine, experimental design, and improved approaches to scientific investigation.

as they are now with substantial reduction in numbers and increased coverage of some of the basic materials of importance for intelligent utilization of the sophisticated technologies employed in the various medical and surgical specialties. This process would be facilitated by the development of special pathways preparing uniquely qualified individuals for research in the various clinical and basic science areas as illustrated in Figure 7-8. This approach would involve the deliberate insertion of material and examples into existing courses or electives to encompass disciplines such as mathematics, physics, and engineering of particular relevance to the various kinds of research and clinical activities represented in modern medicine.

In many other countries, a majority of academic research positions are occupied by individuals with medical degrees (M.D.) supplemented by extensive research training corresponding in depth to the Ph.D. degree. In the United States there is an implied assumption that the medical curriculum provides a background suitable for research or clinical investigation, particularly if some additional postdoctoral experience in research can be acquired in training programs. Unfortunately, the gross deficiencies of most medical students in the academic disciplines of mathematics, physics, engineering, materials science, and experimental design cannot be readily overcome by a year or two of postdoctoral training. This is particularly true when the postdoctoral training is provided by professional preceptors whose backgrounds are also deficient to varying degrees in these same areas. For these reasons, the increasing sophistication and complexity of biomedical research suggests a progressively increasing need for a medical school pathway toward academic research careers for clinicians.

One approach to this requirement involves expanding the number of years so that both an M.D. and a Ph.D. degree are earned in series. Some institutions provide pathways to combined M.D. -Ph.D. degrees attained with somewhat shorter investment in time.

Inserting Essentials into Medical Curricula. The backgrounds of people aspiring to research careers could be strengthened by appropriate insertion of essential materials and utilization of examples in the context of current course offerings. The prerequisites for medical school might be extended to include mathematics through calculus and higher level physics and physical chemistry—at least for those people who wish to pursue a research career pathway.

Some of the material of greatest importance to clinical investigators (and to specialists as well) can theoretically be inserted at appropriate places in existing course offerings as indicated schematically in Figure 7-8. For example, physicians necessarily employ elements of probability and decision theory in diagnosis and therapy whether they know it or not. It appears quite reasonable to insert such material into the medical curriculum as a requirement for certain medical students. Biostatistics, experimental design, and methods of data management could be inserted as electives. The widespread use of computers in medicine requires some minimal level of understanding for students that aspire to research careers or medical management.

Some of the principles of epidemiology and of program evaluation as mentioned in Chapter 6 could profitably be inserted into the medical curriculum in the context of covering disease states or clinical service for which these techniques are relevant to various types of students.

Essential information about the fundamental principles of electronics and wave energies, so widely employed in medical diagnosis, could be inserted into the premedical and medical curricula, as indicated in Figure 7–8. Clearly, physicians responsible for prescribing and interpreting the many sophisticated technologies of modern medicine need sufficient basic understanding of how they work to intelligently evaluate their outputs. The indoctrination of all medical students could be strengthened in these areas to the benefit of all. A more extensive and richer fare could also be provided to individuals aspiring to professional careers in research.

PREPARATION FOR RESEARCH CAREERS

The American educational process is designed to produce highly *competent* graduates who are knowledgeable, conscientious, consistent and capable. These are properties of great value in the practice of medicine or the "scientific method" of research into *technical problems* (see Fig. 3–2). In contrast, innovative approaches to *theoretical* problems, leading to sudden insight or new concepts illuminating conceptual obstacles to progress are much more likely to stem from *creative* individuals having very different characteristics.

OVERCOMING TECHNICAL AND
THEORETICAL OBSTACLES

The distinctions between technical and theoretical obstacles were identified in Chapter 3. The educational experience of physicians does not generally prepare them to engage in the kinds of innovative approaches that lead to intuitive insights or new concepts opening portals for surges of progress. True flashes of insight occur relatively infrequently and appear to be the province of a special breed of individuals who might be characterized as *creative* (20,21). Imaginative ideas are the essential ingredients for overcoming the theoretical problems which have impeded progress in many or most of the disease entities currently under most vigorous attack. The fundamental understanding of cause(s) and cure(s) of cancer, atherosclerosis, chronic diseases of lungs, kidneys, liver, and other organs are still in urgent need of major conceptual breakthroughs. These will probably stem mainly from rare and unpredicatable individuals with unusually creative minds. For these reasons, there is need to consider mechanisms by which both competent and creative individuals can be identified and specifically trained in our academic institutions.

COMPETENCE AND CREATIVITY:
THEIR ROLES IN RESEARCH

COMPETENCE AS A COMMON ACADEMIC OBJECTIVE

All children appear to be endowed with a combination of curiosity, imagination, and creative tendencies to varying degrees. They are comfortable with novel or innovative observations or interpretations which are non-conventional and often amusing in the eyes of adults. Estimates range that as high as 90% of five-year-old children can and should be classed as "creative." When these children become deeply involved in our educational system, much or most of these imaginative and creative tendencies are thoroughly suppressed. From earliest childhood, training is directed toward enforcing uniformity and discipline in preparation for life in a complex society. The recent educational philosophies that stress individuality and liberal attitudes have not succeeded in effectively conserving originality of any but the most recalcitrant and independent spirits (Fig. 7-9).

At home, at church, and in school, the developing child is expected to deport himself in accordance with standards or requirements of adults. In school his social conduct and his intellectual processes are expected to follow traditional lines. Indeed, the pressures of mass education have created schools which are "temples of worship for right answers" (22). Success is achieved most easily by learning what the teacher says and what the books contain and then laying the proper answers on the altar. A student who persists in questioning the traditional views or argumentatively produces a different point of view may be encouraged at first, but soon is suppressed because he is likely to distract the whole class. His performance is evaluated by objective examinations or by intelligence tests which indicate how quickly prescribed answers can be produced without making errors.

Progressing through the grades to high school graduation, the major acceptable expressions of originality and ingenuity are to be found in art classes, woodworking shops, and home economics. In college, students have opportunities to discuss various aspects of politics, literature, and recent history. They are not really encouraged to challenge the "facts and concepts" presented as the body of scientific knowledge. The widespread dependence on textbooks for undergraduates and graduate students of chemistry, physics, astronomy, geology, or biology does not encourage them to read original communications or works in which divergent views could be discovered. Their books tend to present concrete problem-solution combinations which have become accepted by the professions. Problems closely related in method and substance are then solved by students by processes through which the text has led them.

A student graduating from medical school usually winds up in internships and residencies fully equipped with a complete set of "generally accepted concepts." These appear to explain most all the phenomena he is likely to encounter (see Fig. 1-3). Students, interns and residents are well

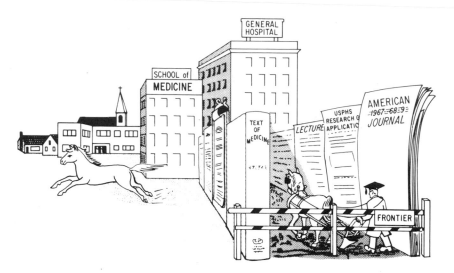

Characteristics of Creative Individuals	Characteristics of Competent Individuals	Characteristics of Scientifically Acceptable Mavericks
Imaginative	Predictable	Consistently imaginative
Adventurous	Conscientious	Concientious but adventurous
Innovative	Orderly	Orderly but innovative
Impulsive	Deliberate	Deliberate when impulsive
Intuitive	Analytical	Intuitive but analytical
Curious	Meticulous	Curious and meticulous
Ingenious	Skillful	Skillful and ingenious
Original	Stable	Original but stable
Independent	Conservative	Conservative and independent
Agnostic	Knowledgeable	Knowledgeable but agnostic
Idealistic	Practical	Idealistic but practical
Visionary	Dedicated	Dedicated but visionary
Unfettered	Traditional	Traditional but free thinking
Questioning	Respectful of	Respectfully questioning
authority	authority	
Flighty	Comprehensive	

Figure 7-9. There is need to recognize and to train larger numbers of creative individuals for academic research. Creativity implies imaginative characteristics prepared to penetrate theoretical obstacles, develop new concepts or innovations leading to progress. Competence can be defined in terms of specific characteristics that describe qualities of special value for the practice of medicine, resolution of technical problems, meticulous collection and analysis of data. Very competent individuals can be rendered more creative by special forms of training that would produce creatively competent academic investigators.

equipped to replow straight furrows under gentle guidance, but not progressing beyond the frontiers of knowledge (Fig. 7-9). Conscientious efforts to bring research and inquiring minds to bear on problems during medical school training are alleviating these problems to some degree. However, the primary thrust of professional education is to produce competent graduates able to conform to the standards of practice and procedure of the day.

The professional and personal characteristics, which are represented by the term *competence*, are well suited to research conducted in accordance with the "experimental method." They are suited to the quest for correlation coefficients and for certain types of analytical research. Competence is also an essential ingredient for overcoming "technical" obstacles, as described in Chapter 3. Investigators with characteristics of competence are not such likely candidates for the sudden flowering of originality or the development of revolutionary new concepts either by intention or serendipity.

CHARACTERISTICS OF CREATIVITY

A brilliant deduction or flash of insight propelling progress beyond the frontiers of current knowledge is more likely to emerge from innovative individuals with lively imaginations and other properties which differ significantly from those listed under competence (Fig. 7-9).

The process of originating new and novel things or thoughts is the essence of creative endeavors. Everyone has his own concept of creativity, so no single definition of the term is generally acceptable. Uniqueness and individuality tend to characterize most creative individuals but there are some traits that appear quite consistently. Creativeness is a kind of mental courage that enables individuals to break with traditional patterns of thought, "think the unthinkable." A sudden flash of insight is a part of the creative process which can be facilitated by engaging in preparatory steps.

The Creative Individual. A creative person can be characterized as one who risks going off in new directions, freed from the ordinary and diverging from the customary. He enjoys the risk and uncertainty of the unknown. The attributes of creative adults were considered by MacKinnon (21) from a number of studies. From the traits listed in Figure 7-9, a picture is constructed of a person who is adventurous, defiant of conventions, disrespectful of traditional ideas or authority, energetic, comfortable in disorder, full of curiosity, independent of thought and judgement, nonconforming, spirited in disagreement, self-assertive, stubborn, temperamental, emotional, visionary, and willing to take risks. A person with these traits would be an unwelcome addition to most classrooms. We have come to associate such characteristics with black leather jackets, long hair, motorcycles, and "dropouts" rebelling against their views of social inequities. Modern society is willing to begrudgingly tolerate some of these unpleasant features in people who manifest demonstrable talents in arts and letters. Even the most brilliant and talented may have serious academic problems when faced with the enforced discipline of mass education.

Very few intractably creative people traverse the long road to an academic career in quantitative science and retain their nonconventional attitudes. Such a person would be hard pressed to find a comfortable niche in a scientifically oriented institution. Clearly the optimal characteristics of a scientific investigator are not found exclusively under the attributes of either the competent individual or the creative individual (Fig. 7-9).

DEVELOPING CREATIVE ABILITY

The pressures to conform are so great that individual curiosity and in-quiring spirit are thoroughly suppressed in most children before they are finished with elementary school. One approach to the development of more creative individuals is to preserve and nurture nonconventional thinking in our educational system. Extraordinarily creative students are often difficult to manage because they tend to resist order and to behave in unpredictable fashion. Much could be done, however, by preserving the intellectual curios-ity and independence of thought of the very bright students who are cur-rently compressed into rather rigid molds.

Identification of Mavericks. The curiosity and creative tendencies so clearly evident in five year old children are well worth conserving and molding into socially and scientifically acceptable channels of great potential value to a society faced with problems that traditional approaches have clearly failed to resolve. Athough the pressures toward conformity are overwhelmingly powerful to many young people, there is still a substantial number who fit well into society and yet display overt evidence of residual creative ability. These traits can be recognized by identifying individuals who are reluctant to accept the traditional views expressed by books and professors. They ques-tion or even challenge authority. Even more significant are the occasions when a student proposes an alternative explanation or new and novel solu-tion to a problem, even though it might be regarded as impractical or incor-rect. These indications of exceptional creativity occurring in intellectually superior students should be recognized more consistently so that these talents could be more effectively fostered in subsequent educational processes.

During the past few decades, a growing number of indicators or tests designed to elicit evidence of creativity have been developed and evaluated (20). Such tests challenge students to display versatility and nonconformity in their responses to specific situations or problems. One important charac-teristic of creative people is their tendency to come up with many and diverse responses to circumstances that ordinarily stimulate stereotyped responses in the average person. The ability to rapidly produce a wide variety of different potential solutions to a proposed problem is also a key criterion.

The number of applicants for entrance into medical schools is large in comparison with the number of available positions. Consequently, the students admitted are selected on the basis of extensive review processes, including not only various tests but also personal interviews. Since this is already a fairly comprehensive review, it would be entirely possible to include the testing of the creative ability of students who might be par-ticularly suited to research careers by virtue of exceptional creative ability. Some of them would likely fail to compete on even ground with less imagina-tive but highly competent students. Their mental capacity may not be as well expressed in grade point averages. The people who perform exception-ally well in tests of creativity might be awarded entrance into special research pathways with curricular content particularly designed for the purpose. If this process proved successful, the testing for creativity could be undertaken during premedical education so that quantitative science, experimental design, biostatistics, instrumentation, and other prerequisites to modern science could be more readily introduced.

Education of Mavericks. There is a large and rapidly expanding literature on creativity, its recognition and development, but this is rarely encountered in most academic disciplines (20-24). These concepts are much more commonly encountered in industry but appear to be beneath the intellectual dignity of most academic faculty. An assumption is implied that genius is born—not made—and that academic faculties are exceptionally endowed with these characteristics. This attitude does not seem entirely warranted. There is no inherent reason why creative ability could not be improved with coaching, training, and practice.

Alex Osborn has published a number of textbooks presenting practical approaches to the development of creativity (24,25). Occasional articles reaffirm the impression that creative ability is widely distributed and is quite independent of the usual measures of qualities such as I.Q. (26). For reasons that are not obvious, one can look in vain in academic curricula of most universities and colleges for courses or educational experiences that are specifically directed toward the enrichment and enhancement of the creative abilities of the students.

If mathematical ability can be developed by solving problem sequences of increasing complexity, surely creative abilities could be sharpened by carefully designed sequences of situations calling for perception, ingenuity, three dimensional visualization, nonconventional approaches, and invention. Courses in experimental design should certainly include the intelligent selection of problems, the identification of key variables, establishing specification for measuring techniques. When the scientific community awakens to the opportunities and need for preserving and developing the ingenuity and nonconventional characteristics of a larger proportion of its mavericks, the rate of progress should accelerate.

The potential rewards for combining the best features of competence and creative ability are very great. Many of these characteristics are not mutually exclusive. For example, a knowledgeable man replete with "facts and concepts" can still retain a healthy agnosticism, questioning the accuracy of the facts, the applicability of their interpretation, and the validity of the resulting concepts. Similarly, a scholarly attitude does not preclude an imaginative approach to experimental design, development of instrumentation, or the analysis of data. A meticulous investigator may sometimes benefit from an intuitive plan of action. Conservative scientists must also be nonconformists at times. The most authoritative expert must be receptive to new and nonconventional ideas. A thoroughly trained investigator still has need for sufficient curiosity to impel excursions into the unknown and to successfully attack theoretical problems as well as technical obstacles.

SUMMARY

1. Medical schools have undergone a major metamorphosis since the Flexner format firmly established the traditional academic disciplines as departmental entities. Academic research, specialization, and empire building have expanded rapidly through research support of medical faculties by granting agencies. Each academic discipline has branched out into specialty and subspecialty groups which have become progressively overlapping. This process obscures distinctive differences and fosters overlapping teaching efforts that leads to the development of core curricula. The budding branch of family practice seems rooted in sterile soil in a somewhat hostile environment that impedes growth.

2. The dominance of clinical specialties in medical schools is also reflected in the preponderance of specialties in practice so that the supply of general practitioners has dwindled. The curricula of medical schools are strongly oriented toward specialties and provide experience that bears little relationship to conditions encountered by family physicians. The extravagant utilization of health services by medical school faculty represent a poor prototype for the role of purchasing agent for patients that now represent a major responsibility of practicing physicians.

3. The scope of medical practice has extended far beyond the management of disease and disability, penetrating many areas for which physicians are ill-prepared in medical schools (i.e., nutrition, aging, psychosocial problems, team leadership, and management).

4. The medical profession so dominates the field that other health professionals with extensive qualifications are suppressed and enforceably underutilized. The training and experience of nurses, pharmacists, optometrists, pyschologists, and many other professionals are sufficient to provide quality services far in excess of current practice, as evidenced by many impressive prototypes scattered over the country.

5. The medical school curriculum as presently constituted is failing to meet the overall needs of modern society. The deficiencies in numbers of family doctors and creative investigators might be overcome by developing three separate pathways specifically designed to train selected specialists, family practitioners, and academic investigators.

REFERENCES

1. Duffy J: *The Healers: the Rise of the Medical Establishment.* New York, McGraw-Hill Book Company, 1976.
2. Tapley DF: Flexner revisited. Medicine on the midway. *Bull Med Alum Assn,* University of Chicago 32:12-14, 1977.
3. Milles JS: *A Rational Public Policy for Medical Education and its Financing.* New York, National Fund for Medical Education, 1971.

4. Griner PF, Lippzen B: Use of laboratory in the teaching hospital; implications for patient care education and hospital costs. *Ann Int Med*, 75:157-163, 1971.

5. Hodgkin K: *Toward Earlier Diagnosis: A Guide to General Practice*. Edinburgh and London, Churchill-Livingstone, Publishers, 1973.

6. Masland DW, Wood M, Mayo F: A data bank for patient care, curriculum, and research in family practice: 526,196 patient problems. *J Fam Prac* 3:25-68, 1976.

7. Kennedy WB, Kelley PR, Hubbard JP: The relevance of National Board Part 1 Examinations to medical school curricula. Report to medical schools. Philadelphia, February 1970.

8. Engle G: The need for a new medical model; a challenge for biomedicine. *Science* 196:129-136, 1977.

9. Kehrer BH: The physician as purchasing agent for his patient, in Eisenberg B (ed): *Socioeconomic Issues of Health*. Center for Health Services Research and Development, American Medical Association, Chicago, 1974.

10. Synopsis of the Education for the Health Professions. Committee of Presidents of the .Health Professions Educational Associations. Edmund Pelligrino, Chairman, Association for Academic Health Centers, Washington DC, 1975.

11. Analysis and Planning for Improved Distribution of Nursing Personnel and Services: Inventory of Innovations in Nursing, Sheila Kodadek (ed), DHEW Pub No (HRA) 77-2, November, 1976.

12. Spitzer W, Sackett D, et al: The Burlington randomized trial of the nurse practitioner. *N Engl J Med*, 290:251-256, 1974.

13. Burack R: *The 1976 Handbook of Prescription Drugs*. New York, Pantheon Press, 1976.

14. Karch F, Lasagna L: *Adverse Drug Reactions in the United States: An analysis of the scope of the problem and recommendations for future approaches*. Medicine in the Public Interest, Washington DC, 1974.

15. Levin T: *American Health: Professional privilege vs. public need*. Praeger Special Studies in US economic, social, and political issues. New York, Praeger Publishers, 1974.

16. *New Members of the Physician's Health Team; Physician's Assistants*; Report of the ad hoc Panel on New Members of the Physician's Health Team of the Board on Medicine. National Academy of Sciences, 1970.

17. Stead E: Conserving costly talents—providing physicians new assistants. *JAMA* 198:182, 1966.

18. Smith R: MEDEX. *JAMA* 211:1843-1845, 1970.

19. Somers AR: Health care in transition; directions for the future. Chicago, Hospital Research and Educational Trust, 1971.

20. Getzels JW, Jackson PW: The highly intelligent and highly creative adolescent, in Taylor C, Barron F (eds): *Scientific Creativity; its Recognition and Development*. New York, John Wiley and Sons, Inc, 1966.

21. MacKinnon DW: The nature and nurture of creative talent, in Wolfle D (ed): *The Discovery of Talent*. Cambridge, Mass, Harvard University Press, 1969.

22. Barron F: The psychology of imagination. *Sci Amer* 199:151-165, 1958.

23. Gerard RW: The biological basis of imagination, in Ghiselin B (ed): *The Creative Process: a Symposium*. Berkeley, Calif, University of California Press, 1962.

24. Osborn AF: *How to Become More Creative*. New York, Charles Scribner and Sons, 1964.

25. Osborn AF: *Your Creative Power. How to Use Imagination*. New York, Charles Scribner and Sons, 1966.

26. Douglas JH: The genius of everyman. Discovering creativity. *Science News* 111:268-270, 1977 and 111:284-287, 1977.

CHAPTER 8

Self-Care as a Health Service: Opportunities for Participative Partnerships

Charlie Lough, Ph.D.
Beckie Stewart, R.N.

The active participation of the individual citizen is an essential component of both health maintenance and health care. This chapter is intended to present self-care as part of health service. Self-care encompasses many opportunities for participative partnerships with health care professionals in the prevention, management, and remedy of health problems. These opportunities are being expanded as the "health care system" is extended into the behavioral and social aspects of life. Further development of health education, incentives for health maintenance, and health counseling are needed to support self-care practices as the health care system becomes increasingly complex.

A working definition of self-care has been proposed by Levin (1) as a process whereby a person "can function effectively on his or her own behalf in health promotion and decision making, in disease prevention, detection, and treatment at the level of the primary health resource in the health care system." The person as the *subject* rather than as the *object* of health care decision action is the important concept in this definition. Such freedom of choice and action in our society carries with it the responsibility to accept the consequences of one's actions. The person must evaluate the usefulness and potential effectiveness of the options and may need guidance in selecting the most appropriate course of action. A partnership between the individual citizen and the health care provider is built around relevant information about presenting problems. Patients and health care professionals require sufficient rapport to effectively exchange the information needed for successful care of health problems, The relationship between personal self-care and professional health services varies with the complexity and severity of the health problem. The salient question is how much professional intervention is required, not how much self-care is involved.

Only on rare occasions is the person excluded from an active role in the management of health problems. As an extreme example, patients brought into emergency rooms unconscious or suffering from life-threatening conditions must delegate full responsibility to the health professionals. Otherwise the cooperation and compliance of patients are of extreme importance in the management of both urgent and chronic illnesses of virtually any degree of severity (Fig. 8-1).

Lacking the necessary cooperation of the patient, the best laid medical plans are ineffectual, a situation commonly called "noncompliance" by physicians. This critical term implies that the patient is at fault if the therapy is not as effective as it "should be." Actually, a failure of compliance by patients indicates that the appropriate level of shared responsibility between doctor and patient has not been effectively established. In many instances such a situation represents a failure of the professional to assume the proper education or interpretive roles, either individually or as a leader of a team.

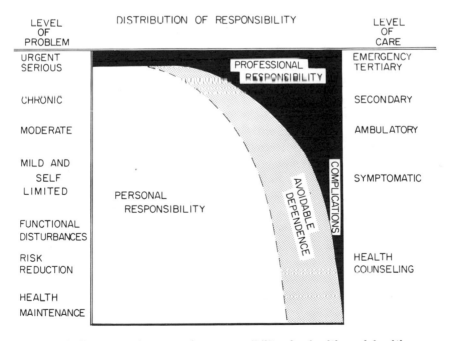

Figure 8-1. Everyone has a major responsibility for health and health care, shared to varying degrees with health professionals. Complete delegation of responsibility to professionals rarely occurs except in extreme emergencies. The shaded region, identified as "avoidable dependence," represents additional opportunities for personal responsibility where professionals currently provide health care.

The role of the patient becomes relatively more important in less serious ailments. Since the least severe illnesses tend to be overwhelmingly common, there are many mild, functional, or self-limited ailments for which the average citizen is fully capable of exercising his own initiative in recognizing the problem and undertaking appropriate therapy. A conceptual relationship between the nature and the severity of various ailments and relative participation by the patient or professional in their management is shown in Figure 8-1. This chapter deals with personal responsibility and particularly the area of avoidable dependence.

Self-care is clearly the predominant mode of health care for the common complaints. Studies by Pratt (2), Fry (3), and Kirscht (4) suggested that as much as 75% of health care is undertaken without intervention by professional providers of health care. There appear to be many and diverse opportunities for self-reliance. In one survey, half the doctors questioned thought that at least 25% of consultations were for conditions people could treat by themselves (5). A similar proportion was reported by Williamson, who further noted that general practitioners in Britain believed an additional 15% to 18% of illnesses would benefit if treatment were supplemented by self-care (1). Medical experience in general indicates that most common illnesses are self-limited and these are effectively managed by independent action in most cases (6). Self-care needs to be more clearly identified as part of health services, inasmuch as the patient is usually an active participant in the process.

General practitioners are often overloaded by patients with "trivial" ailments. Dr. Keith Hodgkin (7) kept track of the seriousness of problems presented to him by thousands of patients during several years of practice. He found that trivial or transient problems were presented 10 to 100 times more frequently than serious ones. Specifically, Dr. Hodgkin encountered over a four year period 6,258 patients with a recent cough of "trivial or transient origin" as contrasted with only 111 patients with a recent cough of "serious" origin. This ratio of trivial to serious cough amounted to 57 to 1. Following are the ratios between "trivial" and "serious" symptoms, as presented to Dr. Hodgkin:

Problem Presented to Doctor	Ratio of Trivial or Functional to Serious Causes
Diarrhea	100 to 1
Headache	65 to 1
Cough	57 to 1
Hoarseness	55 to 1
Constipation	40 to 1
Listlessness and fatigue	25 to 1
Lower abdominal pain	20 to 1
Passage of blood per rectum (piles regarded as trivial cause)	20 to 1
Dyspnea	10 to 1

The National Center for Health Statistics (8) elicited a surprisingly large proportion (60%) of trivial problems presented by ambulatory patients under 25 years of age. This observation suggests that young people may be conditioned by their parents or others to seek medical care for nonserious problems.

Widespread experience has indicated that problems that provoke panic at night turn out to be relatively innocuous the next morning. In this connection Lewis Thomas (9) noted:

> Meanwhile, we are paying too little attention, and respect, to the built-in durability and sheer power of the human organism. Its surest tendency is toward stability and balance. It is a distortion, with something profoundly disloyal about it, to picture the human being as a teetering, fallible contraption, always needing watching and patching, always on the verge of flapping to pieces; . . . The greatest secret, known to internists and learned early in marriage by internists' wives, but still hidden from the general public, is that most things get better by themselves. Most things, in fact, are better by morning.

THE FRAIL BODY FALLACY

Unwarranted fears and phobias represent an important impediment to self reliance. Contrary to common belief, the human body is remarkably sound and resistant to all manner of health hazards. Messages conveyed by mass media suggest that the human body is frail and constantly on the verge of some impending malfunction. However, such misconception is belied by evidence that exists all around us. In the first place, the human species is at the end of a continuous line of living creatures, unbroken since the beginning of life billions of years ago. During the intervening eons, the remarkable adaptability of living creatures has permitted survival through all manner of natural disasters and climatic changes, from drought to ice ages. More immediately, there are groups of people who have adapted and thrived in virtually all the latitudes, at altitudes over 15,000 feet, and in conditions ranging from arid desert to steaming jungle. We take enormous pride in the complexity and performance of the human body, an attitude which is fully justified.

Engineers have not succeeded in developing adequate substitutes that match performance of living organs. For example, the typical human heart beats over 90,000 times a day for periods averaging 70 years without any preventive maintenance. When confronted with an increasing load, the heart is capable of increasing its output automatically. If a chronic load is imposed, the heart can increase its size and power to meet the increasing demands (10). If the load is reduced, it automatically slims down to its previous proportions. Insulted by infection, it can heal itself. Most important of all, the heart represents a self-actuating power package that cannot be approximated by the most sophisticated modern technology.

Equally unique and impressive characteristics can be identified in all tissues at all levels, from cells to organ systems, as exemplified by the brain, the skin, the liver, kidneys, muscles, bones, and joints. The extent to which the various tissues can adapt to stress and recover from damage or heal the ravages of many diseases and disabilities must not be forgotten in our pre-occupation with modern medicine and sophisticated technologies.

HEALTH WITHOUT HEALTH CARE

Health care has come to be regarded as a necessity without which citizens might wither and fail. This exaggerated impression does not consider the number of individuals who survive extended periods without access to health care through geographical or voluntary choice. For example, the maldistribution of physicians and facilities leaves large areas lacking adequate health services. Populations in remote and rural areas with adequate nutrition and housing seem to have fewer health problems. Perhaps the remoteness contributes to healthy living conditions and to self-reliance in health matters. Farmers, lumbermen, woodsmen, and fishermen are not noted for poor health. It is possible that heredity, self-selection, individual behavior, or environmental conditions might preferentially favor the health of individuals electing to live rugged outdoor lives.

Christian Scientists in America are exposed to virtually the same stresses and the same likelihood of minor or severe illnesses as other citizens. They voluntarily avoid the use of health services. Their lives and health do not seem to be jeopardized. At least, they pay the same life insurance premiums as anyone else, with no distinctions. Followers of this faith seek medical care reluctantly, if at all, and then only when their own approach is clearly un-availing. As a consequence, their visits to physicians' offices are rarely for trivial reasons, which is in marked contrast to the behavior of the average American. There is no clear evidence that the health status of Christian Scientists, woodsmen, fishermen, or others working in remote areas is demonstrably worse than individuals with equivalent nutrition and affluence in cities or suburbs.

The nature and extent of the individual's responsibility for his or her own health has been clouded and confused in recent years. With the best of intentions, both the health professions and the various levels of government have progressively assumed expanded functions, often tending to usurp the individual's need to make decisions or initiate actions in support of health status.

DEEPENING DEPENDENCE ON PROFESSIONALS

Sophisticated technologies have undermined self reliance and prompted helplessness in many facets of society. Fifty years ago, the average citizen could be self-reliant in repair of wagons, washing machines, or the simple implements of the time. The inner workings of cars, kitchen appliances, communications instruments, and other necessities of modern life have become "too complicated for the average citizen." The same kind of phenomenon has occurred with relation to health. During our first quarter century, simple remedies prepared at home were clearly competitive with the foul-tasting drugs prescribed by physicians. Few people would have felt it necessary to call upon the services of a physician for the most common kinds of ailments. Today many people have become excessively dependent upon the ministrations of physicians for simple ailments for which self-care is just as effective as professional care for lack of effective therapy (see Chapters 5 and 6).

A large and growing number of people is reacting to the high cost of dependence, particularly among the young. Do-it-yourself approaches to the maintenance of cars, and electrical and kitchen appliances are becoming increasingly popular. A similar reaction in health care has been demonstrated through the growing popularity of self-care practices including diet, exercise, relaxation, stress management, and the large and growing selection of books, manuals, pamphlets, and other sources of information that help people take better care of themselves. Virtually every newspaper and magazine has one or more articles on health matters. Despite the inherent diversity and lack of consistency in the public articles, much of this noncommercial information is basically sound. A number of the social mechanisms for enhancing self-care is already in place. The greatest remaining requirement is to reduce the obstacles and provide positive incentives for citizens to assume more responsibility for health care. Mechanisms by which the typical citizen can safely and effectively manage a large proportion of the common, self-limited ailments represent the most significant approach to improved medical care at a lower cost.

The degree of dependence is also a function of the severity of illness (11). The relationship between the perceived severity of an illness and the degree of dependence on the health care system is illustrated in Figure 8-2. Under ideal conditions the degree of dependence is appropriate for the severity of illness, as indicated by the line at 45°. This means that dependence increases with severity of illness. Excessive dependence on the health care system— exorbitant utilization of health services—is represented by positions above the 45° slope. Inappropriate independence of the health care system is displayed in the lower part of Figure 8-2, representing the people who fail to seek professionals for services, information, skill, or equipment when such steps are warranted by the severity of their illness.

OPERATIONAL OBSTACLES

The health care delivery system encompasses characteristics which tend to discourage self-reliance under many different conditions. The utter complexity and diffuseness of the facilities and services provide varying degrees of access or availability (Table 8-1). Specialization in medicine fosters hierarchical structures in which the physician occupies the apex and yet is frequently the initial point of contact for the system. The mystic qualities ascribed to medicine coupled with relatively unintelligible terminology and jargon erect barriers to mutual understanding between health care profes-

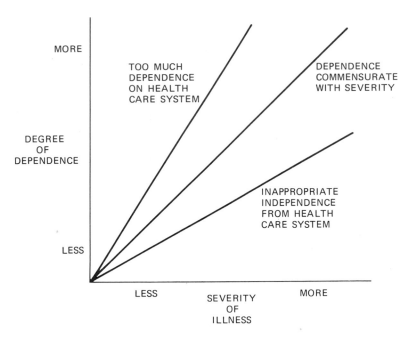

Figure 8-2. The degree of dependence of average citizens on health care professionals should relate to the severity of the illness. The region above the 45° line implies dependence which is not commensurate with illness severity. On the other hand, the region below the 45° line represents inappropriate dependence from the health care system.

sionals and the public. The fee-for-service tradition reimburses the physician on the basis of the procedures employed (process) and not on the outcome of efforts (product). For this reason, there are strong incentives to be generous or extravagant with services and to discourage initiatives by patients.

Health care professionals too often fail to take patients into their confidence and provide understandable explanations of issues vitally important to a person with a health problem. This deficiency is commonly excused on one or more of the following grounds:

1. People don't want to know it.
2. People should not know it.
3. People would not understand it anyway.
4. People won't remember it.

Extensive research is needed to develop and evaluate practical methods for eliminating or overcoming obstacles to a participative partnership in the encouragement and provision of health care. A participatory focus on health care depends upon the utilization or mobilization of the people with knowledge, skills and experience appropriate to the nature and significance of the illness under consideration. The concept of interdependence is preferable to either dependence or independence. Health education and counseling for

TABLE 8-1. Barriers to Self-Care Which are Associated with Some Health Care System Characteristics

Health Care System Characteristic	Barriers to Self-Care
1. Complex, high technology system, operating in diffuse and diverse settings	1. Widely varying degrees of availability, accessibility and personalization in different geographic and socioeconomic sectors
2. Widespread specialization by professionals across many skill levels and practice settings, with preoccupation with roles	2. Hierarchical organizational structure with complicated access and fragmented approach to healing
3. Subject matter of medicine is widely regarded by professionals to be too complex for most laypersons	3. Promotion of excessive dependence on health professionals and discounting of potential contributions of education
4. Patient information base derived from sophisticated technologies and phrased in technical language	4. Reinforces dependence of patients on professions for acquisition of objective data and their interpretation
5. Reliance on orders and prescriptions for access to therapy encourages passivity of patients as the "objects" of management	5. Obscures the potential value of interdependence in the person-professional relationship
6. Fee for service principle coupled with third-party payments represents strong economic incentives for generous use of health services	6. Individual initiatives for assuming responsibility for health and welfare tend to be diminished in favor of "artificially cheap" or "apparently free" health services

many people can best be directed at demonstrating that the average citizen can comprehend important elements of disease and disability and can effectively manage most of them with appropriate access to relevant information.

BARRIERS TO UNDERSTANDING

The average American, exposed to enormous amounts of information about health, remains remarkably illinformed and misinformed regarding the origins and options for management of even the most common illnesses (see Chapter 6). The root causes of this paradoxical situation stem from many sources: the educational exposure in schools tends to emphasize hygiene, social adjustments, and normal function, almost to the exclusion of study of patterns of signs and symptoms or methods of management for common ailments. The deluge of conflicting information about health matters in mass media and in commercial advertising is sufficient to confuse anyone. The diversity of opinion about the best methods for treating certain common ailments is a reliable indication that none is truly effective. The diversity of prescriptions, over-the-counter drugs, nostrums and folk remedies is equally confounding. A similar degree of senseless confusion surrounds the management of most common ailments, for which definitive treatments are not yet available. Such common complaints are among the leading causes of unrewarding encounters with physicians. Interviews with patients following hospitalization have disclosed that patients are more frequently dissatisfied with the lack of communication than with any other element of the health care delivery system (12). A principal difficulty lies with the fact that physicians are not noted for their ability to convey the necessary information in understandable form. At the same time, they are reluctant to delegate responsibility for conveying such information to other people. They are justifiably concerned that information may be inconsistent or incorrect when presented by someone who is not entirely familiar with either the details of medicine or with that particular patient. There is a substantial requirement for development of an ever-increasing amount of authoritative health information packaged in useful forms for distribution to citizens.

A survey conducted by Louis Harris (13) concluded: "The major breakthrough in health will be one that strips away the illusions of invulnerability and the false hopes for miracle cures, and which leads the public to deal responsibly with its own health and embrace more healthly lifestyles." The concept of responsible self-reliance embodied in the above statement includes two ideas that seem important:

1. The individual practitioner of self-care must be willing to accept responsibility for the consequences.
2. Responsible self direction carries an obligation to respect the rights of others in the appropriate utilization of health facilities and services and in assessing the effect of self-care actions on others in the community.

Huber and Patrinos (14) suggested the need for "a new balance between public need and personal desires," including new insight and fresh appreciation of the meaning of the basic ethical principle of freedom with responsibility, "long nourished but frequently forgotten in history."

There are several situations where the promotion of self care might produce undesirable results (15). For example, promotion of self-reliance could be used as an excuse to cut budgets for needed attention or services required by specific social segments such as the poor, the elderly, the disabled. Focus on self-care of symptoms may distract attention from causes of illness. There is need to apply the mechanisms of health service evaluation (as described in Chapter 6) to assess the extent to which self-care might produce unintended side effects.

Interdependence between people and health care professionals also requires new perspectives about traditional relationships. For example, Norman Cousins (15) described the ideal patient as one who:

1. Does not require a prescription to demonstrate he is getting his money's worth,
2. Does not believe that the best medications are necessarily represented by the latest and most powerful chemical concoctions,
3. Does not feel insulted if he is told by the doctor that his problem is psychogenic and not organic,
4. Does not dump his symptoms on the doctor's table and expect the doctor to accept full responsibility for cure,
5. Does not panic at the first sign of pain.

An important point for policy development in the area of individual responsibility for self-care includes the development of guidelines for promoting individual responsibility for self-care and the use of self-care, while at the same time protecting social rights from being jeopardized. The perceived roles of professionals are not clear concerning the extent to which they could or should foster self-care decision-making and screening, recognizing the probability of false-positive and false-negative indications. The mechanism for enhancing informed decision-making and the necessary incentives to do so are important research questions.

The concept of a participative partnership between the individual citizen and various health care professionals requires a reexamination of the idea of a "health care delivery system". It is unrealistic to consider some people inside a system delivering some kind of a product to people outside the system.

Encouragement of interdependence always and independence often are preferable to utter dependence in health care. Such an approach could contribute to the confidence of the average citizen that health and illness are not beyond comprehension, nor is correct treatment necessarily beyond his/her competence. People encouraged to practice self-care will become more confident of the healing power of their own bodies, which in itself may have a beneficial placebo effect. Carefully controlled experiments are needed to evaluate the extent to which self-care is comparable to conventional health care with respect to costs and benefits for a similar set of common ailments.

OPPORTUNITIES FOR PARTICIPATIVE PARTNERSHIP

Across the range of health problems presented to health professionals there are numerous opportunities for participative partnerships which encompass the continuum from independence to utter dependence. They include inducements for individual initiatives in risk avoidance, adoption of healthy living habits, and specific therapy of chronic illnesses (i.e., diabetes). A number of these opportunities have already been widely employed and could be tested by rigorous research methods. They include means for meeting the goals of health care without increasing the demand for health services and means of improving availability and accessibility to health care while containing or reducing the cost of health care.

INDIVIDUAL RISK AVOIDANCE

The greatest threats to life and health of persons from the ages of 1 to 35 is included under the general heading of violence. High on the list of threats are highway accidents, crime, and suicide. It is not generally recognized that by far the most common site of accidents is in the home. Data from the National Center for Health Statistics indicate that 42% of all accidents occur in the home in contrast to 13.6% in streets and on highways. It is true that the severity of the home accidents is relatively slight compared with automobiles, but the overall effect is enormous.

People who are "accident prone" are often required to pay higher insurance premiums than those with good records of performance. The same principle might be applied to individuals who intentionally engage in activities that have a high probability of resulting in injurious accidents. In one sense, complete comprehensive medical coverage for individuals who are ardent participants in dangerous activities actually tends to encourage injuries by removing this part of the economic restraint. It would seem desirable to exclude from medical insurance coverage certain dangerous and indiscrete voluntary activities. Mountain climbers who get into trouble because of lack of training or equipment or good judgment often cost large rescue teams a great deal of time, money, injuries, or even life. In many instances, foolhardy undertakings jeopardize the lives and health of others. There is a growing tendency to require responsible parties to make payments under such circumstances. Such instances are rare and are more like penalty payments than full reimbursement. However, such approaches may ultimately help inhibit some portion of unnecessary risks. A slight extension of this concept now justifies imposing higher health insurance premiums on smokers since use of tobacco is recognized as a health hazard.

The health professions have been increasingly assuming an improbable role of a substitute or supplement for the conscience and common sense of many citizens. The process of medicalizing society has tended to expand the scope of health care to encompass voluntary indiscretions and excesses. Thus, physicians become involved in "managing" problems of obesity, sloth, and unhealthy habits such as drinking and smoking. Obviously, the individual is the only one who can control such behavior. All the powers of persuasion or propaganda by the doctors or health agencies have proved to be rather inefficient. Surely these are conditions that can and should be regarded under self-care as responsibilities solely of the individual.

There is a growing awareness that effective therapy or cure of most chronic diseases are not imminent because the causes remain veiled in mystery (see Chapter 4). Consequently, current efforts are being directed toward reducing risk factors that have been identified and that might be avoided. An obvious result has been the added emphasis on healthy personal habits, in the form of diets, exercise, antismoking measures, and reduction of other excesses, including drinking, drugs, and environmental hazards. The current jogging and food fads are obviously encouraging the public to be more responsible for their own health status. Even exercise can be carried beyond reasonable limits and result in strains or injuries. The current trends toward increased interest and awareness of health problems has not yet demonstrably diminished the tendency for the average American to seek professional intervention for common complaints which are just as effectively managed by simple home remedies as can be provided by the most highly trained specialist.

Emphasis on healthy habits is generally accepted as being a valid approach to improved health status. The concept has been supported by various kinds of studies that are generally retrospective. Breslow and Bellock (17) conducted a longitudinal study on 7,000 adults for 5½ years to assess the significance of seven health habits:

1. Three meals a day at regular times (avoiding snacks)
2. Breakfast every day
3. Moderate exercise two or three times per week
4. "Adequate" sleep (seven or eight hours per night)
5. No smoking
6. Weight moderation
7. Alcohol abstention or moderation

They concluded that a 45-year-old man regularly conforming to none, one, two, or three of these "healthy habits" has a predicted life expectancy of 21.6 (to age 67) and compliance with six or seven of the habits would increase expectancy 11 years (to age 78).

Dr. John Knowles (18) has emphasized that greater self-discipline is needed by an American public that spends more than $30 billion a year for cigarettes and whiskey. Benefits of healthy habits have emerged from unlikely sources. For example, a recent study of 78 United States Navy pilots who had been prisoners of the North Vietnamese for several years were compared with a matched control group of equal size. The study demonstrated that an austere diet with no alcohol, limited smoking, and rigorous physical fitness was actually conducive to "good health." The prisoners were found to have one-fourth the incidence of heart disease or high blood pressure.

ENHANCING INDIVIDUAL INITIATIVES FOR HEALTH: RECOGNITION AND MANAGEMENT OF SELF-LIMITED AILMENTS

The educational process is one of the most important services provided by the state in America, but some of the fundamental information required to play an important participatory role in self-care has not been forthcoming for developing rational restraint or avoiding known health hazards.

Educating people to take care of themselves is a much broader process than simply providing information about home remedies for common illnesses. It is a process whereby individuals become more independent and competent to perform maintenance and therapeutic activities on behalf of their physical, social, and emotional welfare through their own knowledge and experience. They should be able to evaluate their own health status, to seek outside sources as needed, and to provide important elements of primary care. Most importantly, they learn to be self-reliant in caring for their own needs. These self-initiated actions can perhaps best be learned as part of the more general educational objective of reasoned independence.

Education about self-care can take two such forms. The most basic is education for promotion of health maintenance, healthy habits, and risk avoidance. Another dimension is health information encompassing descriptions of diseases and their effects, as well as community resources for information and referral.

Another important and yet usually neglected aspect of self-care involves the "lay education" about the roles, capabilities, and expectations of physicians, specialists, nurses, and other members of the health care profession. The public has given power to the health care professional, especially the physician, by expecting unlimited abilities and performances from him. Numerous surveys reflect a common belief that most disease/illness conditions can be cured. Excessive expectations can lead to disappointment with performance and disenchantment with the "system." Obviously access to the health care system does not assure good health or "wellness."

SELF-CARE AS A VIABLE OPTION

Most people are able to make sound decisions when supplied with information about diseases, forms of health care delivery, and capabilities of doctors, nurses, and other health professionals. They do it every day. The value of self-care lies in the fact that it is an *option* or supplement to the traditional health care system, even for those who are dissatisfied with traditional health care.

Rational Responses to Common Complaints. The general public exhibits little interest in matters relating to health as long as they feel well. The mass media bombards us all with barrages of information in commercial advertisements, the credibility of which is strained to the utmost by conflicting claims for various products. Premature promises of imminent cures or control of major diseases fail to materialize and therefore undermine public confidence in the scientific community. There is need for a national effort to reestablish credence. An excellent starting point would be to establish and publicize authoritative consensus regarding signs, symptoms, and suggested management of common self-limited conditions. Widespread agreement already exists among medical experts regarding the identifying indicators for common complaints and also the most appropriate means of management. Part of the agreement stems from awareness that most of the most common ones are not significantly influenced by treatment so that supportive or symptomatic measures are all that can be reasonably justified. We need not sacrifice placebo effects of medical intervention for these common ailments because most people are aware of the extent to which treatments are effective (Fig. 8–3).

The medical profession generally encourages the teaching of innocuous things like normal function or hygiene, but physicians often express concern that a little information about diseases may be dangerous. There is little to lose and much to be gained by educating young people to understand the origin and potential significance of common symptoms, the recognition of common complaints, and indications for seeking professional help. Middle school and high school students can easily comprehend information about such common ailments as colds, flu, sore throats, bronchitis, diarrhea, and similar problems. They must make decisions about these and more pressing problems throughout their lifetimes. A growing proportion of the public is showing signs of desiring more practical information on health-related issues as evidenced by the widespread appearance of such issues in the popular press.

HEALTH ADVOCATES: A PROTOTYPE

Innovative programs have been designed to explore the prospects of encouraging self-care among college students. At the Hall Health Center of the University of Washington, a demonstration program has been developed involving training of peer health advocates. These are volunteers among the residents in selected dormitories who are given intensive training and serve as counselors in health matters for the students in their residence halls. They also serve as interfaces with the student health center, which is fully equipped for ambulatory care. Such guidance mechanisms help students recognize the significance of their symptoms and appropriate next steps. These include the use of descriptive protocols like those in Figure 8-4 for both preliminary recognition of some of the most common problems and recommended steps for their alleviation.

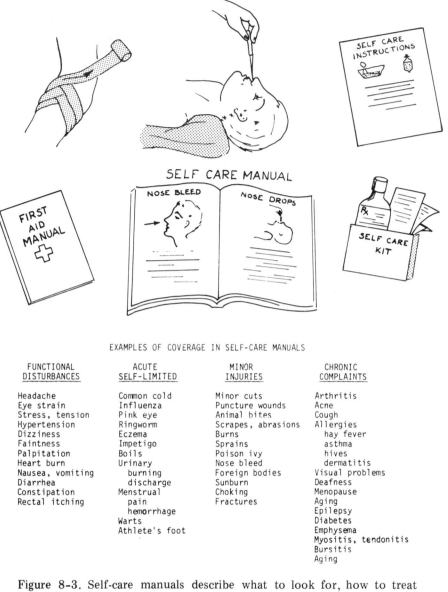

SELF CARE MANUAL

NOSE BLEED

NOSE DROPS

FIRST AID MANUAL

SELF CARE INSTRUCTIONS

SELF CARE KIT

EXAMPLES OF COVERAGE IN SELF-CARE MANUALS

FUNCTIONAL DISTURBANCES	ACUTE SELF-LIMITED	MINOR INJURIES	CHRONIC COMPLAINTS
Headache	Common cold	Minor cuts	Arthritis
Eye strain	Influenza	Puncture wounds	Acne
Stress, tension	Pink eye	Animal bites	Cough
Hypertension	Ringworm	Scrapes, abrasions	Allergies
Dizziness	Eczema	Burns	hay fever
Faintness	Impetigo	Sprains	asthma
Palpitation	Boils	Poison ivy	hives
Heart burn	Urinary	Nose bleed	dermatitis
Nausea, vomiting	burning	Foreign bodies	Visual problems
Diarrhea	discharge	Sunburn	Deafness
Constipation	Menstrual	Choking	Menopause
Rectal itching	pain	Fractures	Aging
	hemorrhage		Epilepsy
	Warts		Diabetes
	Athlete's foot		Emphysema
			Myositis, tendonitis
			Bursitis
			Aging

Figure 8-3. Self-care manuals describe what to look for, how to treat ailments at home, and suggest what conditions require professional attention. The common complaints listed are generally recognized and effectively managed by individual initiative in the general population.

    A self-care facility has been developed for students who wish to perform simple self-care diagnostic procedures independently, such as screening eye tests, blood pressure checks, urine pH and glucose tests, throat examination, and height/weight measurements.

    For conditions that are not covered by the standard decision sequence, additional instructions and guidance are provided to channel the student into the appropriate medical clinic. This program is a logical extension of a current trend toward the development of self-care manuals, which are based on the same kinds of systematic approach to common ailments.

POPULAR SELF-HELP MANUALS

Books intended to provide basic information on health matters for popular consumption are not new or novel. A variety of valuable books, many paperbound, have appeared in recent years that are specifically intended to improve self-reliance.

Donald Vickery and James Fries (19) have written a very popular manual entitled *Take Care of Your Self*. It includes instructive protocols and also provides important background information that would help alert an individual to the indications for seeking professional help if needed. Dr. Keith Sehnert (20) not only published a book *How to be Your Own Doctor—Sometimes* but also supplemented it with a course intended to produce "activated patients." The popular *Well Body Book* appeals to members of the younger generation (21). A large and growing list of such books provides useful information intended to help people take better care of their own health problems. Their readers are encouraged to seek professional help more appropriately and avoid presenting trivial problems to their physicians. Despite some obvious differences in the details presented by such books, there is rather remarkable consensus in their procedures and approaches to diagnosis and treatment. The best of these manuals or a combination of their best portions could provide ideal textbook material for class presentations at various stages in the educational process.

The books by Sehnert and by Vickery and Fries employ simple decision trees or algorithms to guide the reader through a series of decisions. They cover most of the common ills that account for 60 to 70% of the reasons for seeking visits with doctors, pediatricians, internists, obstetricians, or gynecologists during a typical year. The instructions also supply indicators for seeking professional services to avoid complications from the illness. Finally, these texts improve the process of intelligible communication between patient and physician regarding common ailments.

DECISION TREES

The use of simple sequences which the average citizen can employ to arrive at rational courses of action has been developed and subjected to rather rigorous evaluation. The basic concept derives from a process of identifying the kinds of analysis utilized by experienced physicians during the diagnostic process and expressing these steps in terms of branching logic trees. By this means, the diagnostic and therapeutic approaches of highly qualified physicians can be analyzed to arrive at reasonable consensus and converted into a standard format that can be readily used by individuals with much less training than required of health professionals.

Colds are caused by viruses finding a suitable environment in the nose and throat. The body protects itself by trying to float the virus away in a bath of mucous. Blood flow increases to the nose and throat to bring in white blood cells and antibodies to kill the virus. The result of the increased blood flow is the red, swollen, mucous membranes of the nose and throat which are commonly observed with a cold.

Colds often start with a scratchy throat, followed by sneezing, a runny or stuffed up nose (from the virus-fighting mucous) and general, achy feelings of illness. Early action on your part when you get the first signs can help limit the severity of the cold and can help avert possible follow-on infections from bacteria (which grow well in the mucous).

If your cold isn't unusually persistent lasting more than 14 days, isn't coupled with unusual symptoms, and isn't settling into a single location, such as your throat, ears, or sinuses (along with other signs of bacterial infection), be confident you can handle it yourself.

SELF CARE DECISION PROCESS

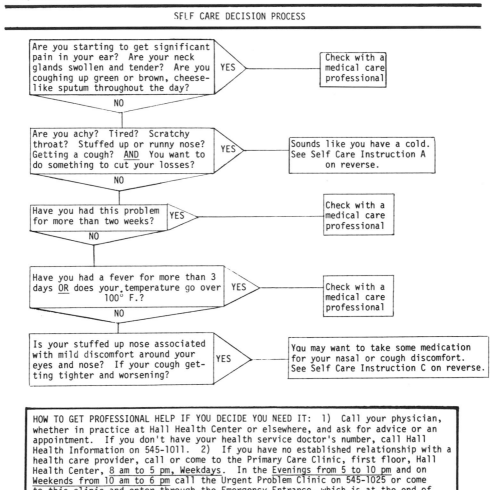

HOW TO GET PROFESSIONAL HELP IF YOU DECIDE YOU NEED IT: 1) Call your physician, whether in practice at Hall Health Center or elsewhere, and ask for advice or an appointment. If you don't have your health service doctor's number, call Hall Health Information on 545-1011. 2) If you have no established relationship with a health care provider, call or come to the Primary Care Clinic, first floor, Hall Health Center, 8 am to 5 pm, Weekdays. In the Evenings from 5 to 10 pm and on Weekends from 10 am to 6 pm call the Urgent Problem Clinic on 545-1025 or come to this clinic and enter through the Emergency Entrance, which is at the end of the driveway on the south side of Hall Health Center.

Figure 8-4. (a) Decision trees or protocols provide effective guidance in identifying and managing many typical ailments. An example for the common cold is typical of such organized instructions. Identification of malfunction follows rationally from step-by-step decision processes.

314

A CUT YOUR LOSSES WITH ACTION NOW!

Rest and relax. Conserve your body's healing energies.

Avoid exposure and fatigue. Take a hard look at your current life style. What is it that you are doing - overwork, tension, stress, worry, diet, etc. - that is setting the stage, providing a suitable environment for the cold virus? Adjust your life and get some action going to keep that cold from getting worse.

Monitor the progress of your cold. Is it hanging on or are you going to fight it off? If cough seems to be increasing or signs are hanging on, turn back to the Decision Process on the other side.

B HEAD OFF POSSIBLE COMPLICATIONS FROM YOUR COLD!

Keep doing step A, above.

Drink large quantities of fluids, about 8 oz. every couple of hours to thin the mucous and ease your coughing.

Steam inhalations or a steamy shower can also help thin the mucous to help your breathing and before you lie down to sleep.

Take your temperature 3 times a day. Thermometers are available in the Hall Health Self Care Clinic or from your Student Health Advocate if you live in Haggett, McCarty or Sand Point.

Rest in bed with a fever

Monitor the progress of your cold. Is it improving or does it seem to be settling into a specific part of your body, such as your ears, nose, throat, or chest? If cold is not improving, turn back to Decision Process on reverse.

C NEED RELIEF FROM THOSE SYMPTOMS?

Keep doing step B, above.

Try aspirin or acetaminophen (Such as Tylenol) for muscle aches and fever. Read the information circular supplied with these drugs to decide if they are right for your body. In reading the circular pay special attention to the "Warnings", "Contraindications", "Precautions", and "Adverse Reactions" sections.

Try cough medicine for severe cough not helped by steam. Dextromethorphan hydrobromide is the ingredient that suppresses a cough. It is found in non-prescription drugs such as Robitussin Cough Syrup.

Nose drops or oral nasal decongestants may help your runny, stuffed up nose, although there may be some side effects, such as wakefulness, increased blood pressure, and faster heartbeat. Check your information circular. Sudafed, ARM and chlortrimeton decongestant can be obtained without prescription.

Still have problems? If so, turn back to Decision Process on reverse.

Figure 8-4. (*b*) The reverse side of a self-care instruction sheet may indicate treatment options related to each stage in the decision process.

315

This approach was used with significant success by Sherman and Komaroff (22) in a large cooperative program involving MIT and Beth Israel Hospital in Boston. They demonstrated that both the diagnosis and treatment decisions by health assistants using carefully constructed decision trees (protocols) were entirely consistent with those of highly qualified physicians and could be used effectively without hazard to the patients. This should not be surprising since the sequential steps were specifically derived from careful evaluation of the processes by which these and other trained physicians approached these same problems. Use of decision trees for specific ailments, rather than a collection of such protocols in a manual, also needs testing to determine their efficacy in facilitating recognition and self-management of common, self-limited ailments. Perhaps a given decision tree could be explained on spot television announcements and made available in newspaper ads in a large scale single city epidemiological-type study of its utility for various population segments.

SELF-CARE KITS

The information and symptomatic treatment for common complaints can also be easily packaged into highly informative kits to be dispensed by pharmacists. The packets could include specific and accurate information covering current knowledge regarding the cause(s), signs, symptoms, and possible indications of complications in understandable language, and supplemented by informative illustrations. A typical self-care kit might include some or all of the following:

- Characteristics of the presenting problem: signs, symptoms, typical course and illustrations indicating what to look for.
- The nature, origin, and significance of these signs and symptoms.
- Recommended types of supportive action, symptomatic treatments, and reasonable expectations regarding the results.
- Cautions regarding the interactions with drugs the patient might be taking for other reasons.
- Specific and illustrated instructions regarding how to perform essential procedures (i.e., instilling nose drops, enemas, simple bandaging, etc.).
- Questions for the health professional, should a contact be needed.

The role of the certified pharmacists could be extended to include responsibility to show each kit user how to gain maximum benefit from the material in the packets (see Chapter 7). They could supplement this information by answering specific questions or dispensing more comprehensive booklets on the subject. In this way, pharmacists could become the natural channel for dispensing information as well as appropriate medications to people at the very time when they are most interested and responsive to information about their own specific problems. Pharmacists trained in recent years are among the most overtrained and underutilized health professional team as evidenced by their extensive education (see Chapter 7, Table 7–1). A statutory authorization of this extended role of pharmacists would greatly improve the quality of care for the self-care sector with substantial reductions in health care cost, if the frequency of needless visits to doctors could be correspondingly reduced.

HEALTH COUNSELING AND SUPPORTIVE SELF-CARE

Health counseling is communication in the form of guidance, information-giving, and reassurance for the purpose of helping people achieve satisfaction from their own decision-making and action-oriented health processes. The range and scope of health counseling has broadened in recent years as the number of categories of counselors, media of communication, and content of counseling have increased.

Health counseling does not attempt to meet all the needs of the public, but it can help guide people toward the mode of health care they feel is best suited to their needs. In some instances, health counseling provides people with need for reassurance to act independently in selecting their own home remedies. In others, health counseling provides specifically needed community-based home health service. In many instances, guidance is more effective if it stems from within the community whose population it serves.

A relatively small proportion of the general public displays complete self-reliance and self-confidence in self-care without consulting a professional. However, the numbers of people who are buying popular self-care manuals, eating natural foods, exercising, and demonstrating concern for their health are quite obviously growing spontaneously. An important obstacle to enhancing self-reliance is the common requirement for reassurance that any particular health concern is not a harbinger of something serious and that a chosen approach to eliminate symptoms is correct and safe. The widespread impression that only doctors can provide this important element of guidance and counseling is being dissipated for many individuals and communities by the rapid growth of many different types of new health professionals and health aides.

There is need for a major increase in the numbers and sources of reliable health information to facilitate the public's health care selection process. Some of the opportunities and options for providing reliable and effective guidance and advice concerning particular health-related problems are worth consideration.

CATEGORIES OF HEALTH COUNSELORS

Advice and guidance about health-related problems is by no means confined to doctors, despite the widespread tendency to expect and demand such service. For example, many patients with well-established relationships with a primary care physician often find it efficient and effective to seek advice from their doctor's office nurse. This approach produces desired results in many instances without the need to wait for a return call. Substantial confidence and reassurance results from awareness that the nurse will consult the doctor in case of doubt. Receptionists with long experience in a doctor's office often become extremely effective and dependable as sources of reliable health information with the same kind of general backup by the nurse and physician.

Health counseling is a major function of all participants in the health care delivery process to varying degrees and in various settings. For the solo practitioner, the receptionist serves as a gatekeeper and makes appointments, depending in part on the perceived urgency of the problem. Instructions are conveyed about steps that might be needed, such as bringing in specimens, and so forth. Each individual contributes instructions or explanations if the system is working correctly. Despite the enormous diversity of health professionals, there is inadequate provision for a readily visible information channel except through the personal physician.

HEALTH INFORMATION CENTER CONCEPT

The quality and distribution of health care could be greatly enhanced with little additional expense by providing immediate access to a source of reliable information and guidance. For this purpose, health information centers could be established within communities or neighborhoods to provide an exceedingly valuable service. The operational scope of a potential health information center is illustrated in Figure 8-5. Such a center may not now exist, but the specifications might be envisioned as follows:

Consider a central location within a community of 5–10,000 people containing a data bank for which a full-time health counselor is responsible. This data bank would include a detailed listing and description of the available sources of health care over a very wide range of problems. For example, a roster of pharmacies organized by their zip codes could be continually kept up to date, including the names of the pharmacists who would be on call or available at various hours of the day or night. Similarly, the availability of physicians, nurses, and paramedics could be maintained for ready reference, not only in terms of their location, but also of their availability. The location and services available in drop-in clinics in the area should be detailed. The community hospitals in the immediate vicinity or at greater distances should be known, along with the particular kinds of services they are prepared to render. For both legal and practical reasons, this information center would need to have the supervision of a qualified physician to whom problems could be immediately transmitted if the patient did not have a regular physician. The responsible physician could also answer questions or give advice about issues beyond the competence of counselors.

A health information center could serve as a valuable source of reassurance to people who are home-bound and are otherwise dependent upon others in the event of an accident. A valuable referral outlet could be provided for individuals who need to talk to someone about problems which are

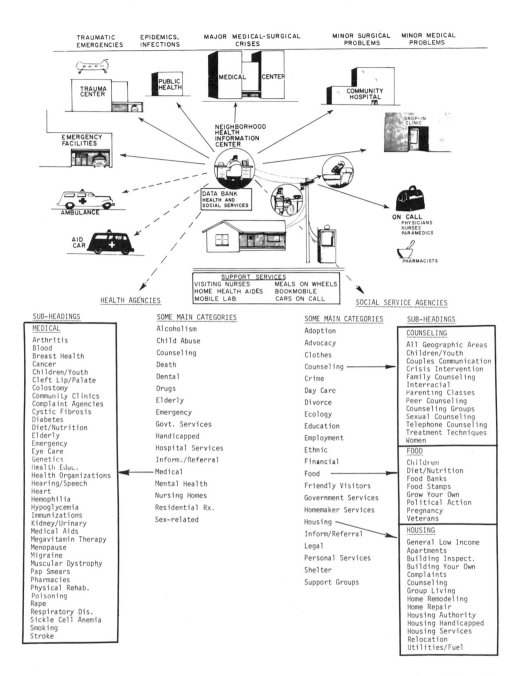

TRAUMATIC EMERGENCIES EPIDEMICS, INFECTIONS MAJOR MEDICAL-SURGICAL CRISES MINOR SURGICAL PROBLEMS MINOR MEDICAL PROBLEMS

TRAUMA CENTER

PUBLIC HEALTH

MEDICAL CENTER

COMMUNITY HOSPITAL

DROP-IN CLINIC

EMERGENCY FACILITIES

NEIGHBORHOOD HEALTH INFORMATION CENTER

AMBULANCE

DATA BANK HEALTH AND SOCIAL SERVICES

ON CALL PHYSICIANS NURSES PARAMEDICS

AID CAR

PHARMACISTS

SUPPORT SERVICES
VISITING NURSES   MEALS ON WHEELS
HOME HEALTH AIDES   BOOKMOBILE
MOBILE LAB.   CARS ON CALL

HEALTH AGENCIES   SOCIAL SERVICE AGENCIES

SUB-HEADINGS	SOME MAIN CATEGORIES	SOME MAIN CATEGORIES	SUB-HEADINGS
MEDICAL	Alcoholism	Adoption	COUNSELING
Arthritis	Child Abuse	Advocacy	All Geographic Areas
Blood	Counseling	Clothes	Children/Youth
Breast Health	Death	Counseling	Couples Communication
Cancer	Dental	Crime	Crisis Intervention
Children/Youth	Drugs	Day Care	Family Counseling
Cleft Lip/Palate	Elderly	Divorce	Interracial
Colostomy	Emergency	Ecology	Parenting Classes
Community Clinics	Govt. Services	Education	Peer Counseling
Complaint Agencies	Handicapped	Employment	Counseling Groups
Cystic Fibrosis	Hospital Services	Ethnic	Sexual Counseling
Diabetes	Inform./Referral	Financial	Telephone Counseling
Diet/Nutrition	Medical	Food	Treatment Techniques
Elderly	Mental Health	Friendly Visitors	Women
Emergency	Nursing Homes	Government Services	FOOD
Eye Care	Residential Rx.	Homemaker Services	Children
Genetics	Sex-related	Housing	Diet/Nutrition
Health Educ.		Inform/Referral	Food Banks
Health Organizations		Legal	Food Stamps
Hearing/Speech		Personal Services	Grow Your Own
Heart		Shelter	Political Action
Hemophilia		Support Groups	Pregnancy
Hypoglycemia			Veterans
Immunizations			HOUSING
Kidney/Urinary			General Low Income
Medical Aids			Apartments
Megavitamin Therapy			Building Inspect.
Menopause			Building Your Own
Migraine			Complaints
Muscular Dystrophy			Counseling
Pap Smears			Group Living
Pharmacies			Home Remodeling
Physical Rehab.			Home Repair
Poisoning			Housing Authority
Rape			Housing Handicapped
Respiratory Dis.			Housing Services
Sickle Cell Anemia			Relocation
Smoking			Utilities/Fuel
Stroke			

Figure 8-5. An easily accessible neighborhood health information center would provide information and counseling on a wide variety of service categories typically available in most regions. Such a center could provide information on the full range of social and health services and could include counseling for self-care at certain levels of management.

319

not necessarily medical. Such service could be offered by selected physically handicapped individuals who would be particularly sensitive and responsive to the needs of individuals for "someone to talk to." They could carry on conversations that would tie up a health information center for extended times if the main counselor were the only one available to handle them.

The aided access to physicians, pharmacists, and clinics as illustrated at the right of Figure 8-5 could serve as a valuable backup to anyone who wishes to engage in self care. However, for serious medical and surgical crises or emergencies, additional facilities need to be available. For this purpose the health information center would have available not only the names and capabilities of the various medical centers, but also direct telecommunication access to trauma centers, emergency facilities, ambulances, and aid cars, as required. The services described thus far would appear to overlap those of emergency numbers such as 911, through which people can gain access to emergency services or hospitals for a major medical/surgical crisis. However, the conception of a health information center would include information and guidance into a much broader selection of health and social services than is ordinarily encompassed at the present time.

There are two contexts in which a health information center might be conceived. In an affluent neighborhood in a suburb, such a service could be developed to provide a valued service that would be economically self-supporting, despite the fact that individuals are perfectly prepared to pay for their medical care. The most important attribute of such a center would be that it would be immediately accessible without delays to provide necessary health guidance. It would be supplemented in most cases by a health professional in the form of a nurse-consultant or a paramedical person (see Chapter 7). Such a person would be in a position to provide immediate health counseling about the proper management of simple self-limiting illnesses, or advice regarding whether or not a particular complaint requires prompt medical attention. In addition to the medical problem, the health information center could also be a source of valuable information regarding other kinds of nonmedical services that are health-related.

Almost all population centers are now endowed with very large numbers of social and health service agencies, both voluntarily and governmentally supported. In large metropolitan areas, these are so numerous that the selection or access becomes exceedingly complex. For example, in the Seattle area, there are some 3,000 health and social service agencies covering a very wide range of personal needs and requirements of the sort which are illustrated at the bottom of Figure 8-5. Included in this formidable selection of agencies are potential answers for a very wide spectrum of problems that might affect most anyone in a modern society.

The categories of social and health agencies illustrated at the bottom of Figure 8-5 include many subheadings, and each of the subheadings contains a wide selection of different agencies. Obviously, several different specific agencies are prepared to deal with problems related to arthritis, blood, breast, health, cancer, children and youth, cleft palate, and so forth. The current deficiency is a lack of clear understanding on the part of most people regarding what kinds of services are available in these various agencies, where they are located, how to get access to them, and how they relate to the health services provided by a physician or other health professionals. The average citizen is quite unaware of the nature, scope, and services rendered by these various agencies, and physicians are not very much better informed. There is a need for a readily accessible entrance into this huge and valuable resource. Information and referral services have been set up in large communities but the problem has mushroomed so rapidly that now there is a plethora of information and referral services, so that it is even difficult to decide which of these should be contacted. The concept of a health information center could facilitate the process of deciding which agency would be most appropriate for a specific kind of problem with possibilities for feedback on which are most effective in the provision of desired services.

The resources available through social service agencies are also very large. Many provide help to people coping with the problems of modern society in terms of clothing, counseling, food, and housing, as indicated at the right of Figure 8-5. The main categories contain substantial numbers of subheadings, and each subheading contains multiple listings of individual agencies. It seems obvious that patients with health-related psychosocial problems could more properly be referred to carefully selected agencies rather than to continue to rely solely on physicians to provide advice about such problems. The health information center concept described above is primarily a guidance mechanism by which people with problems might be aided in their efforts to gain appropriate access to health services. An expansion of the concept would provide an even more valuable supplement to individual efforts at self-reliance and self-care.

The health information center is a concept that has another potentially valuable connotation. Medically deprived populations of the country (i.e., central cities) could derive considerable benefit from a central source of information of this sort. It would enable individuals who need guidance into the complex health care system to obtain the kind of help which could both reduce unnecessary demands on the system and at the same time provide rapid response to specific problems with the kind of services which are most relevant.

AIDED SELF-RELIANCE

The aids to access described in the preceding paragraphs do not cover diagnosis or therapy. They are intended to facilitate access to the necessary kinds of health care. However, if the person manning the health information center were a trained health professional of one sort or another, with access to a physician, an enormous amount of very useful information could be conveyed on the telephone to help individuals take care of their illnesses. For example, a nurse practitioner or a consulting nurse in such a situation is capable of providing a wealth of information that will tend to resolve a very large proportion of the minor complaints and concerns which beset any family several times a year. This is the operational equivalent of relying upon the clinic nurse of a family physician for such information and has therefore a long tradition.

Nurse Consultants. A very successful prototype of health counselors was set up to provide valuable information over the telephone by nurse consultants at Group Health Cooperative of Puget Sound, a prepaid comprehensive health plan that serves 250,000 enrollees. A room next to the emergency clinic of this organization has been set aside as a small office in which three highly qualified nurses rotate around the clock, 24 hours a day, answering questions by telephone for many of the enrollees. The diversity of questions encountered is utterly enormous. On the other hand, the warmth and sympathy with which these nurses explore the problems, counsel and advise appropriate action, is exceedingly reassuring. From this central location, the nurse consultants are equally able to respond to emergency situations by arranging for ambulance service if that is necessary. They routinely alert doctors in the emergency clinic as to the types of cases which are being referred in. If the question appears to be relatively straightforward, these nurses discuss the symptoms and their significance, recommend courses of action, and then arrange for check-backs at appropriate intervals. This is one health service that has received unanimous and unqualified approval throughout the entire organization.

A simple survey indicated that the nurse consultants receive some 10,000 calls a month, at an average overall cost of about 56¢ per call. It is estimated that approximately 60% of the problems presented during the calls are handled over the telephone without the necessity for an encounter with a physician. Those problems requiring a clinic visit are more effectively managed in the interval between the initial call for assistance and the ultimate encounter with a physician. If the problem is sufficiently puzzling or serious, the nurse consultant has ready access to a specific physician for additional advice and counsel, but this is required only on rare occasions. Listening to a sequence of these calls over a period of a few hours leaves a lasting impression that the simple home remedies that are commonly recommended are greatly welcomed by the concerned patients or their parents. Furthermore, the reassurance that is provided by this contact with a health professional is an extremely valuable asset for the health cooperative. This health counseling function has been so successful, that it is now being extended by establishing health counseling procedures in the nine ambulatory clinics, and in some cases, in the clusters which compose them.

During recent years there has been a rapid emergence of a wide variety of new health professionals. These represent expanded roles for nurses, nurse practitioners, physicians' assistants (Chapter 7). They have been trained to relieve physicians of some of the more routine aspects of medical care, in accordance with their particular levels of training, experience, and competence. Persons selected to play the role of the health counselor in a health information center could be selected from this broad selection of health personnel, depending on the particular situation, the nature of the population to be served, and the type and proximity of supervision. In some instances, persons living within the neighborhood could be specifically trained to establish a health information center at home after intensive training in the process. This approach is reminiscent of the development of village health aides for the native villages of Alaska, which has proved to be very successful in providing valuable health services in exceedingly remote and inaccessible areas (Chapter 7).

Technologies in Home Care. Specialized technology of modern health care can effectively support and supplement individual initiatives. Biomedical engineering has produced many home health aides, assistive devices, and handicapped self-help equipment to be used in homes. Hospitals and hospital supply companies once had control over this type of equipment, but through clinical evaluation programs and consumer feedback, appropriate changes toward simplicity, functional ease, and compactness have been made, thus making more feasible the use of biomedical equipment in the home. A prime example of family care and modern medical care working together to provide health care is seen in the home peritoneal dialysis program. At the kidney centers sponsoring home dialysis, patients and families of patients are intensively trained by a team of health professionals to render patients and families self-sufficient in the complex process of routine dialysis for kidney failure.

The management of most chronic diseases (i.e., diabetes, arthritis) necessarily requires a collaborative effort among health professionals, patients, and their families. For example, the home hypertension program cannot be simply managed by daily blood pressure readings. The person's diet, exercise level, and emotional levels are all important to hypertensive management as well as blood pressure readings. Evaluating these additional parameters may be performed by family members, with guidance by health care professionals. The skills and knowledge to perform the various required roles and activities are transferred from professional to patient and family.

Educational services of this kind are numerous and include hospital patient education programs, outpatient programs, clinic-based classes and courses, health maintenance organizations, health education classes, and industrial and occupational health education programs. In all these instances the public receives information to help them more actively participate in self-care activities ranging from decision making to physical care skills.

Rehabilitation encourages and requires self-initiated behaviors. The successes of patient-education programs for chronic illness stem from the patient's generally obvious need to assume responsibility and undertake initiatives in hospital and at home.

Such programs could be rendered more effective by a number of steps such as:

1. Including family/friends in their development and implementation.
2. Encouraging patient independence in care activities.
3. Practicing self-care, to the extent of the patient's capability and desire while in the hospital. Learning through experiencing and evaluating one's performance is more effective than description or demonstration. In addition, hospital-based self-care practice could render more gradual the transition from hospital to home.

In Philadelphia, patients at the Pennsylvania Urban Health Maintenance Program (23) and, in Seattle, patients at the University of Washington are under "contract" to be a responsible partner in their care. The contracts at the University of Washington specify the procedures agreed upon (i.e., daily muscle strengthening exercises, regimented dietary intake), with specific rewards contingent on conforming to contract. In some cases, noncompliance results in sending the patient to another hospital program (24).

Mutual Aid Groups. Certain chronic ailments are more amenable to management by nonprofessional peers than by fully trained health professionals. A notable example is alcoholism, for which Alcoholics Anonymous has compiled a very impressive record of success. There is a bond of sympathy coupled with personal experience which can be supportive and effective in helping deal successfully with personal experience which can be supportive and effective in helping deal successfully with persistent problems. For example, patients with colostomies are confronted with unique problems which can be relieved by gaining skills to surmount both the practice and psychological problems of managing excreta. Such mutual aid groups have been expanding in numbers, diversity, and scope as an indication that they serve an important role in the overall health care delivery system. The exchange of information, experience, and support through mutual aid groups could be actively encouraged by the health professions to the benefit of all concerned.

SUMMARY

1. Self-care is still the predominant mode of health care, despite the progressive assumption over time by health professionals and the government of functions which are properly the responsibility of individual citizens.
2. A working definition of self-care needs to emphasize the concept of the individual citizen as *subject* initiating action rather than the *object* of health professionals' actions.
3. There is opportunity for even more self-care, given the large number of trivial and self-limiting ailments for which people unnecessarily consult physicians.
4. Reliance on "experts" fosters dependence. The idea of a participative partnership between providers and citizens can foster a socially desirable *interdependence*, which avoids costs associated with the other two extremes while still providing their benefits.
5. The quality of treatment for common ailments has not kept pace with the quantity of expenditures for their diagnosis. Thus, a major challenge for health education is to find ways to help people learn that most illnesses which they bring to doctors are rarely serious and that their bodies are fully capable of overcoming most problems without reliance on sophisticated technologies.

6. Responsible self-direction in health care implies that people accept responsibility for the consequences of their self-care decisions. The participative partnership in this case requires a reassessment of "provider" and "consumer" roles.

7. The health care system contains many effective obstacles to self-care such as specialization, high technology, jargon, and current economic incentives. Intensive and extensive research efforts should be encouraged to identify and test means for eliminating barriers to self-care now extant within the health care system.

8. Opportunities for participative partnerships exist and require evaluation to determine the extent to which they meet the goals of health care and improve accessibility without increasing cost. These concepts need to be tested as part of the process of health services assessment (see Chapter 6).

9. The preceding discussion is intended to convey the impression that the traditional reliance of the public on physicians as the ultimate arbiter on health matters is undergoing significant revision. The average citizen is now much better informed on health matters than all previous generations. There are opportunities for diversifying and improving health care delivery which should be pursued despite the impending development of National Health Insurance.

REFERENCES

1. Levin LS, Katz AH, Holst E: *Self Care: Lay Initiatives in Health*. New York, Prodist, 1976.
2. Pratt L: The significance of the family in medication. *J Fam Studies*, 4:13-31, Spring, 1973.
3. Fry J: *Self Care: Its Place in the Total Health Care System*. A Report to the Copenhagen Conference on the Role of the Individual in Primary Health Care, in Katz AH, Holst E (eds): *Lay Initiatives in Health*. New York, Prodist, 1973.
4. Kirscht DP: The health belief model and illness behavior, in Becker MH (ed): *The Health Belief Model and Personal Health Behavior*. Thorofare, NJ, Charles B Slack, 1974.
5. Dunnell K, Cartwright A: *Medicine Takers, Prescribers, and Hoarders*. London, Routledge and Kegan Paul, 1972.
6. Levin LS: Forces and Issues in the Revival of Interest in Self Care: Impetus for Redirection in Health, in Fonaroff AL and Levin L (eds): *Issues in Self Care. Health Education Monographs*, vol 5, no 2. pp 115-120, 1977.
7. Hodgkin K: *Toward Earlier Diagnosis*. London, C and S Livingstone, 1966.
8. Ambulatory Care Utilization Patterns of Children and Young Adults: National Ambulatory Medical Care Survey, National Center for Health Statistics, 1978.
9. Thomas L: *The Lives of a Cell: Notes of a Biology Watcher*. New York, Viking Press, 1972.
10. Rushmer RF: *Cardiovascular Dynamics*, ed. 4. Philadelphia, WB Saunders Co, 1975.

11. Becker MH: *The Health Belief Model and Personal Health Behavior.* Thorofare, NJ, Charles B Slack, 1974.
12. Gordon G, Anderson OW, Brehm HP, Marquis S: *Disease, the Individual, and Society.* College and University Press, Publishers, New Haven, Conn, 1968.
13. Harris L and Associates: *Chicago's Health. A Study of Health Beliefs, Knowledge and Behavior Among Residents in the Chicago Area.* Vols I, II. October 1976.
14. Huber MJ, Patrinos D: Preliminary thoughts on the concept of health as an obligation. *Futures Conditional* 5:18-19 (3), November 1977.
15. Cousins N: *What You Owe the Doctor, Seattle Times.* vol 4, p A12, September 24, 1978.
16. Guttmarcher S: A critique of self help and self care. *Futures Conditional* 5:20-21 (3), November, 1977.
17. Breslow L, Bellock NB: *Futures Conditional* 5:19 (3) November, 1977.
18. Knowles J: The responsibility of the individual, in Knowles J (ed): *Doing Better and Feeling Worse,* New York, WW Norton and Company, 1977.
19. Vickery D, Fries J: *Take Care of Yourself; A Consumer's Guide to Medical Care.* Reading, Mass, Addison-Wesley Publishing Company, 1976.
20. Sehnert K: *How to be Your Own Doctor—Sometimes.* New York, Grosset and Dunlap, 1975.
21. Samuels M, Bennett H: *Well Body Book.* New York, Random House, 1973.
22. Sherman H, Reiffen B, Komaroff ALAL: Aids to the delivery of ambulatory medical care. *IEEE Trans Biomed Eng* BME-20, 165-174, 1973.
23. Lanberg L: Patient, help thyself. *Fam Health* 7:34-8, January, 1975.
24. Anderson R: Seattle Programs Involving Our City's Elderly. 815 4th Avenue North, Seattle, Washington, 1976.

CHAPTER 9

Alternatives From Abroad: Prototypes in the World Laboratory

The requirements for forward planning have become increasingly urgent with the growing complexity of the biomedical research enterprise and of the health care delivery systems. The emergence of program evaluation (Chapter 6) and technology assessment (Chapter 5) illustrates the recognized need for assessing the consequences of decisions about both services and facilities by the most relevant and reliable analytic procedures that can be mustered. In each case, the ultimate evaluation is generally based on analyzing feasibility studies, demonstration units, clinical trials, or introduction of innovations into routine practice. All these options have become inordinately expensive to the point that there is really no prospect of comprehensive evaluation of the many changes appearing in rapid succession. Important additions to our fund of knowledge and experience can be obtained from the actual experience of other countries or cultures. The world can be viewed as a vast complex of social laboratories in which corresponding problems have been addressed by very different approaches.

The international dissemination of scientific and technical literature is rapid and effective among research communities in various countries. Strangely enough, exchanges of information between countries is relatively deficient with respect to favorable or unfavorable consequences of various organizational and operational approaches to biomedical research and practice. For example, the countries of Western Europe have many decades of experience with various forms of nationwide health services, supported by government appropriations. They have many similar features but represent a variety of policies, priorities, strategies, and procedures. Among these diverse approaches there exists an enormous body of information and experience covering some of the sources of uncertainty confronting this country as we attempt to forecast the consequences of various versions of National Health Insurance. The differences in their social, economic, and cultural backgrounds may complicate extrapolation from their experiences to the conditions obtaining in the United States. On the other hand, many of the myriad approaches can be regarded as feasibility or demonstration programs of potential value in planning for our own plunge into this complex morass.

Awareness of consequences and costs of various prototypes in other countries could have great value in avoidance of irreversible miscalculations, that could represent enormous waste of time, energy, and resources. A comprehensive review of the many examples could not be approached in this kind of publication. However, some specific examples derived from on site observations in selected countries can serve to illustrate opportunities that deserve consideration. For this purpose, Great Britain, Sweden, and Canada have been selected as representative of comprehensive commitments to National Health Services in very different geographical and political environments.

CHARACTERISTICS OF HEALTH SERVICES IN SELECTED COUNTRIES

The United States has lagged behind other developed countries of the world in commitment of government to equitable access to health services by all segments of the population. Legislation authorizing federal funds to facilitate access to health services for the senior citizens (Medicare) and for the disadvantaged (Medicaid) are relatively recent in comparison with developments in all other countries of Western Europe. The initial experience with health insurance began in Germany under Bismarck. The Swedish National Health Services were introduced nearly 40 years ago after an intensive study of requirements. The National Health Service of Great Britain was introduced by Aneurin Bevan directly after World War II and is probably the most familiar form of "socialized medicine" to American citizens. Although we can learn from successes and complications encountered in any culture, Great Britain, Sweden, and Canada have been selected as representative of the kinds of approaches toward equality of access worthy of consideration for adoption or modification for the American people (Table 9-1).

Only about one-third of the American people have insurance against major medical problems (generally restricted in duration or amount). More than half (65%) have some degree of coverage for hospitalization. The coverage is incomplete for all but the very wealthy or very fortunate. The populations of Great Britain, Sweden, and Canada have attained a far greater equality of access than these figures indicate for the United States (Table 9-1A).

The availability of health services is limited by resources in Britain, and deficiencies are represented by waiting periods (Table 9-1B). In Sweden, high-quality services are more generously supported and available as needed

TABLE 9-1. Health Care Comparisons: Potential Prototypes

Characteristics	Great Britain	Sweden	Canada	United States
A. Prime objective: Equality of access	Almost 100%	Almost 100%	Almost 100%	Major medical 35% Regular med. 65% Hospital 85%
B. Utilization	As available	As needed	"Medically necessary"	As covered or affordable
C. Physicians' income	NHS scales or Contracts	Uniform pay scales	Fee for service	Fee for service
D. Hospitals	Government owned	Regional and county owned	Private, nonprofit	Private, nonprofit
E. Cost controls	80% central 9% NHS payments 6.5% local	75% county councils, 10% cities, 20% federal	Provincial, 50% central govt. 50%	(See Figure 5.7)
F. Planning	Regional health authorities	Regional, county councils	Provincial	Health systems agencies
G. Quality of care Metropolitan Rural, remote areas	 ++ ++++	 ++++ ++++	 ++++ +++-0	 ++ +++-0
H. Public attitudes	Generally satisfied (except for delays)	Generally satisfied	Generally satisfied	Satisfied but critical of costs and primary care
I. Prime priorities	Aging Mental illness Handicapped Child health	Alcoholism Handicapped Aging Integrated care	Heart Disease Accidents Resp. Dis. Suicide	Cancer Heart disease Chronic disease Environmental hazards
J. Research support	Medical Research Council	Institute for Rationalizing Health and Social Welfare (SPRI)	National Research Council	National Institutes of Health and related agencies

329

with relatively few unmet needs. The Canadian approach is to provide health services as medically necessary. In the United States the services are most effectively used by those who are covered by third parties or are relatively affluent. The funds supporting health services are predominantly from the central government in Britain (1) and primarily by local governments (County Councils and cities) in Sweden (2) (Table 9-1E). Costs are shared between the provinces and the central government in Canada. In the United States there is a strong tendency toward centralization of health care in Washington by large funding sources (Medicare, Medicaid, VA, Department of Defense, etc.).

The National Health Services of Sweden were developed in a deliberate and orderly process after a great deal of planning, organization, and with generous financial support (Table 9-1F). In contrast, the British, Canadian, and American systems have developed by a process of spontaneous evolution strongly impelled by political pressures and expediency with powerful influences exerted by the medical professions.

In Britain the quality of care in outlying areas is widely regarded as superior to that available in metropolitan areas. It is uniformly good in Sweden except for the remotest areas of the north. In Canada and the United States the quality of care is nonuniform, ranging from good (+++) to none at all (0) in rural and remote areas and in central cities (Table 9-1G).

The public is generally satisfied with the health services delivered in all four countries. The British are pleased with their acute care but are critical of long waiting periods (i.e., for elective surgery). The Swedish and Canadian systems are generally approved by the public. The segment of the American public that gains access to health services is generally satisfied with services but disturbed by the high and rising costs and deficiencies in primary care (Table 9-1H).

The prime priorities for current and future developments are distinctly different in the four countries (Table 9-1I). These priorities are reflected in the allocation of resources for both health services and research, as indicated below. The mechanisms by which research is supported in the four countries have much in common. The Medical Research Council of Great Britain is an interesting counterpart of the NIH of the United States (Table 9-1J).

BRITISH BIOMEDICAL RESEARCH

The medical research enterprise of Britain is widely acknowledged as of the highest quality. The magnitude and significance of British contributions to current knowledge seems out of proportion to the magnitude of the budgetary allocation. To be specific, the United States medical research budgets are about 20 times the amount of support provided the British effort. Indeed, the total biomedical research support in Britain is approximately the amount of money spent by the NIH in *administering* its research programs. The underlying factors which are responsible for the unquestioned excellence and productivity of the Britsh research effort deserves careful consideration, particularly with current constraints imposed in the United States.

National pride has always been directed toward fine academic institutions, notably Oxford and Cambridge, creating a tradition of scholarship and popular respect for learning. Governmental support of pure science has been extremely generous and unquestioning up until relatively recent times. Recognizing that the total number of people who make major contributions in scientific efforts is relatively small, generous support is provided the most illustrious talents on the cutting edge of science. It is also reinforced by longer periods of training, which provide opportunities for observation of upcoming scientists while they are in subordinate positions. Britain is a relatively small country and the total number of research positions is small enough that senior members of the research community are intimately familiar with virtually all other colleagues in the same areas of interest.

Until recently, the governmental priorities for science were relatively nonspecific and tended to allow for somewhat more basic and balanced attack on problems than is generally manifest in the United States.

The Medical Research Council is the British counterpart for the National Institutes of Health. A medical Research Committee was set up in 1913 as part of the National Insurance Act of 1911 with £53 thousand accumulated by setting aside one penny for each insured person. This function was encorporated by Royal Charter as the Medical Research Council (MRC) in 1920 as a responsibility of the Privy Council. By 1976–1977, the Council was responsible for expenditure of £52 million (3). Consistent and conscientious efforts have been expended to allocate federal financial resources by mechanisms that assure quality, maintain academic freedom and avoid governmental involvement.

FUNCTIONAL MECHANISMS OF THE MEDICAL RESEARCH COUNCIL

The basic mechanisms of the Medical Research Council resemble a small version of NIH in many respects. The Medical Research Council consists of about 20 members with policy-making groups maintaining oversight over four Research Boards and a committee on Environmental Medicine (Fig. 9-1).

There are two main ways in which research is supported through the Medical Research Council:

1. Directly by staff employed in research institutes and units;
2. Indirectly by supporting the staff of other organizations, especially universities, by
   a. three-year project grants
   b. longer-term program grants in fields where Council policy has defined a special need
   c. block grants to independent research institutions

MEDICAL RESEARCH COUNCIL: ORGANIZATIONAL RELATIONS

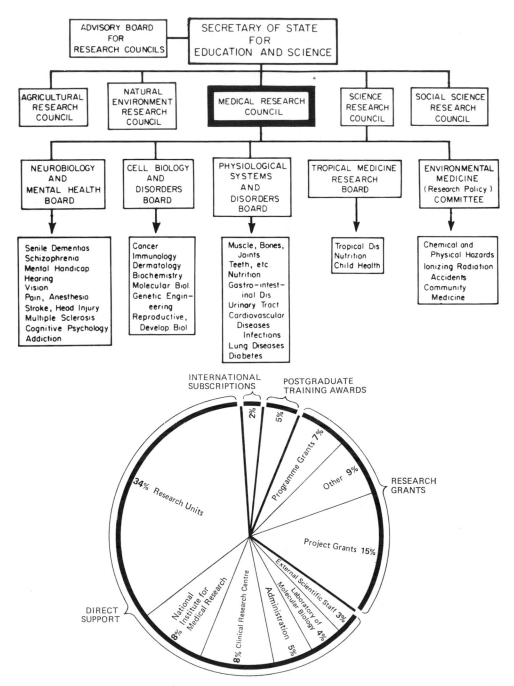

Figure 9-1. The Medical Research Council of Britain is one of five research councils under the Secretary of State for Education and Science. The Medical Research council plays a role for Britain similar to the Institutes of Health in the U.S. Investigator initiated projects represent only about half the allocation to research units which resemble major program projects or centers in the NIH. The National Institute for Medical Research and the Clinical Research Centre are roughly equivalent to the NIH intramural programs.

d. fellowships, studentships, and other awards for training for research careers.

Project Grant Review Processes. Each of the Boards has two project grant committees meeting about five times a year to review project proposals. As a first step, the staff studies the proposals and sends each one to referees (2-4) for review. Two members of the committee are designated to engage in special homework on each grant. The chairman digests the reports of the referees and the material is presented to the committee as a whole. All members of the committee score each grant request on a scale of one to six. The process is rendered most effective by the intimate acquaintance between the applicants and review bodies in the tight community of scholars in Britain. The allocation of funds is influenced to a significant degree by the priorities established by the leadership and membership of the Medical Research Council. Examples of priorities as of 1976-1977 are listed in Table 9-1I. These priorities exhibit a pronounced orientation toward the problems of the aging, the handicapped (physical, emotional, and mental), and the developing child. These priorities are representative of national research goals in Britain which differ greatly from those in the United States (see Prime Priorities in Table 9-1).

Program Grants (7% of Budget). The research boards also review long-term program grants for research, ordinarily of five years' duration and awarded generally to well-established investigators. The program proposals are circulated to reviewers, and interviews are commonly conducted with the principal investigator(s). These awards tend to cover two to five research assistants and perhaps three or more technicians, ranging in value from £100-300,000 over a five-year period.

Research Units. Once or twice a year, each of the boards may identify one or more "Research Units" by selecting some area(s) deserving more intensive research effort, or promising rapid progress. The size of units can vary from relatively modest to very large programs. Ordinarily, the suggestions for new units come from universities. Once a unit is established, a search for an appropriate director is instituted. In general there is a fairly vigorous response because universities tend to covet units. The selection of the director is regarded as crucial; in fact, if an appropriate one is not identified, the unit may be cancelled. As a result of this activity, 30-40 units may be operative at any particular time, supported by about 35% of the MRC budget (Fig. 9-1).

Intramural Programs. The Medical Research Council also supports two major Research Institutions, each receiving about 8% of the budget (Fig. 9-1):

1. The National Institute for Medical Research
2. The Clinical Research Center

These are both very large organizations with permanent staffs and organized by divisions. Each division is a responsibility of one of the three boards, with on-site monitoring on alternate years. At the end of each four-year period, a more extensive review is undertaken. An example of the current level of activity and the scope of its enterprise is indicated by some sample innovative approaches to care of the aged (see below).

Policies and Priorities of the Medical Research Council. The annual reports to Parliament by the Medical Research Council tend to emphasize the relevance of the various research efforts to categorical diseases or malfunction. According to Sir Harold Himsworth (4a) and Dr. J.L. Gowans (4b), the underlying philosophy of the MRC is based on the following considerations:

1. The operational priorities of the Medical Research Council are based very largely on previous research programs and experience.
2. The most important consideration is the identification of good research talent, based largely on previous performance in the development of promising and innovative ideas.
3. The support of quality is the most important consideration in establishing priorities.
4. Selection is based on confidence that good scientists are as interested and concerned with relevance as are the public and their representatives in government.
5. There is an underlying conviction that real advances in science are made by a relatively few people in any society, so that you can't "buy progress" with a flood of funds.
6. Finally, the limiting factor in scientific progress is the quantity and quality of the talent.

RELEVANCE REQUIRED BY THE ROTHSCHILD REPORT

The biomedical research efforts in most developed countries have encountered increasingly strident criticism of scanty return on large investments in basic research. The very high quality and relatively cost-effective research efforts in Britain have not spared the Medical Research Council restraints imposed for the announced purpose of assuring greater applicability of the overall research effort. The manifestations of discontent took the form of budgetary constraints and the insertion of an additional layer of bureaucracy in the sequence of allocating research resources.

The essential requirements for basic medical research as a prerequisite to mounting major campaigns against disease were recognized in Britain and in the United States alike (4a). The anticipated cure and control of the major diseases of the day have failed to materialize at the rate anticipated by the public servants that control the federal funds. All five of the major research councils, illustrated in Figure 9-1, have been under increasing attack with allegations that their research was not sufficiently relevant to the needs of the corresponding departments. During the four decades before 1970, the five research councils shared a common approach, characterized by deliberate policy of supporting scientists with proven research records. Judged in terms of scientific achievement, this approach was highly successful. In general, the most eminent scientists were engaged primarily in basic research, and therefore they tended to win in open competition against others oriented toward more applied objectives. The fundamental attitude of the research councils could be accurately described as elitist in the sense that they did not bend to political pressures readily. From 1966 to 1970 the successive Ministers of Health criticized policies of the Medical Research Council in the belief that the output lacked emphasis on needs of the Department of Health and Social Security. Successive surveys and investigative reports displayed that there was actually a larger percentage of applied research than most people recognized, but these data failed to satisfy critics.

In response to many pressures, the Central Policy Review Staff was delegated the responsibility of conducting a review of government strategies for research and development. Lord Rothschild, the chairman, announced a new scheme for enhancing the relevance of research being conducted by the research councils in general and the Medical Research Council in particular. The report (5) incorporated the concept that applied research and development must be done on customer-contractor basis.

> The customer says what he wants; the contractor does it (if he can); and the customer pays. Basic, fundamental, or pure research, called basic research in this report, has no analogous customer-contractor basis, though those engaged in such work may and sometimes too often, do, become involved in applied R & D. . . . The country's needs are not so trivial to be left to the mercies of a form of scientific roulette, with many more than the conventional 37 numbers on which the ball may land.

The Rothschild report also contained some specific recommendations regarding the means of enhancing the prospects that the research supported by the MRC would have more tangible relevance to the nation's health. The Medical Research Council's involvement in applied research and development was estimated to be about 25% of the total budget. On this basis, it was recommended that about one quarter of the MRC budget be removed and allocated to the Department of Health and Social Services to be disbursed to projects selected by the Department of Health and Social Services (DHSS). The chief scientist of the DHSS was expected to establish mechanisms for developing priorities and allocation procedures to meet more effectively the needs of the department.

The undesirable consequences of this approach to research management were reviewed after five years in a report of a Nuffield Working Party (6). According to this analysis, the attempts to establish an adequate customer organization appear to have failed. The chief scientist did not set up an adequate organization. The accountability seemed no better than was provided by the Research Councils. The net effect has been to add an additional layer of bureaucracy in the path of allocating some 25% of the Medical Research Council's budget. The areas of research do not appear to have been significantly changed, in part due to the fact that the DHSS advisory bodies tended to be composed of roughly the same individuals as had been advising the Medical Research Council in the first place.

As one manifestation, "research liaison groups" were formed to be the customer organization of the DHSS. Unfortunately, these liaison groups were composed very largely of nonmedical, administrative civil servants whose basic jobs were to maintain health and personal or social services under extremely difficult conditions. They were under heavy political pressure and confronted by a bewildering number of subjects and areas for consideration. Some of the liaison groups have performed well, but most of them have been lacking in visible evidence of success.

The pressures for payoff for the generous investments in basic research in the United States have many of the same elements as the problems arising in Britain. It is hoped that the current efforts by Congress to increase the applicability of our research can take cognizance of the dangers inherent in approaches like those recommended in the Rothschild report.

Disquieting Trends and Portents for the Future. The British research establishment is undergoing a period of serious trial with potentially disastrous effects in the future. The most clearly evident problem is the effect of financial constraints. Britain is having much the same kind of problem facing up to the contraction of funding as has occurred in the United States. In Britain, the universities expanded rather continuously for about 20 years. In the 1960s, a substantial number of new positions opened up and were filled by the young scientists at that time. The number of positions is now relatively fixed, causing a serious shortage of open positions for newly trained scientists. With increasing frequency, highly trained people are required to pursue many nontraditional avenues in search of professional careers, despite credentials that would have easily assured them a promising career in the past (4c). Many such individuals are unsuccessful in obtaining positions in academic institutions—often after as many as 10 years of successful research on federal grants. An example of the financial stress is represented by changes in sources of support. Some university laboratories that had only 5% of their budgets from grants in 1969 are now deriving some 60% of their budgets from research grant sources. This condition was encountered within Oxford University, where funding in the past has been quite generous. The conditions in other academic institutions must be even more serious.

Disincentives for Research Careers. In the past, careers in basic research in prestigious academic institutions were extremely attractive to young people graduating from their schools of medicine. At the present time there is a growing shortage of fellowship funds which will support young students interested in academic careers. As mentioned above, the number of positions available is also highly restricted and provides a high level of uncertainty regarding future professional opportunities. Research funds are limited from both the universities and the grant sources. Finally, the financial rewards for engaging in basic medical research have been seriously undermined. The salary scales for various levels in universities are established on a nationwide basis. They have been increasing at an average of about 10% a year during times when the inflation rate was as high as 20%. It is now estimated that the academic salaries have effectively declined about 20% during the past three years, and current efforts to bring equity back are only partially successful.

Financial rewards for engaging in clinical medicine have been increasingly attractive. Income and conditions of practice have been greatly improved for the general practitioners through the active efforts to encourage and support group practice and to provide additional fringe benefits for special kinds of services. More recently, the junior house officers and registrars have received considerable improvement in their income, including mechanisms by which they can actually supplement their income to levels above that of their supervising consultants (7). The income of consultants is being negotiated upward due to this pressure from below. All these trends toward more favorable income and career opportunities in clinical medicine are causing shifts of basic medical research activities to clinical departments, with some depletion in the activities in basic medical science departments.

These factors all militate against the recruiting of high quality young investigative personnel into the training required for academic positions. If these trends persist, the future of quality research in Britain is very much in doubt.

The basic medical sciences in the United States have been examining their future with evident concern, just as have the corresponding investigators in Britain. Pressures for curtailing or cutting back predoctoral and post-doctoral training by congressional action also tends to reduce the number of opportunities for young, enthusiastic investigators to enter these careers. The concerns expressed by congressmen that training more basic medical scientists will only increase the costs of research without corresponding benefits in terms of improved health status of the people is certainly a short sighted view. However, it could ultimately affect the total research capability of the United States in much the same way that the future in Britain appears threatened.

PROTOTYPE: A NATIONAL HEALTH SERVICE (BRITAIN)

The United States is progressively moving toward some form of national health insurance. The economic impact of greatly expanding the access to "artificially cheap" health care (see Chapter 6) could be so threatening that every effort should be made to anticipate the kinds of problems that might be encountered. For this purpose, it is wise to look at the experience, both positive and negative, of countries that have had a long-range experience with nationwide health programs supported by public funds.

The British population is confronted by health problems similar to those encountered in America, but an attempt is being made to meet the public needs by different mechanisms, organized in accordance with a different set of priorities. In the United Kingdom, equality of access is the foremost goal. Top priorities are assigned to the aged, handicapped, and developing children. In the United States, quality of care is provided with benevolent extravagance to patients who can afford the costs (directly or through third parties). Use of sophisticated equipment and progressive specialization are the predominant trends in the United States, with emphasis on comprehensive diagnostic efforts. In the United Kingdom, emphasis is on continuity of primary care by teams comprised of general practitioners and health professionals supported by a nationwide network of paramedical and social services.

The advanced state of "socialism" precludes wholesale adoption of the British approach to the conditions prevailing in the United States. The costs of the compassionate health care in Britain represent a heavy burden on a relatively weak economy. Any attempt to provide correspondingly comprehensive care, superimposed on the extravagant and open-ended utilization of sophisticated resources in America would rapidly result in economic collapse of the system. Despite these profound differences in organizational and operational objectives and mechanisms, there are features of the British system that deserve our consideration as potential prototypes that might be modified for use in the United States. Some of the manifestly successful efforts at meeting human needs with different emphasis and approaches can serve as feasibility studies which may be applicable to appropriate situations in the complex patchwork that is America. The size, diversity, and dispersion of the American people across this broad land demand correspondingly diverse, adaptable and imaginative mechanisms for meeting the needs of the people. A brief review of the evolution of the national health service of Great Britain can expose some of the problems that are almost inevitable in any enterprise of this magnitude.

Historical Perspective. The requirements for health care are always greatest among the poor who are least able to afford it. Public relief of the poor in England dates from the Elizabethan Poor Law Act of 1601, which provided the only public service concerned directly or indirectly with the needs of sick and disabled citizens unable to support themselves.

A National Health Insurance Act of 1911 provided a limited range of medical services and a weekly sum paid to insured persons who were sick or disabled, but it was applicable only to the insured person and not to any dependents. Other people had to pay for their medical care and many did by voluntary insurance or through "friendly societies." These arrangements were obviously inadequate, as evidenced by a large proportion of army recruits unfit for service. The commonest reasons were poor physical development, defective vision, and certain chronic illnesses. Inferior health and physical conditions of school children were equally disturbing. Both the unemployment and health insurance arrangements of the 1911 Act were a distinct advantage over the provisions of poor laws, but were unacceptable as a final solution to the problem.

The Beveridge Report (1942) was a document of historical importance, attempting to deal comprehensively for the first time with the problem of poverty. Under the leadership of Sir William Beveridge, social services were expanded in accordance with certain principles (8).

· The relief of need should be only one facet of a social policy concerned with the five major problems of want, disease, ignorance, squalor, and idleness.

· The state should provide security to the individual in response to service. In other words, individuals should work and contribute when they can; the state would provide for them and their dependents when they cannot. The method proposed was a flat rate of benefit with a constant rate of contribution by the individual and the unification of the administrative responsibility, with the inclusion of all workers, either employed by companies or self-employed.

This "ideal" plan for health service was conceived to provide full treatment for every kind of ailment for all citizens without direct payment and without economic barriers to access. During the postwar period, Winston Churchill strongly supported this program as follows:

> Disease must be attacked wherever it occurs, in the poorest or richest man or woman, simply on the ground that it is the enemy . . . Our policy is to create a national health service, in order to secure that everybody in the country, irrespective of means, age, sex, or occupation, shall have equal opportunities to benefit from the best and most up-to-date medical and allied facilities available. (9)

The political advocates of the time were not worried about the cost of a national health service, because of a fallacious concept. It was firmly believed by Aneurin Bevan, that by providing generous health services, the overall health status of the country would improve to the point that the rising costs would reach a peak, then drop. The postwar progress in medical technology was not foreseen. Instead of costs rising to some level of expenditure and then dropping, the demand has continually increased without respite. As a result, increasingly rigid control of health care costs became necessary and was achieved by placing ceilings on the total national health service expenditures.

REGIONAL ORGANIZATION OF NATIONAL HEALTH SERVICES (BRITAIN)

In 1948 the National Health Service was created from the following elements: two different hospital systems (one voluntary and the other public), personal health and sophisticated services administered by local specialists, and general practitioner services financed partly by national health insurance and partly by private payments. A proposal to consolidate all these elements into a single, comprehensive service was effectively resisted by the physicians. Both general practitioners and consultants were opposed to administration of health services by local government. The ultimate decision, in 1948, was to assign to the Ministry of Health responsibility for the central administration of the national health services. Local and regional responsibilities were for:

· Hospital facilities and consultant services
· General practitioners
· Personal health services were divided between three authorities.

Hospital services were planned and regulated by hospital boards for each of 14 regions in England and Wales. Teaching hospitals were administered separately by boards of governors directly responding to the Ministry of Health. Arrangements were slightly different in Scotland and Northern Ireland. Other governmental departments outside of the National Health Service had responsibilities for health, particularly the Ministry of Education (health of school children), the Ministry of Labor (factory hygiene and occupational hazards), the Home Office (Care of Deprived Children), the Board of Control (Lunacy and Medical Deficiency), and the Privy Council (Medical Research).

The Reorganized National Health Service (1974). Organizational consolidation was accomplished in 1974 by incorporating the several components into a more streamlined system, as illustrated in Figure 9-2. Accordingly, the Secretary of State for Social Services is responsible for national policies related to health and for National Health Service under the Department of Health and Social Security. Regional health authorities administer the 14 regions, with advice and guidance from regional advisory committees. Each region is subdivided into areas administered by area health authorities, some of which are divided into two or more districts. (Some areas are composed of single districts.)

Area health authorities are responsible for the 72 areas outside of London, of which 38 correspond to nonmetropolitan counties and 34 to metropolitan districts. The area health authorities are involved in both planning and the operation of services. For those areas containing more than one district, there are district management teams consisting of a consultant, a general practitioner, a district community physician, district nursing officer, district finance officer, and district administrator, who are jointly responsible for district management. The district management team receives direct input from district medical committees representing general practitioners and specialists (including dentists) working in the district. This brief review of the organizational relation of the National Health Service is incomplete, neglecting differences in the mechanisms prevalent in Wales, Scotland, and Northern Ireland.

Wales was a principality of England in 1948, with a degree of autonomy that was partially preserved when the National Health Service was created (10, 11). It is now included as one of the 14 regions and contains about 3 million people. Thus, it has a larger population than other regions and is generally less affluent than many regions in England. It receives an appropriation from the British budget which is apportioned among the various districts by the Secretary of State for Wales. It is widely conceded that the health services of Wales, Scotland, and Northern Ireland have fewer

THE REORGANIZED NATIONAL HEALTH SERVICES

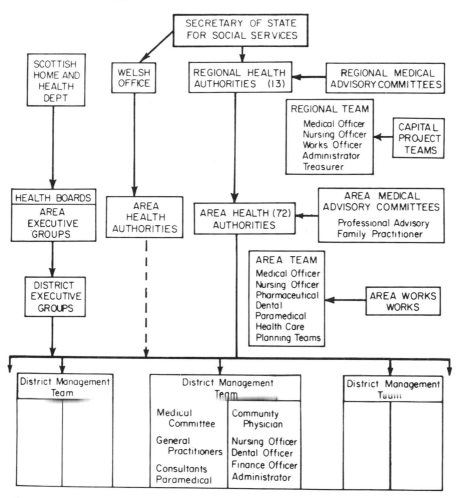

Figure 9-2. The National Health Services of Britain are illustrated after reorganization in 1974 designed to clarify and formalize the roles of regional (13), area health authorities (72) and district organizations covering the British Isles. This organizational hierarchy engages in long range planning efforts as well as provision of health services.

tiers of organization and are more efficiently managed than in England. Thus, they were not affected as profoundly by the reorganization of 1974. One innovation of interest was the development of a more coordinated approach to the provision of sophisticated medical services (i.e., clinical chemistry, chemical pathology, hematology, radiology, and radiotherapy, medical physics, nuclear medicine, etc.). A Welsh Scientific Committee was established with subcommittees representing these various elements of medical technologies to develop policies and priorities for capital equipment, evaluation, purchases, and maintenance, quality control, education and training requirements, use of computers, and so on (4h). By this mechanism, Wales developed mechanisms for more effective utilization and equitable distribution of its capital equipment and sophisticated services than occurred in England. The comprehensive Department of Medical Physics at the University of Cardiff played an important advisory role in relating to the available types of instrumentation.

Scotland and Northern Ireland have preserved a considerable degree of autonomy and retained some distinctive differences in their approaches to health service delivery and organization. The Scottish Home and Health Office deals with health problems in Scotland, while social services are provided by a separate arm of the ministry. Unlike England, Scotland is not divided into regions but is served only by area health authorities (and some district organizations). This substantially reduces the amount of administrative load on the system and is envied by many administrators in England. The financial base of Scotland is less affluent than England despite the North Sea oil development. Sir John Brotherstone (4i) attributed the superior quality of health care in Scotland as due in part to the higher ratio of doctors to the general population, even in highland and island areas. In Scotland, as in other parts of the United Kingdom, the health care provided in outlying areas is substantially better than in metropolitan areas (i.e., Glasgow), where environments are not attractive. In cities, the lists of patients tend to be extremely long and demanding for the available general practitioners who are not uniformly of the highest caliber. In the islands (i.e., Outer Hebrides), physicians are isolated and often lonely. There is growing conviction that these islands might be better served by nurses or other health professionals rather than disgruntled physicians (see Chapter 7).

The Scottish Home and Health Office has its own Chief Scientist, Sir Andrew Watt Kay (4k), encouraging research, development and evaluation programs on a somewhat smaller scale than that of the Medical Research Council and the DHSS in England.

Sir Andrew has succeeded in developing a very effective staff, including twenty professionals, in contrast with the small number of corresponding positions in London. A substantial program in health services research and evaluation has been developed under their initiatives (i.e., studies of cost/effectiveness of various kinds of medical and surgical services). A large number of health centers are being constructed in Glasgow, which has the most highly concentrated and deprived population in Scotland. These health centers are designed to accommodate groups of general practitioners, supported by a variety of other types of health professionals and practitioners (i.e., registered nurses, health visitors, midwives, social workers, etc.). The health centers are designed solely for ambulatory patients and lack beds. Inpatients are accommodated almost exclusively in hospital services under consultants and their attendant "firms."

PROBLEM: PROFESSIONAL PAYMENT POLICIES

General practitioners are the point of initial contact with the National Health Service and are acknowledged as key figures in the system. Their numbers (22,015 in 1974) are reported to exceed the ranks of medical consultants (11,485 in 1976). Except in emergencies, patients are referred to specialists by general practitioners as the main means of gaining access to sophisticated diagnostic facilities and hospital services. Much of the consultant's (specialist's) work load is carried by assistants or "juniors."

A balance is maintained between the numbers of general practitioners and specialists in Britain and other countries of Western Europe. General practitioners are not generally provided staff privileges in hospitals but must refer their patients requiring hospitalization to appropriate specialists. In Britain, the specialists are called consultants and their numbers are limited to fixed numbers of positions for each specialty in each hospital. Each consultant is the leader of a "firm" or a retinue of junior staff physicians, registrars, and others aspiring to attain the exalted position of consultant at some future date. Only a small proportion of these aspirants ultimately achieve a position in a hospital, even after serving periods as "juniors" for a dozen years or more. Since the number of consultants is stringently limited, the remaining graduates of medical school become general practitioners, junior staff physicians, or emigrate to other countries.

The problem of providing equitable and satisfactory remuneration for both consultants and general practitioners has always posed serious problems. In 1948 the general practitioners were not well represented in the negotiations for the NHS. For many years, they were poorly rewarded for heavy and unremitting medical responsibilities. As a consequence, large numbers of these practitioners emigrated, mainly from the areas that needed them most (i.e., underserved metropolitan areas).

Since 1973, the net outflow of United Kingdom and Irish-born doctors has increased and in the last two years has more than doubled, but these are partly replaced by doctors from other countries. One mechanism designed to stem the flow of British doctors is to increase their remuneration which is substantially below those of the other common market countries. The review body of remuneration (7) for 1976 recommended an average increase of £312 per year up to a ceiling of about £8,500.

Because of the very intense competition for positions, consultants are extremely well qualified by any standard. They generally held principal positions of power at the time when the National Health Service was introduced. In order to encourage the consultants to join in the National Health Service, Aneurin Bevan promised them the privilege of practicing private medicine, fee-for-service, in some percentage of the beds in the National Health Service hospitals. By this means, income from private patients supplemented specialists' income and provided important tax deductions which indirectly increased the take-home pay of the consultants. In addition, consultants benefitted from merit or distinction awards, which ranged from very slight to substantial (i.e., £8,000) (1).

Most consultants are affiliated with the NHS and are remunerated by salary, either full time or part time, according to a number of weekly sessions they provide. They have been entitled to two half-days of private practice per week, even when employed "full time." There is widespread suspicion that many of the consultants devote considerably greater proportion of their time to private practice and leave the management of many National Health Service patients to the junior staff.

General practitioners provide primary care for lists of patients who select and sign up with them. At the outset most of these family physicians were in solo practice. The geographical distribution of the general practitioners has been uneven in Britain (as in the United States). In many parts of large metropolitan areas, the number of general practitioners is grossly inadequate. Estimates run as low as 1:100,000 population at the extreme. Thus, the quality of care in many metropolitan areas is manifestly deficient, as indicated below. On the other hand, most general practitioners are conscientious and provide good or excellent levels of care, particularly in smaller communities and rural areas. Many are not inclined to depend upon sophisticated diagnostic technologies for their routine primary care. However, they can refer patients for laboratory work at the hospitals in the vicinity or refer patients to consultants as the conditions warrant.

Despite common misconceptions, the general practitioners are not on salary, but have individual contracts with the National Health Service with reimbursement based on a complicated formula involving the number of people enrolled on their list, plus a number of other factors (nowadays including such services as obstetrics, family planning, and home visits).

The National Health Service has been financed mainly by taxation and only marginally by insurance contributions. During the economically favorable years of 1950s and 1960s, health services expanded both in magnitude and diversity of the services provided, so the level of satisfaction was quite high. The need for delivering health services often took precedence over budgetary allocations for capital improvements and construction. Hospital construction costs increased from less than 3% of total in 1951 to 6.5% in 1970 but the average age of hospitals was reduced only from 70 years to an average age of 50 years (1).

Technological developments have greatly increased the cost of facilities for both diagnosis and therapy, further diluting the available funds for maintaining the integrity of the facilities. For this reason, many of the National Health Service hospitals are in a serious state of disrepair. A disquieting number of new hospitals have not been opened for lack of money to run them, and many valuable facilities are underutilized for lack of staff (i.e., technicans or nurses). The situation has become progressively more intense during the recent downturn of the British economy.

Complications of Providing Equitable Compensation. The incomes of general practitioners have been substantially improved in recent years. Junior staff members in consultant "firms" succeeded in obtaining overtime payments for the long hours that they worked. Some claimed to be working as many as 100 hours per week. The cost of this increase was more than twice as much as expected because the "juniors" working under the consultants discovered that they could greatly increase their income by remaining on call in the hospital rather than being at home. Under these circumstances many of the junior staff obtained incomes higher than their supervising consultants.

Most recently, negotiations with the consultants appear to be producing corresponding complications. Consultants may receive extra fees for emergency calls requiring a recall to the hospital (equivalent to one-half day's pay being on call). According to one proposal, consultants would be eligible for the "recall fee," even though still on the hospital premises carrying out routine work when called. It is anticipated that many of the currently full-time consultants may elect to undertake more private practice, since penalties are reduced for doing so. All these examples are cited to indicate the serious problem of attempting to arrive at equitable distribution of resources to widely varying kinds of professionals engaged in very different forms of practice. An interesting approach to the problems of compensation is to be found in Sweden where virtually all physicians are paid according to the same pay scales (see the section on contrasts between Swedish and American hospitals, below).

PROBLEM: MALDISTRIBUTION OF METROPOLITAN MEDICINE

The citizens that live in cities and are on the lists of conscientious general practitioners receive excellent primary care. They can be referred, as necessary, to consultants of the highest caliber in academic hospitals in the large metropolitan centers in Britain. However, the highest quality services are very much in demand and often involve intolerably long waiting periods, except in emergencies. Everyone agrees that the emergency care is prompt and extremely effective. Access to many consultant services is delayed for months or years by long waiting lists which are a source of great frustration to most citizens.

In many parts of the large metropolitan areas, the living conditions are undesirable and general practitioners are extremely scarce. These general practitioners can earn comfortable incomes by serving long lists of registered patients. The resulting heavy patient load generally produces extremely brief encounters with doctors, averaging 6 minutes' duration, and ranging from 1-15 minutes. As a consequence, pressures and low morale may lead doctors to deliver minimal and mechanical health care. Most patients seeing general practitioners depart with a prescription that was hastily written, or a referral to a consultant that removes the responsibility from the general practitioner and places the patient on a waiting list.

As British physicians emigrated toward brighter professional futures (i.e., in Canada or the United States), some of the resulting vacancies were occupied by an influx of foreign doctors. By 1975, the number of foreign physicians rose to represent 35.2% of the total, with some 14.3% of consultants educated in foreign medical schools (7). Concern reached a peak in 1975 when qualifying examinations were required of foreign physicians (for the first time) and two-thirds of them failed.

Deputizing Services. Many metropolitan practitioners function alone with very large lists, sustained pressure, and little free time. When such physicians need to be away from their practices, they can turn their practice (list) over to a deputizing service which functions temporarily as a surrogate for the practitioner in his absence. The deputizing services respond to practitioners' calls by dispatching physicians from their own lists to see patients with which they are unfamiliar. A substantial proportion of the deputizing service physicians are moonlighting junior staff or foriegn doctors, many of whom have difficulty with English. This mechanism is particularly prevalent in metropolitan areas and is the cause of considerable dissatisfaction.

Constraints on Diffusion of Technologies. At a time when the major concentration of interest, effort, and resources in the United States are trending toward ever-increasing high technology encompassed within large hospitals, priorities are quite different in Great Britain. The consultants and many of their patients continue to argue for inclusion of high technology devices such as CAT scanners, advanced models of gamma cameras, artificial kidney services. Their diffusion into widespread use has been curtailed by financial constraints. As an example, CAT scanners, offered as donations by philanthropists, have been refused by hospitals lacking funds for the necessary support personnel to operate and maintain these costly instruments. The first CAT scanners were built by an English firm (EMI) but only a few (1-2 dozen) of these costly devices are in use in Britain. There is a growing suspicion on the part of administrators in the NHS that the high technologies do not in fact contribute sufficiently to the health and welfare of the population to warrant these very heavy expenditures that could cause neglect of other higher priority items (i.e., primary care).

It is not difficult to discover rather glaring defects in the NHS of Britain for three fundamental reasons. The objectives were extremely ambitious and based to some extent on the fallacious concept that an investment in health would ultimately reduce the demand for health services. Second, the National Health Service was necessarily built upon the preexisting and entrenched mechanisms for the delivery of health services by physicians and facilities. Finally, the organizational mechanisms devised to deliver the services were fragmented, producing both complex bureaucracy and a deficiency in comprehensive planning mechanisms for prioritizing utilization of resources. The net result has been a system which is generally satisfactory to the general public for primary care and emergencies, but involve discouragingly long waiting lists for some kinds of medical care and surgery in hospitals. It is worth noting that the original goal of equality for all to access to health care was abandoned at the outset by provisions for private practice by consultants. Furthermore, uniform access was further diluted because of long waiting lists due to insufficient facilities and personnel. In large teaching hospitals in cities and in the well-organized health centers in outlying areas, the quality of care is exceedingly good. This is not the case in many of the deprived areas.

The extent to which health services meet the perceived needs of the public depends upon the total amount of resources allocated to the effort and to the priorities assigned to the various categories of health services. In the United States, the dominant thrust toward sophisticated technologies and highly specialized services has depleted access to primary care in many areas of the country. Increasing pressures for improved access to primary care by the American public affords ample justification for exploring and assessing the mechanisms being employed in a system where such personal services have a top priority.

COMPREHENSIVE AND COMPASSIONATE PRIMARY CARE (BRITAIN)

General practitioners are the initial point of patient contact and are responsible for continuity of care in the National Health Service. They are more prominent in both relative numbers and roles than in the United States. Their contribution to health care is being actively upgraded in the United Kingdom by a number of mechanisms.

GROUP PRACTICE BY GENERAL PRACTITIONERS

The very heavy responsibility and unremitting pressures on family physicians in solo practice have been recognized so they are being actively encouraged to form group practices by financial support of renovations. Increasing numbers and diversity of health personnel are available to support the groups of general practitioners and to contribute to the care of the "lists" of patients (see the section on health centers and team development, below).

ADDITIONAL "VOCATIONAL" TRAINING OF GENERAL PRACTITIONERS

The National Health Service (Vocational Training) act of 1976 enables the Secretary of State to require from a date to be decided, that all new physicians in general practice in the NHS shall be "suitably experienced." At present this implies a period of some three years in "vocational training." The first year a "house officer" divides his time between medicine and surgery. The second year is spent as senior house officer in two selected areas (obstetrics and pediatrics are most popular). The third year is devoted to training in general practice (13). The program is roughly equivalent to family practice residencies being expanded in the United States. The legislative intent is to develop increased competence among the next generations of general practitioners in various combinations of clinical disciplines. Such postdoctoral experience will raise the status of solo general practitioners and also encourage members of group practices to concentrate on special areas of interest so that reliance on consultants will be reduced.

GENERAL PRACTICE HOSPITALS

When the NHS was first introduced, the country was divided into regions containing approximately 1.5 million population, with each containing at least one large regional hospital plus smaller district general hospitals located strategically throughout the region. In addition to these general hospitals, there are many small hospitals under the control and supervision of general practitioners. To be specific, there are approximately 350 general practitioner hospitals averaging about 24 beds in each. These hospitals constitute only about 3% of the acute beds in England and Wales, but they provide initial hospital care for large segments of the population. In addition, these general practitioner hospitals cope with some 13% of all casualties, 6% of operations, 4% of x-ray examinations. According to a survey by Dr. A.J.M. Cavenaugh (4g), 16% of the general practitioners provide services to patients in these general practitioner hospitals. Even larger numbers of extremely small cottage hospitals are operated with considerable economic inefficiency and are gradually being phased out despite local opposition.

HEALTH CENTERS

Group practice by general practitioners is encouraged and enhanced by encouragement and support of newly developed health centers, particularly in underserved areas. Health centers are ambulatory care clinics staffed by general practitioners and supplemented by a variety of other health professionals and support personnel as mentioned in connection with the developments in Scotland above. In 1976 there were 705 health centers staffed by about 3,600 general practitioners, and an additional 120 were being built (13). The responsibility for planning, developing, and supporting these centers was delegated to the various health authorities. A minimum of £25,500,000 were allocated for such capital expenditures to health authorities.

HEALTH TEAM DEVELOPMENT

The concept of developing teams of health professionals and support personnel to provide comprehensive and integrated services for groups of patients is much more highly developed in Britain than in the United States. A panel on primary health care teams was convened by the British Medical Association (14) to include the full spectrum of services with unusually broad definition and delegation of responsibilities. The general practitioner assumes the ultimate responsibility in the clinical sphere but "all members of the team are free to initiate and are responsible for activities within their own fields." The full exercise of nursing competence and skills was encouraged including the assessment of patients, counseling, and even initiation of therapy under some conditions. The enhanced scope of nursing in provision of primary care in Britain is more general than expanded roles described in a few settings in the United States (see Chapter 7).

Health care teams are envisioned as a "nucleus" composed of doctors, nurses, social workers, and medical secretaries (Fig. 9-3). The teams interact with appropriate departments of medical schools, area health authorities, local government, and voluntary agencies. Patients are referred to consultants for hospital care as necessary.

PRIMARY TEAM

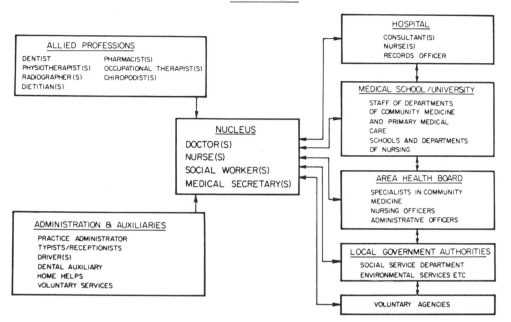

Figure 9-3. Primary health teams represent an extremely high priority developmental objective of present planning in Britain. Each primary team is envisioned as comprised of a central nucleus of health professionals and practitioners supported by a variety of essential health personnel and administrative support people. The exact composition of the primary teams and their organizational relationships are adjusted to meet the needs of particular communities and locations.

The increased demand for primary care has encouraged the development of health care teams which are designed to encourage the development of group practice by general practitioners supported by state registered nurses, home nurses, health visitors, midwives, and professionals. About 60% of all general practitioners now work in practices with three or more doctors, and some 80% of the home nurses and health visitors are attached to general medical services. In some areas, social workers employed by local authorities are also attached to primary health teams. The government is clearly intent upon encouraging and supporting the development of group general practice as an important refinement in the methods of delivering primary care to the general public. A major growth rate of 6% per year for home nurses and health visitors has been proposed to support the compassionate components of medicine.

NEW NURSING FUNCTIONS

The State Registered Nurses in Britain play the familiar role of clinic nurses, and in addition, may serve as district nurses which correspond with public health nurses in the United States (4i). They may go out to the homes and treat patients on site. In the past, midwives delivered a majority of babies in the homes with little involvement by physicians. This autonomous role of the midwives has substantially changed, due to a major trend toward deliveries in hospitals. Governmental support and fetal monitoring mechanisms in hospitals have drastically altered the approach to obstetrics. At the present time it is estimated that more than 90% of all deliveries are carried out in hospital, many of them are still carried out by midwives under supervision of consultants in obstetrics.

A major nationwide effort has been expended in attempting to improve the health status of the young. The midwives are responsible for the initial prenatal care in collaboration with the general practitioner or consultant obstetrician. However, two weeks after delivery, a specially trained health professional, known as the health visitor, is usually involved automatically.

Health Visitors. Most health visitors are state registered nurses with additional training in preventive care, nutrition of children, and geriatrics, with heavy emphasis in health education. The reporting of a birth automatically triggers a series of visits by a health visitor to the home (4i). The sphere of interest encompasses early infant care, with particular reference to the home condition, nutrition, hygiene, and other obvious health problems. They are also responsible for checking visual and hearing abilities at seven months. Health visitors are expected to educate the mothers in the care of their children—not only the newborn but older children as well. Their responsibility extends to the encouragement of preventive care and immunization. Many provide lectures and coursework in the schools on subjects such as "parentcraft." In addition to the care of the young, and the health education for the whole family, a major role is the care of the elderly. Health visitors are particularly concerned with the older individuals who might be mentally confused, living alone or with relatives. They will tend to assess the situation and the extent to which old or infirm people have support from the family and from their neighbors. They frequently engage in supportive activities such as cleaning, shopping, helping to cook, assuring the nutrition, even paying bills.

Community Psychiatric Nurses. Most districts have at least one large psychiatric hospital to provide domiciliary care for the mentally ill. Some 55% of the total hospital beds are occupied by the mentally ill. A major effort is now being mounted to reduce the number of individuals who must remain chronically in hospitals, returning many of them to the community. One part of this effort is the provision of community psychiatric nurses. Many of these nurses are male, based on a long tradition that the staff of mental hospitals have been largely male. General practitioners are rarely able to spend sufficient time with emotionally disturbed patients, but the psychiatric nurses typically spend the initial hour assessing patients' needs and arriving at appropriate decisions regarding the best management. The training of the community psychiatric nurse extends for three years (or 18 months added to the senior registered nurse training). The ultimate responsibility for the mentally ill remains in the sphere of the psychiatrist, but the community psychiatric nurses see patients in outpatient clinics as referred by general practitioners or by their psychiatric consultants. District nurses or health visitors may also refer patients after checking with the appropriate physician. Approximately 80% of the patients requiring this kind of service are categorized under geriatric psychiatry. Furthermore, it is estimated that some 50% of the patients who visit general practitioners have some degree of psychosomatic or psychological problem currently treated mainly by drugs. Many of these are expected to benefit from the services of a psychiatric nurse. General practitioners welcome the kinds of help that can be provided by such a psychiatric nurse because it relieves them of very difficult problems they have insufficient time to handle in their busy schedules.

Day Hospitals. Adjacent to geriatric hospitals or psychiatric hospitals, most counties have one or more day hospitals staffed by one or two qualified nurses and a few auxiliaries to provide a site for day treatment of the mentally ill and at the same time to relieve the family of the continuing nagging responsibility for older people in the home. At these day hospitals patients may receive medications and have an opportunity to engage in social exchange and occupational therapy.

Home Health Services. Home help aides provide services to patients in their homes (i.e., washing, shopping, cleaning, cooking, fetching, etc.). They were formerly a part of the local health departments, but have recently been transferred to Social Services. This has led to a certain amount of overlap and duplication of services under certain circumstances. Nursing aides provide health services in the home under supervision of state Registered Nurses. There is a recognized need for improved integration of the services provided by health visitors, midwives, and home health aides.

SERVICES USED MAINLY BY THE ELDERLY

The 6.5 million people over 65 in England comprise about 14% of the total population. This is an increase by more than 25% since 1961. Services used mainly by the elderly (and often by physically handicapped people) are a very high priority at the present for future planning (3). About 95% of all elderly people are living in the community, and family doctors are meeting their most important medical needs. Their continued ability to live in the community is dependent upon the availability of community services, such as:

· *Home Helps.* In 1974, about 41,000 wholetime equivalent home helps were available (6 per 1,000 elderly).
· *Meals.* Many meals are served each week through Meals on Wheels services (about 200 per week per 1,000 elderly).
· *Home Nursing.* Over half the time of home nurses is thought to be spent on elderly. In 1974 there were about 11,000 home nurses in all—slightly

less than 1 per 4,000 total population. The projected guideline is 1 per 2,500–4,000, depending on local needs.

- *Day Centers.* In 1974 23,000 day center places were available to the elderly and younger physically handicapped (2 places per 1,000 elderly; projected guidelines: 3 to 4 places per 1,000).
- *Chiropody.* Such services do a great deal to prevent immobility; these are particularly relevant to the elderly (1 per 5,000 elderly).
- *Residential Facilities.* There are about 125,000 "local authority places" which have been made available particularly for elderly people and for the younger physically handicapped and others (about 18.5 places per 1,000 elderly).
- *Hospital Facilities.* Over 50% of all hospital beds are used by people over 65. For general medical conditions, old people are admitted to general medical beds or to beds designated for geriatric medicine. It is estimated that 80% of persons admitted to geriatric beds remain there for less than three months. However, those who refuse to leave for lack of adequate home facilities present a very serious problem.
- *Day Hospitals.* Most local authorities have waiting lists for admission to residential homes for the elderly and the mentally infirm.

For these reasons, a major expansion of the facilities and services for the elderly is required to keep up with their increasing numbers.

Innovative research and development efforts are oriented toward the development of technologies needed for care of the elderly and the physically handicapped (4f,4m). Examples include monitoring and alarm systems by which older persons living at home could summon help. An interactive environment is under consideration to accommodate the shorter memory span of older persons by means of devices that automatically trigger tape recordings to remind older folk of necessary steps in day-to-day living alone (i.e., remembering to take the key when venturing out of doors). The causes and treatment of pressure sores of the aged and also prosthetic devices of use to handicapped are also featured (4m). A prime motive is to develop technologies that would permit a larger proportion of older people to remain safely and securely in their own homes rather than in institutional settings.

AN INTEGRATED HEALTH TEAM (WALES)

The Brecon War Memorial Hospital is a notable example from among the 350 general practitioner hospitals. It is located in the small community in Powys, a remote mountainous area of southern Wales. A group of seven general practitioners, each with special areas of particular interest, function in a clinic and at the hospital. They are supported by an impressive array of district nurses, health visitors, and others. The composition and organization of this health team is indicated in Figure 9–4. The general practitioners are supplemented by visiting consultants coming at regular intervals from more distant cities in the environs. Conversations with many citizens in the

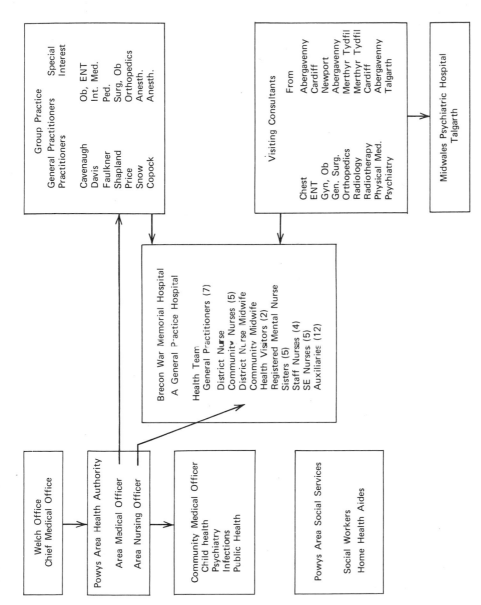

Figure 9-4. An exceptional example of an integrated team practicing in both a clinic and a general practice hospital is found in Brecon, a small remote community in the mountains of southern Wales. This comprehensive health service demonstrates mechanisms for delivering of health care by mutually supportive health personnel.

353

town of Brecon amply confirmed that the hospital was a source of great pride and confidence among the general population. Perhaps the most impressive aspect of the health services was the effectiveness with which continuity of care was provided by the district nurses, midwives, health visitors, and other members of their team. A visit to this facility and to the Powys Area Health Authority (4i) provided an indelible impression of competent and dedicated professionals providing compassionate health care to a widely dispersed population. The quality could serve as a standard for corresponding situations in the United States.

A HOSPITAL SPECIFICALLY PLANNED
FOR PRIMARY CARE (OXFORDSHIRE)

The Oxford Regional Health Authority is one of the most advanced and respected in Britain. It is the source of some notable innovations, particularly related to Oxfordshire but potentially relevant to other situations. The area around Oxford is well supplied with general practice hospitals (about 35 in Oxfordshire). These are generally situated in relatively affluent communities of small size. In addition, very small "cottage hospitals" of 5–25 beds are present in large numbers but appear to be uneconomic and are probably not viable. The larger district general hospitals are more widely dispersed in population centers of some 250,000 about 20 or more miles apart. The need for a more rational distribution of health services oriented toward primary care has been actively addressed by the Regional Health Authority.

As a product of continuing program planning, a new hospital at Wallingford was meticulously designed as a prototype purposefully and expressly organized to provide health services by a primary care team (15,16). According to Dr. Rosemary Rue (4d), "Oxford was unique in recognizing the principle that the hospital might serve as supportive of primary care instead of the other way around."

The "ideal model" of a community hospital was seen to comprise a health center with accommodation for general practitioners, their staff, local health authority services, consultant clinics, and certain diagnostic services, day treatment facilities, and some inpatient accommodations. A full range of integrated facilities was provided in the conviction that general practitioners with adequate facilities can serve as an alternative to the more expensive district general hospital care. The concept that inpatient and day care could more effectively be provided as an extension of primary care, rather than as an appendage to sophisticated hospital services was an important consideration (17). This approach gives meaning to the principle that primary health teams should be provided with the necessary facilities and staff to deliver comprehensive and integrated primary care of high quality. The specialist hospitals could provide sophisticated "tertiary" care more effectively if they were unencumbered by a large volume of primary or continuing health care (18).

The Wallingford Hospital is the product of a long-range planning effort conducted with a wide variety of interdisciplinary committees to provide an optimal community hospital serving a small city of about 8,000 population (15). This is specifically *not* a "mini-district hospital" and does not provide surgery except for minor accidents. It is primarily a hospital that is supportive of the primary care functions of general practitioners. It serves large groups of patients who do not need all the facilities provided by district general hospitals, but do require some hospitalization at lower levels of sophistication.

One main wing of the hospital contains six single rooms, two 4-bed wards, and four 6-bed wards, a total of 38 beds, devoted primarily to long-stay chronic care of patients. The other main wing is a 20-space day unit that averages about 24–25 patients per day; most of these patients come in two or three times a week. They are older senior citizens for the most part, coming in by ambulance or by private car, beginning at about 9:30 in the morning. Most of them begin to leave about 3:30 in the afternoon. They come to the hospital both for ambulatory treatment and for a social environment in which they can remain for most of the day. There is a large occupational therapy room where many of the older people are engaged in hobbies and manufacture of small items. A physical therapy program with three physical therapists serves both outpatients and inpatients. In addition, there are three single, one four-bedded, and two five-bedded wards for the accommodation of older senior citizens on a longer-term basis. There are numerous outpatient clinics for children, for eye problems, and for many other problems, for which consultants come in at regular intervals.

The hospital is heavily involved in the management of senior citizens, many of whom are seriously disabled, mentally disturbed, and pose problems for management outside the hospital environment (16). A universal problem in all developed countries is the occupancy of acute hospital beds by patients with chronic ailments. The continually expanding numbers of both the elderly and the parents of families with children who require help has greatly accentuated the recognized need for provisions for the elderly, the mentally ill, the mentally handicapped, and the physically handicapped. The priorities for these services have been elevated over those of general and acute hospital services (18). The unsatisfied needs of the aging and handicapped appear to call for expenditures increasing more rapidly than the more traditional health requirements (see the section on long-range planning, below).

HEALTH SERVICES RESEARCH

Mechanisms for evaluating the outcome of investments in various alternative health services are of great interest whenever public demand greatly exceeds the available resources (See Chapter 6). In Britain, the importance of assessing the ultimate benefits derived from investments is keenly felt because of the rather fragile economy of the country. During the first decades of the NHS, sequential decisions regarding the most beneficial directions of effort and resource allocations were based more on political pressures, expediency, and intuition than on relevant data or analytical approaches.

The development of the necessary data base and analytical approaches for program assessment has been tardy, deliberate, and beset with uncertainties in Britain as in other developed countries. In recent years these deficiencies have been recognized more generally and a freshet of publications attests to awakening of widespread interest in developing a sounder foundation for allocation of resources.

According to Gordon McLachlan (19), "The one thing that is certain is that the health departments are now virtually in a monopoly position with regard to health services research and development in the United Kingdom and the whole style of approach in this field in the future is likely to be conditioned by the department's attitudes and their actions in the next phase." The conclusions reached from such studies can be converted into action through the governmental controls on budgets more readily in Britain than in the United States. For this reason, the ultimate usefulness and consequences of various approaches to health care can be more easily appreciated in countries with powerful governmental influences on health services and also active research programs in the field.

A significant step taken in Britain was a comprehensive study of the Health Services Research programs in adjacent members of the European Common Market (i.e., France, West Germany, Belgium). The similarities in the research objectives and targets indicate that outcome analysis in one of these countries might be extrapolated to others (20). There is growing awareness that gathering information alone is not sufficient in a system as complex as health care delivery. There are so many social variables complicating any intervention that traditional data may be useful as a beginning for research but are not sufficient to provide the necessary answers. The British are aware of the American experience with supplementation of demographic data with experiments involving epidemiological observations and analysis (see Chapter 6). All the developed nations of the world are heavily engaged in devising effective methods for exploring three issues:

1. Assessment of need, demand, and utilization
2. The effects of alternative resource allocations
3. The evaluation of services provided

The approaches to these questions are remarkably primitive considering the size and complexity of the system under study. Progress will be accelerated and more soundly based if the information gleaned from the various efforts can be assembled in formats that permit us all to learn from others' successes or mistakes. Such information is of the greatest importance in developing rational long range plans.

LONG-RANGE PLANNING PRIORITIES

The National Health Service has emerged by an evolutionary process that involved little long-range planning in terms of setting goals, objectives, and priorities of the sort discussed in Chapter 6. Efforts at providing health and social services inevitably encounter demands that outstrip capacity to provide resources. A major new approach to planning was presented as a consultative document on priorities for health and personal social services (21). This document is strongly reminiscent of the forward plan for health of the NIH discussed in Chapter 2. However, the objectives and priorities are very different in the two countries, despite the many similarities in their antecedent history and common cultural characteristics.

Priorities for the elderly, the handicapped, and for child development are reflected in adjustments in the rate at which the annual budgets were expected to increase as follows:

Services for	Yearly Increase
Elderly	3.2% per yr.
Mentally ill	1.8% per yr.
Mentally handicapped	2.8% per yr.
Children and families with children	2.1% per yr.
Acute and General Hospitals	1.2% per yr.
Hospital Maternity Services reduced by	-1.2%-1.8% per yr.

The level of growth for acute services was regarded as posing serious problems without rationalization and required increased efficiency through provision of day-surgery units, short-stay wards, and shortened hospital stays. The reduction in support of maternity services was a response to a discrepancy revealed by data indicating that the costs were continually rising despite a lowering of the birth rate. The special care for newborn babies has been assigned a top priority. The past, current, and projected growth of the various categories of services (21) are displayed in Figure 9-5.

New planning systems were introduced in April 1976 by which regional and area health authorities initiated preparation of ten-year strategic plans for the development of the services taking into account both local needs and national priorities. The first of the long-term plans were submitted to the Department of Health and Social Security early in 1977. Areas and districts began drawing up three-year operational plans, including the needs for social services (13). The importance of joint planning to achieve a proper balance of services for the elderly, children, the disabled, mentally ill, and mentally handicapped was stressed (21).

ROYAL COMMISSION ON THE NATIONAL HEALTH SERVICE

In accordance with long tradition a Royal Commission has been appointed under chairmanship of Sir Alec Morrison to undertake comprehensive evaluation of the NHS and make appropriate recommendations regarding mechanisms for its improvements. The mandate of the commission is to consider the best use and management of the financial and manpower resources for benefit of patients and for those who work in the National Health Service of England, Scotland, Wales, and Northern Ireland. The

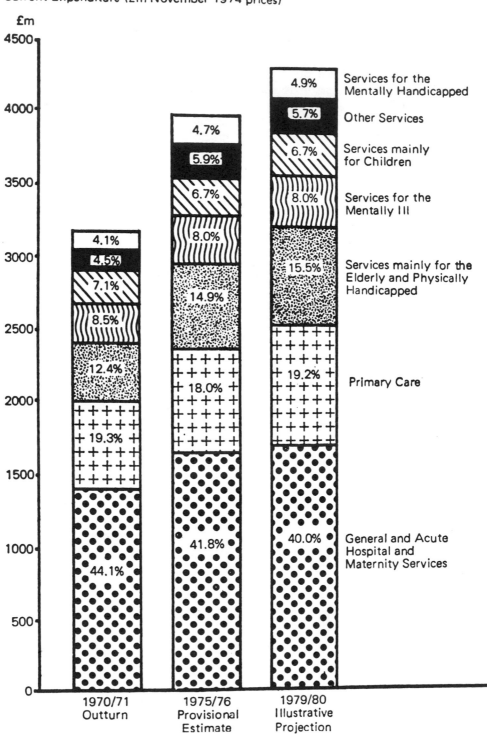

Expenditure by programme as a percentage of Total Expenditure
Current Expenditure (£m November 1974 prices)

£m

Figure 9-5. The National Health Service budgets, past, present, and projected, demonstrate that funds for general hospital and maternity services have leveled off. Primary care retains a high priority but the greatest expansions are in the services for elderly, physically handicapped, and mentally ill.

358

stated objectives of the commission are to assess the quality of service against goals and expectations. The likely developments over the next 20 years will be considered in terms of a wide range of matters such as demographic change, technologies, and alterations in lifestyle and living standards. The Commission announced in advance its interpretation of the task and invited comments or statements with respect to present services, future projections, services of family practitioners, hospitals, community services, private practice, management, and allocation of resources.

Superficially, Royal Commissions appear to be roughly equivalent to the profusion of commissions that have conducted studies on similar topics in the United States. Two substantial differences deserve mention:

1. Royal Commissions are composed of highly respected persons whose backgrounds enable them to receive and evaluate evidence of experts but who have little or no proprietary interest in the subject under study. This approach is at variance with the American propensity of setting up commissions composed of "experts" who are professionally and personally involved in the questions being analyzed. It is almost axiomatic that a commission composed of individuals with strong proprietary interests will recommend support and expansion of their chosen line of endeavor.
2. Recommendations of Royal Commissions are very likely to become expressed in legislative and administrative actions directed toward implementing them within a reasonable period of time. In contrast, the natural history of most commission reports in the United States is to defuse hot issues, divert attention during the period of study, and create a temporary flurry on release and then quietly occupy file space.

The contrasting characteristics of Royal Commissions and corresponding United States counterparts are vividly displayed in the case of recombinant DNA. A Royal Commission developed guidelines for the conduct of experiments involving Recombinant DNA quietly and efficiently in Britain. During the same period a major nationwide controversy raged in the United States. The conscientious efforts of dedicated scientists trying to take responsible action was rapidly converted into a long series of emotional debates in an adversarial atmosphere involving both the scientific community and emotionally charged citizens and public servants. Experience of this sort suggests that we could profitably employ the Royal Comission Approach to evaluate and recommend appropriate courses of action in many important issues in the United States.

CONTRASTING CHARACTERISTICS: UNITED STATES AND UNITED KINGDOM

A synthesis of the many diverse impressions gained from interviews with many people in the United Kingdom has revealed some informative and provocative differences between the health services in Britain and those from the United States. These can be summarized as follows:

In the United Kingdom, the development of the health services has been a component part of an overall trend toward the socialization of many components of society under the control of the central government. As a consequence, the principal driving force in the United Kingdom stems from federal control which determines priorities, establishes budgetary levels, and generally controls the kinds and amounts of services delivered. In contrast, the driving forces in the United States are doctor-oriented and directed toward providing ample facilities and services for health care. Sir John Brotherston (4j) described the process as "providing all the facilities and services needed to make happy doctors."

PRIME OBJECTIVES

The stated objective in the United Kingdom is to provide equity or equality of access to adequate health care systems. In constrast, the American approach is to provide highest quality, sophisticated facilities and services, delivered to individuals who have third-party coverage or can afford direct payment, with little concern over total costs.

THE PRINCIPAL APPROACH

The control over the magnitude, type, and distribution of facilities and services is exerted by means of budgetary constraint in the United Kingdom. In contrast, the resolution of perceived problems in the United States is mainly by expanding old or developing new programs by addition or allocation of resources (appropriating funds).

STRATEGIES

The traditional trends and efforts in Britain have been directed toward the provision of primary care, with great reliance on the availability of distribution of general practitioners as the initial contact for entrance into the system. In contrast, the principal emphasis in the United States has been on tertiary care, as evidenced by the predominance of specialization among the practicing physicians in this country.

DOMINANT PRIORITIES

Throughout the United Kingdom, the top priorities for consideration in the development of new programs and in the allocation of resources is in recognition of the problems of the expanding aged population, the problems of the handicapped (both mental and physical), and the problems of providing for healthy child development. Obviously, these are not the priorities of the consultants who are engaged in specialty practice in the various teaching regional and district general hospitals, but they are the primary priorities of the authorities who are managing the budgetary allocations. In contrast, the problems of cancer, cardiovascular disease, and chronic diseases of the lung, kidney, liver, and other internal organs, have been peak priorities for allocation of resources in the United States.

GEOGRAPHICAL DISTRIBUTION

The highest quality care available for the average citizen is to be found in the outlying areas and away from the central cities of Great Britain. While it is true that excellent facilities and talent are to be found in the large and prestigious medical institutions of the country, they do not provide primary care. Metropolitan areas tend to contain deficiencies in the availability of first contact health care for general population. In contrast, metropolitan and suburban areas of the United States are the areas in which the health care is predominantly superior. The central cities suffer from the same kind of neglect in both countries.

COMMUNITY SUPPORT SERVICES

In the United Kingdom, the emphasis on the provision of care for the aging population and for the handicapped and the growing children have led to the development of extensive and widespread community services in the form of health visitors, district nurses, and psychiatric nurses who are becoming very numerous and more uniformly dispersed throughout the country. In contrast, such community services are available in a spotty fashion throughout the United States.

LONG-RANGE PLANNING

Both the United States and the United Kingdom have health care delivery systems which have evolved with very little long-range planning or rationalization of resource allocations until very recently. Responding to political pressures and shifting demands and opportunities, the resulting organizational and operational mechanisms have contributed to extravagance, inefficiency, and rather abrupt, spontaneous shifts in objectives and strategies. In rather sharp contrast to this approach, the Swedish Health System was initiated after several years of study and evolved in accordance of forward-planning efforts in a much more rational and organized approach.

AN INTEGRATED REGIONAL HOSPITAL
SYSTEM (SWEDEN)

The Swedish system of health care is a part of a broad program of social welfare which is based on carefully drawn long-range plans. Equal access of all citizens to health services of the highest quality has been attained to a remarkable degree. The system is widely regarded as the best in the world in terms of comprehensive, integrated, and efficient utilization of resources. By traditional measures, the Swedish nation can boast a population that is healthier and more heavily taxed than virtually any other country. Despite the allocation of a very substantial proportion of the gross national product to health care, the demands for health services still outstrip the available resources. Delayed access is encountered whenever services are in short supply. To some extent, waiting lists are utilized to indicate the need to shift priorities and expand services. Efficiency and effectiveness of care are achieved by organization, centralization, and integration of services which render the services somewhat impersonal (the most common complaint). Overall, the Swedish people are proud and generally satisfied with their system of health care despite such sources of dissatisfaction. The high priorities for health services managed under local control (County Councils) has provided facilities and services of such high quality and profusion that it is difficult to envision such a well integrated system in a country less organized or socialized than Sweden.

THE SWEDISH SETTING

Sweden is slightly larger than California and contains a generally homogeneous population of about 9 million, approximately the population of California in 1940. The country has enjoyed 150 years of peace, having retained neutrality through two devastating world wars. Its emergence as a prosperous industrial country lagged other European countries, but rapidly developed a very high standard of living. It was governed by the Social Democratic Party with virtually no interruption for about 40 years, during which an ambitious social program increasingly assured financial security, plus generous health and social services from cradle to grave. Before 1955, health insurance was voluntary throughout the country. In that year, the Swedish National Health Insurance became a national compulsory tax-financed health insurance which was combined with various pensions in 1963. The government increasingly assumed responsibility for organizing and financing insurance against sickness, disability, and aging, under a compulsory National Social Insurance. All Swedes have equal coverage and equal access to needed services.

The government services are financed by very high taxes which amount to some 41% of a $4,000 salary per year, 60% of $10,000 per year, and up to 80% of higher income brackets. The population continues to pay such high rates (with some grumbling) because of the large quantity and high quality of services received. This degree of satisfaction appears to depend heavily upon a key characteristic; namely, the authority and responsibility vested in local government (the County Councils).

Local government in Sweden is vested in 25 county councils, plus five borough councils ("free" city governments in Stockholm, Gothenburg, Malmo, and Norrköping). The population of the counties varies but averages around 250,000 to 300,000. In the 1950s, each county contained at least one central hospital and numerous smaller ones serving populations of 60-

90,000 people. Anticipating the impending sophistication and cost of modern medicine, a survey was instituted to develop recommendations for a national plan. A deficiency in the number of physicians available to serve the people was recognized. The improved efficiency with which care could be rendered in hospitals led to reliance on major hospital development as the backbone of Swedish health care. For this and other reasons, the Swedish hospital system is superior to any other in the world with respect to the planned integration, quality, and distribution of facilities and personnel, and effective utilization of the resources.

ARTHUR ENGEL'S MASTER PLAN
FOR A REGIONAL SYSTEM

In 1956 Dr. Arthur Engel was appointed as a "one-man commission" to study the needs for resources and to advise on a suitable organization to provide optimal care on a nationwide basis (22). A comprehensive study of the health services of Sweden, Britain, the United States and other countries consumed four years of his time and resulted in a masterplan that served as the fundamental blueprint for development over the past two decades.

In Sweden, local communities or catchment areas of about 10,000 to 15,000 people were found to be commonplace. These served as the natural base for primary care by ambulatory health centers. Larger communities of 60,000 to 90,000 populations require the greater diversity of personnel and facilities provided in "normal" hospitals. Each Swedish county required at least one central hospital to serve about 250,000 people. The county councils were directly responsible for the development and maintenance of all these facilities. The county councils are elected officials empowered to levy taxes and to manage the social and health services in their geographic area of responsibility. Their reelection depends upon consistently providing health and social services of sufficient quantity and quality to their local constituency being served. They have direct control over the central and normal hospitals and health centers within the county borders. It was recognized that such small population bases could not effectively support the large and growing requirements for the increasingly sophisticated and expensive diagnostic and therapeutic technologies.

To implement Dr. Engel's plan, a professional geographer was empowered to develop dividing lines for seven regions of about equal population (around 1,000,000 each) with appropriate economic, social, and political components to support an integrated and comprehensive health and welfare program. Each geographic region was specifically designed to include or accommodate at least one large regional hospital. Most of these were also academic hospitals incorporating medical schools of high quality. Thus, plans took into account metropolitan areas, the industrial and financial bases, and location of key academic and health services institutions. From the outset, county councils have been called on to participate voluntarily in the support of the huge regional or academic hospitals from which the people of their county derive services.

Since both the authority and responsibility for health care resided in the county councils under direct view of their constituency, the quality and quantity of health and social services became prime political platforms of candidates for these offices. There developed a healthy competition between County Councils and regional populations to outperform neighbors in provision of the finest possible services. The local option for health and social services which was so successful in Sweden is not applicable to the United States or the United Kingdom, where the power resides largely in central government (23).

THE REGIONAL PYRAMID

The basic concept of the Swedish Regional Hospital system is displayed in Figure 9-6. In principle, facilities, and services are planned according to ideal bed-to-population ratios for each different medical, surgical, and other specialties. The basic system is comprised of three levels of hospitals, each level serving a larger population base as indicated in Figure 9-6.

The huge regional or academic hospitals are all magnificently supplied with comprehensive complements of highly trained professionsls and support personnel utilizing the most sophisticated and modern of available technologies. Typically, these magnificent facilities have large central blocks surrounded by groups of individual buildings housing various medical and surgical specialties and other relevant health and social services. The planning of the facilities and services is quite frequently based on extensive studies sponsored by the Institute for Rationalization of Health and Social Services (SPRI).

Within each county, at least one large fully-equipped and staffed central hospital is situated to conveniently serve a population of about 250,000 people. The district hospitals contain at least four specialty departments, typically internal medicine, general surgery, radiology, anesthesia, and often including pediatrics and obstetrics. The exact complement of professionals and services varies with geographic location, proximity to other facilities, and other factors.

The underlying principle of Swedish planning has been an organizational hierarchy to provide the individual patients with optimal levels of care at the right place and at the right time (22). Obviously, such an idealistic aim cannot be fully realized but the effective utilization of services and resources has been greatly enhanced by easy and frequent referral of patients to the appropriate level of service or from one level to another. Transfers depend on the nature and severity of illness at the outset and on the course of the disability. Patients in any part of a county can gain access to primary care in their own neighborhood except in the sparsely populated regions such as the northern reaches of the country. The district medical officers in the health centers treat the bulk of the presenting problems and can refer patients to the higher level hospitals in accordance with the specific needs of the patients (23). Efficient ambulance services are widely used to convey patients to hospitals and return. The relatively free flow of patients from one hospital to another in accordance with need for sophisticated services

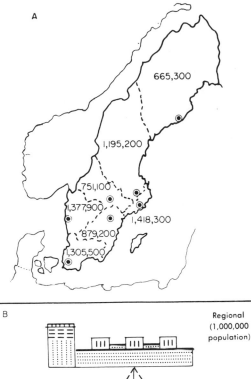

A

665,300

1,195,200

751,100

1,377,900

1,418,300

879,200

1,305,500

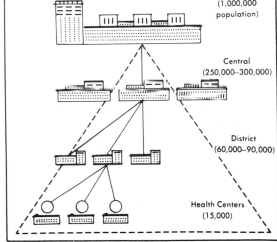

B

Regional
(1,000,000
population)

Central
(250,000–300,000)

District
(60,000–90,000)

Health Centers
(15,000)

Figure 9-6. The Swedish National Health Services
have been developed in accordance with long-range
plans centered around integrated hierarchies of
health facilities. In each of seven regions, the
counties cooperatively support magnificent regional hospitals (generally incorporating medical
schools) that contain the most sophisticated technologies and highly qualified personnel to fully
utilize them. Each county contains one or more
central hospitals, surrounded by district hospitals
and health centers under the local administrative
control of County Councils. (Adopted from Engel,
ref 22.)

365

is an option which rarely is utilized in the United States. Analysis of cost/effectiveness has provided convincing evidence that hospitals designed to provide a rich spectrum of medical and surgical specialties must be larger than 400 beds (24). On this basis, most small hospitals in Sweden have been either converted into district hospitals or phased out altogether. This process has encountered expected opposition in communities containing small hospitals but has generally prevailed. The concentration of resources in the central and regional hospitals has provided Sweden with an integrated system unrivaled anywhere else in the world.

The efficient utilization of facilities is often achieved at a sacrifice of intimate doctor-patient relations. On entering a hospital patients have little or no choice of physicians, but receive care from the doctor serving the ward to which they are assigned, almost always a specialist. Thus, the complaint commonly voiced is that Swedish patients "have many doctors but no doctor," because successive encounters in a hospital or outpatient clinic may involve different physicians. The shuttling between specialty wards and clinics interferes with the development of a warm and personal relationship between patient and doctor.

Evolutionary Trends. The reliance on hospitals to enhance the efficiency of scarce physicians inevitably resulted in patients occupying beds for conditions that could effectively and more appropriately be managed in ambulatory clinics. As many as half the hospital beds have been unavailable for acute care because they were occupied by patients with chronic conditions. Some of the wards were not used for lack of adequate numbers of physicians. Recognition of these problems has prompted a number of remedial actions:

· The number of physicians has been increased through an ambitious expansion in medical school graduates. Physicians numbered 5,000 in 1950 and were projected to reach 20,000 in 1980. This means that the number of inhabitants per physician in Sweden was projected to decrease from 1:1450 (1950) to only 1:450 in 1980 (2).
· Continuing care of patients under the same doctors during recovery periods is being enhanced in some regions by establishing domicilary rooms and apartments adjacent to the large regional hospitals where patients (and their families) may be maintained at greatly reduced cost during the transition from acute care to ambulatory care at home.
· Nursing home facilities are being intensively developed to accommodate patients with chronic ailments that have occupied expensive acute care beds in the larger hospitals.
· Ambulatory health care clinics are being established in conjunction with general hospitals for more efficient utilization of both personnel and facilities. This trend has the advantage of contributing to continuity of care and improved doctor-patient relationships by extending the encounters into and through the ambulatory period of care. The sophisticated laboratory and therapeutic facilities of the hospitals are also rendered accessible to ambulatory patients.

· Health centers are also being expanded as independent units. These are designed to accommodate three to five physicians in most instances, but ranging up to 15 physicians depending on population requirements. Generalists with special interests will be supplemented by selected specialties in these settings. These facilities will function like group practices in the United States but are "owned" by the county council. However, they will include a much larger commitment to social workers, new health professionals, and support personnel than can be found in most group practices in the United States.

The current trends in Sweden are closely related to developments in Britain and other developed countries of the world. The increased emphasis on expanding and improving ambulatory care, chronic care, and personal services is a very general phenomenon, responding to rather universally recognized importance of primary care with provisions for chronic ailments and paramedical support. Such requirements are increasingly recognized in the United States, but progress in these directions is appallingly slow. The autonomy and political power of the health professions is so great in this country that it impedes adaptation and change.

Contrasts Between Swedish and American Hospitals. The integrated hospital hierarchy in Sweden bears little relationship to the competitive autonomous facilities in the United States. American hospitals, large or small, aspire to provide the maximum possible number and diversity of sophisticated health services. Physicians have little or no inclination or incentive to refer patients from one hospital to another to match the needs of the patient to the level of sophistication of the institution. Most American hospitals are much smaller than 100 beds, partly a reflection of the Hill-Burton legislation that supported the development of hospitals in smaller communities. The number and distribution of specialists in Sweden are determined by the positions allocated by County Councils in the various hospitals. Private practice is small and dwindling in Sweden, largely because physicians engaged in fee-for-service practice have no access to the hospital system. Some of the older physicians persist in private practice in their offices, but they are gradually disappearing.

The County Councils are in extremely strong positions to introduce change. Virtually all Swedish physicians are on salaries at prescribed levels. The salary schedules of all the various specialties have been standardized to the point that differences in income are determined primarily by seniority (i.e., years of service). The more sophisticated specialties have the advantage of somewhat more free time and other fringe benefits but financial rewards are now remarkably uniform among all the physicians in the country. It is difficult or impossible to conceive of a set of circumstances by which a corresponding situation could develop in the United States. Thus, there is no prospect of introducing major components of the Swedish system into this country. However, the commitment and quality of the planning and health service evaluation in Sweden is so outstanding that we could derive considerable benefit by using their data in forward planning in this country. A much more relevant prototype for a national health service lies in our neighbor to the north.

A FEE-FOR-SERVICE, INSURANCE-BASED NATIONAL HEALTH PROGRAM (CANADA)

Canada shares many prominent characteristics with the United States. The country is very large (3,560,000 square miles) with large expanses occupied by sparse populations. The 1976 census revealed a population of 22,992,640, of which a very large proportion is concentrated along a narrow band within 100 miles of the border with the United States. The Canadian people share a common British heritage with the United States, but incorporate many diverse ethnic groups, including some vocal minorities (i.e., the French in Quebec). The national health programs of Canada have developed along lines that appear closely related to the current trends in the United States. Canadians have succeeded in instituting universal "free" health care while retaining elements perceived as essential in the United States.

In contrast with the European approach, more than 90% of Canadian health services are provided by fee-for-service physicians rather than by salaried physicians. Physicians are free to set up practice where they please and to bill the central medical plan for their services. The patients retain their rights to choose a family physician. Hospitals are mainly private, non-profit corporations that derive financial support from the government insurance program. The Canadian program demonstrates that easy access to health services without payment out of pocket need not lead to a vast and expensive bureaucracy, a decline in health care standards, overuse of physician and hospital services, or a major disruption of patient-doctor relations. These dire predictions have not materialized for the most part. In fact, the standards of medical care appear to have been well maintained and substantially improved for those who were formerly underserved by virtue of low incomes. Extensive surveys conducted by Edward A. Pickering, a retired industrialist, demonstrated that despite certain recognized deficiencies, the health needs of the Canadian people are being met in a generally satisfactory manner (25). A shortage of doctors was perceived by 56% of the people, ascribed to difficult access to general practitioners. Another complaint was impersonal service and assembly line methods. A superficial impression is gained that Canadians are more fully satisfied than their American cousins.

Surveys indicate that Canadians visit physicians more frequently than Americans, and that access is far more equitable and universal. Hospital beds per capita outnumber those in the United States and the costs-per-day are roughly equivalent. Despite these factors, Canadians spend proportionately less than Americans on medical services. Regional planning of health facilities has developed in many areas through combined efforts of government planning agencies and regional hospital boards. Obviously, the installation and refinement of a nationwide system has not been accomplished without criticism or controversy (including doctor strikes). The net result has been well received in general and the 10 years of Canadian experience appear relevant to the situation in the United States.

THE CANADIAN EXPERIENCE

The evolution of the personal health services in Canada can be traced to recognition of health needs in sparsely populated areas such as Newfoundland and the Prairie Provinces. Immediately after World War I, workmen's compensation made its appearance in all the provinces. Several provinces adopted health insurance legislation between 1935 and 1945, including a draft bill for national health insurance. Saskatchewan proceeded on its own to develop a hospitalization plan financed by a combination of compulsory premiums and taxation. A locally administered medical care plan provided doctors' services for all citizens of Saskatchewan financed by personal property taxes and provincial grants. Similar developments occurred in Alberta and British Columbia. In 1948 the federal government provided grants-in-aid to the provinces for a wide range of services, in anticipation of national health insurance.

Between 1956 and 1961, basic agreements were concluded between each province and the federal government for health plans administered by the provinces to provide all health services for all citizens, excluding payment to private physicians. The federal government provides approximately 50% of the revenues with additional funds going to the poorer provinces, according to a complex formula. Contributions by the federal government were subsequently provided for a variety of developments such as public assistance programs, planning, construction of approved projects and renovation of teaching and research facilities. The organizational and operational mechanisms vary in the different provinces, but net effects are quite similar.

By tradition and current practice, the primary responsibility for health services resides principally with the provincial governments. The federal government has direct responsibility for health services for certain special groups (i.e., armed forces, native tribes, etc.). It also provides extensive financial support through cost sharing and grants-in-aid to programs initiated in provinces. The leverage provided by cost-sharing is used by the federal government to exert pressure for cost containment, for maintaining standards, and for engaging in planning efforts. In many areas of responsibility controversy persists regarding the balance of power leading to jurisdictional disputes despite successive conferences over the years.

PERSISTENT PROFESSIONAL PROBLEMS

The introduction of universal health insurance in Quebec was found to have some unexpected results. The work-week appeared to shorten from 54.8 to 46.3 hours—a reduction of about 8.5 hours per week. Average daily contacts with patients by way of telephone, home and the number of hospital encounters also declined. The numbers of patients seen in the doctor's office increased. A slight increase in "unnecessary" visits was accompanied by a reduction in the numbers of persons who should have sought advice sooner.

A key question always revolves around the reactions of the physicians in such a system. The average incomes have been generous for both general practitioners and specialists, averaging about $40,000 and $50,000 respectively. These levels are sufficiently high so that physicians do not get much sympathy when relatively small raises are proposed in times of fiscal constraints. Physicians' strikes were quite prominent during the early stages of development and are still threatened on occasion, when doctors are asked to bear the brunt of cost-control campaigns. The fees for various services are fixed in accordance with established scales. In some provinces, physicians may charge fees higher than those provided by the health insurance plan and patients are expected to pay the difference. This mechanism has not gained much ground nationwide. There is some exodus of Canadian doctors to the United States where the fees are higher and taxes lower. However, their losses tend to be offset by immigration from Great Britain or other countries where the physicians fare worse than in Canada. A Canadian doctor can double his income without increasing his workload by coming to the United States and reduce his exposure to some of the more stringent government regulations. There is some uncertainty regarding how long such a differential will persist.

Maldistribution of physicians and facilities is a major problem in Canada as in all other countries in the free world. The people in lower income groups in cities and in remote areas of the north have obtained adequate health services only with considerable difficulty. The gravitation of physicians toward metropolitan centers is more a matter of human nature than of the health care system.

COST CONSIDERATIONS

The common concept that utilization of a service is a function of public demand leads to the common conclusion that offering a "free" health service will lead to a flood of demand that can swamp the existing services. Accordingly, a gross oversupply of hospitals and doctors was created in Canada preceding introduction of national health insurance. For example, Saskatchewan built almost seven hospital beds per 1,000 people, built a medical school, and admitted many foreign doctors before instituting its universal health insurance program. This is a general phenomenon, which is readily demonstrable in Europe and in the United States. It may be attributable to a perceived shortage of doctors despite evidence of oversupply in some categories. The public never perceives a doctor surplus, even in suburbs with the greatest over-concentration of physicians. Under these conditions physicians are likely to limit their scheduled working hours or are reluctant to add new patients, thereby retaining leisure time. This process is particularly prevalent among specialists and subspecialists.

The health care system of Canada provides more equitable access for all its citizens at lower cost per capita than the United States system. Apparently the single, comprehensive government insurance program is cheaper to administer than multiple overlapping public and private health insurance plans with various packages, exclusions, and copayments. Such an approach was tried in Canada and abandoned.

Control of health care costs emerged as a major public policy in the 1970s. The concept of requiring patient payments as a deterrent was considered and largely abandoned as being directed at the wrong target. It is much preferred to provide physicians an incentive and an economic stake in conservative approaches to health care. Thus far mechanisms for achieving this desirable goal have not been found to be universally effective. Other mechanisms are currently employed and planned.

COST-CONTROL MECHANISMS

In 1969 seven federal task forces made sweeping recommendations regarding the cost control for health services (26). Their recommendations centered on the desirability of increased reliance on ambulatory services rather than hospitalization. In addition, ceilings were placed on capital and operative expenditures, particularly in hospitals. Group and health centers were encouraged as extensions of home-care plans. Cost-containment measures have taken numerous forms, including:

- Certificate of need for facilities and capital expansion through regional and provincial planning with leverage by the federal government through its participation in footing the bills.
- Controls over costs and utilization through an annual hospital budget review system (and through planning alternatives to hospitalization).
- Negotiations of fees and computerized monitoring of physicians' utilization profiles to identify evidence of gross overuse (see below).
- Referral of instances of aberrant patterns of practice to medical review boards.
- Claims review processes.
- Health manpower planning designed to improve distribution of services geographically and maintaining balance between general practitioners and specialists.

It is worth noting that each of these activities is represented in the United States but generally by a variety of different agencies and authorities which are largely uncoordinated and commonly lacking in the necessary leverage to institute the kinds of changes that are required to rationalize such a complex system.

PATTERNS OF PRACTICE

Equity rather than cost control was the principal objective when the government-administered health insurance was introduced (27). British

Columbia and Manitoba have negotiated medical insurance fee arrangements that would provide physicians an economic interest in controlling utilization. Indeed, modification of physician behavior is a key factor in efforts at controlling utilization while maintaining quality. "Medically necessary" care is the basic commitment by the national health insurance program. In certain provinces quality assurance has become more advanced than in the United States. Practice utilization profiles for individual physicians are maintained by means of computerized data systems (28). These can provide objective evidence of overutilization of services, excessive surgery, use of drugs, and so on. Physicians whose practice profiles fall far outside the normal distributions are subject to further screening to identify persons whose professional activities warrant more intensive scrutiny. There is widespread recognition that the methods of payment of physicians has an influence on the frequency with which surgery is performed in different settings (29). In general, physicians on salary have lower rates of surgical operations. The same kind of process can be useful for assessing the utilization of other kinds of services from reliable data bases. By linking practice profiles with hospital and medical insurance claims and drug prescriptions, opportunities are presented for new approaches to assessment of individual physician performance.

Marc Lalonde, Canadian Minister of National Health and Welfare in 1974, has presented a "new perspective" for future trends in health for Canadians (30). A "Health field" concept was proposed as a conceptual framework for dividing complex health problems into manageable segments. For this purpose, the health field was subdivided into four components:

1. Human biology
2. Environment
3. Lifestyle
4. Health care organization

Human biology includes physical, physiological, and mental aspects that comprise the basic biology of man. This element is regarded as contributing to many kinds of ill health, including chronic diseases, genetic disorders, mental conditions, and so forth.

Environment includes those health related factors outside the body that have influence on health status.

Lifestyle represents the aggregate of decisions made by people that may affect their health. These are potential health hazards over which individuals have some measure of control.

Health care organization represents quantity, quality, organization, and relationships among people and resources committed for the provision of health care. This element is generally considered to be the health care system.

Heretofore, major emphasis has been directed at the health care organization. However, this proposal would elevate the other three factors to higher priority as a means of mounting a more comprehensive attack on the health problems of Canadians. This proposed organizational framework is strongly reminiscent of the changes proposed in forward plans by NIH. Indeed, the same kinds of considerations have surfaced in most other developed countries. This is a fitting reminder of the fact that the world has shrunk to the point that the approaches in different countries are progressively turning toward commonality in many of their most crucial features. It would be a tragedy if we failed to profit by the experience of others in the development of American health services because of misplaced pride or arrogance.

SUMMARY

1. The developed countries of the world have all embarked on various mechanisms for meeting the health care needs of their populations over many decades. Since the requirements of the people are essentially the same, the widely varied approaches employed in different countries can be regarded as prototypes for many alternatives, some of which are potentially applicable to the United States. Many experiences, successes, and problems encountered in other parts of the world could serve as extremely expensive experiments in a world laboratory which could help guide our entrance into the complexities of National Health Insurance to which this country is committed.

2. The Medical Research Council of Britain represents a prime example of policies and mechanisms by which first class research can be accomplished on budgets that are very much smaller than those available to the NIH. The reliance on quality rather than quantitiy of research activity appears relevant to the continuance of *fundamental* research in the United States. The grave consequences of an ill-considered requirement for relevance (the Rothschild Report) should serve as a warning of the potential impact of the inappropriate pressures for payoff in the United States.

3. The National Health Service of Great Britain is an ambitious program that a shaky economy can ill afford. The American economy would also be badly shaken if such a program were superimposed on the extravagant system that prevails here. Certain components of this system represent prototypes that deserve attention as mechanisms for greatly enhancing the compassionate and personal health services, particularly for their areas of highest priorities; namely, the elderly, the handicapped, and children. Some of the consequences of cost constraints on a national health service also warrant our attention to avoid stumbling into similar pitfalls.

4. Prototypes of health services available to British populations outside of metropolitan areas represent examples of well-integrated health teams providing compassionate, comprehensive, and quality care that outshines corresponding services in the United States. Specific elements of organizational and operational mechanisms employed for the provision of such care might be adapted for communities in America.

5. Hospitals specifically designed for providing primary care by health teams led by general practitioners have evolved through extensive planning and are being critically evaluated to assess their utility and effectiveness. The outcomes of such ambitious efforts should be examined to determine

the extent to which such approaches can be extrapolated to conditions in America.

6. In Sweden an integrated regional hospital system has emerged through a prolonged process of long-range planning on a national scale, with iterative evaluation of facilities and services. The result is an integrated hierarchy of health centers and hospitals that is unrivaled anywhere else in the world. An important element in the success of this effort is the local control through county councils of long and stable tradition which have no corresponding counterpart in the United States. For this reason, we could not expect to duplicate such a system here, but there is an enormous experience and body of information that could provide goals and guidelines for specific elements in our hospital facilities.

7. Canada has developed a national health service that appears generally applicable to conditions in the United States. The retention of fee-for-service and free choice of physicians, along with private, nonprofit hospitals seems quite compatible with current trends in this country. The system is not without problems but in general has achieved a nearly equal access to quality services at lower costs per capita than prevails in the United States. The utilization of a single nationwide insurance program (governmental in this case) has demonstrated far greater efficiency than that attained by the diversity, overlapping mechanisms, and autonomous control agencies that characterize the American way.

8. The body of experience that has accumulated in other countries corresponds to the body of scientific literature and deserves to be considered as a store of knowledge from a huge number of feasibility studies so complete that they could not and should not be duplicated here. They should serve as the foundation or platform from which our explorations of options can proceed with more rational approaches than could emerge from our own limited experience.

REFERENCES

1. Forsyth G: United Kingdom, in *Health Services Prospects; an International Survey*. (Published for the Nuffield Provincial Hospitals Trust.) Boston, Little, Brown, and Company, 1973.
2. Wennstrom G: Training of health workers in the Swedish Medical Care System. *Ann NY A Sci* 166:985-1001, 1970.
3. Annual Report, 1976-77, Medical Research Council. London, Her Majesty's Stationary Office, (ISBN 0 10 256677 1), 1977.
4. Personal interviews with the following (among many others):
    a. Sir Harold Himsworth, Secretary of the Medical Research Council, 1949-1968.
    b. Dr. J.L. Gowans, Secretary of the Medical Research Council.
    c. Dr. Geoffrey Dawes, Nuffield Institute for Medical Research, Oxford.

d. Dr. Rosemary Rue, Chief Medical Officer for the Oxford Regional Health Authority.
e. Dr. Alex Gatherer, Chief Medical Officer for the Oxfordshire Area Health Authority.
f. Dr. H.S. Wolff, Head, Division of Bioengineering, Clinical Research Center.
g. Dr. A.J.M. Cavenaugh, President, Association of General Practice Hospitals. Brecon War Memorial Hospital, Wales.
h. Dr. Alwyn Smith, Deputy Chief Medical Officer for Wales.
i. Nurse Mary McCarthy, Chief Nursing Officer, Powys Area Health Authority, Wales.
j. Sir John Brotherston, Member, Medical Research Council, Usher Institute, Edinburgh, Scotland.
k. Sir Andrew Watt Kay, Chief Medical Scientist, Scottish Home and Health Office.
l. Gordon McLachlan, Secretary, Nuffield Provincial Hospitals Trust.
m. Professor R.M. Kenedi, Director, Biomedical Engineering Unit, Wolfson Centre, University of Strathclyde, Glasgow, Scotland.

5. A Framework for Government Research and Development: The Organization and Management of Government R & D. A report by Lord Rothschild, Head of the Central Policy Review Staff, November, 1971, (ISBN 10 148140 3).
6. Five Years After: A review of health care research and management after Rothschild. Published for the Nuffield Provincial Hospitals Trust by the Oxford University Press, 1978.
7. Woodroofe Sir E: *Review Body on Doctors' and Dentists' Remuneration* (sixth report). London, Her Majesty's Stationary Office (ISBN 0 10 164730), 1976.
8. McKeown T, Lowe CR: *An Introduction to Social Medicine*, ed 2. Oxford, London, Edinburgh, Melbourne, Blackwell Scientific Publications, 1974.
9. Gemmell PF: *Britain's Search for Health*. Philadelphia, University of Pennsylvania Press, 1960, p. 20.
10. Ryan M: *The Work of the Welsh Hospital Board; 1948-1974.* Ferndale, RI, WT Maddock and Company, 1974.
11. Bevan RT: *Report of the Chief Medical Officer.* Cardiff, The Welsh Office of Health Services, 1976.
12. Schwartz H: The infirmity of British medicine, in Tyrell RE (ed), *The Future That Doesn't Work; Social Democracy's Failures in Britain.* Garden City, New York, Doubleday and Co, 1977.
13. Annual Report, Department of Health and Social Security. London, Her Majesty's Stationary Office, (ISBN 0 10 169310), 1976.
14. Primary Health Care Teams. Report of a panel, Board of Science and Education, British Medical Association, 1974.
15. The Pattern of Medical Working. Wallingford Community Hospital Research Project, Oxford Regional Hospital Board, January, 1973.
16. Day Care in the Community Hospital. Report of a Study Group, Community Hospital Research Program, Oxford Regional Hospital Board, January 1973.
17. Community Hospitals; progress in development and evaluation; Community Hospital Research Programme. Oxford Regional Hospital Board, AE Bennett, Director, January 1974.
18. The Strategic Plan in Outline to 1991. Oxford Regional Health Authority, February, 1978.
19. McLachlan G: *The DHSS; Comments in Positions, Movements, and Directions in Health Services Research,* (Published for the Nuffield Provincial Hospitals Trust.) New York and London, Oxford University Press, 1974.

20. Douglas-Wilson I, McLachlan G (eds): *Health Service Prospects; an International Survey*. Boston, Little, Brown, and Company, 1973.

21. Priorities for Health and Personal Social Services in England; a Consultative Document. Department of Health and Social Security. London, Her Majesty's Stationary Office, (ISBN 0 11 320654), 1976.

22. Engel A: In Tottie M, Bengt J (eds): *The Swedish Regionalized Hospital System in Regional Hospital Planning: Current Trends in Health Services*. Stockholm, The National Board of Sweden, 1967.

23. Andrews JL: Medical care in Sweden; lessons for America. *JAMA* 223:1369-1375, 1973.

24. Lindgren SA: Sweden, in Douglas-Wilson I, McLachlan G (eds): *Health Service Prospects; an International Survey*. (Published for the Nuffield Provincial Hospitals Trust.) Boston, Little, Brown, and Company, 1973.

25. Pickering EA: The Pickering Report (Part III). *Can Med Assn J* 109:1160-1165. What the public thinks. *Can Med Assoc J*, 110:81-93, 1974.

26. Department of National Health and Welfare, Task Force Reports on the Cost of Health Services in Canada (3 vols), Ottawa, Ontario, Canada, Queen's Printer, 1969.

27. Royal Commission on Health Services, vol. 1. Ottawa, Ontario, Canada, Queen's Printer, 1964.

28. Utilization Profiles for Physicians Services Developed in Saskatchewan (1964). The Second Castonguay Commission Report, Quebec, 1970.

29. Vayda E: A comparison of operations and surgeons in Canada, England, and Wales. *N Engl J Med* 282:1224, 1973.

30. Lalonde M: A New Perspective on the Health of Canadians; a Working Document, Department of Health and Welfare, Ottawa, Canada, April 1974.

Index

Accountability, administrative, 37, 42
  special oversight hearings on, 34
  institutional, examples of, 33, 42, 47
Agencies, social and health services, in
    communities, 320
  categories of, 320
Aging, Institute on, forward plan of, 76
Alcohol, Drug Abuse, Mental Health
    Administration (ADAMHA), 60
Ailments, self-limited, 300
Allergy and Infectious Disease, National
    Institute of, forward plans for, 67-68
Alternative approaches to health care,
    examples from abroad, 327-373
American Cancer Society, 15
American Heart Association, 15
Analyzers, gas, 104
Angina pectoris, surgery for, 151
Anti-science movement, 42
Arteriosclerosis, see Atherosclerosis
Arthritis, Metabolism and Digestive
    Diseases, National Institute of,
    forward plan for, 68
Atherogenesis, mutation in, 148
  recurrent "injury" in, 147
  proliferation, arterial smooth muscle in,
    147
  senescence in, 149
  smooth muscle cell proliferation in, 147
  Virchow, Rudolf, and concept of, 146
Atheromatous plaques, 144. See also
    Atherosclerosis
Atherosclerosis, characteristics of, 144
  coronary, surgery for, 151
  epidemiology of, 145
  risk factors, 145-146; reduction of, 151
  therapy in, 150

Basic research, relevance of, 32. See also
    Research, basic vs. applied

Beck, Claude, and coronary surgery, 151
Beri-beri, etiology of, 129
Bevan, Aneurin, 339
Beveridge, Sir William, 339
  and Beveridge Report (Britain), 338
Biomedical concepts, observation-
    explanation coupling, 8
Biomedical nomenclature, 8
Biomedical research, President's panel
    report on, 35. See also National
    Institutes of Health
Biomedical sciences, delayed development
    of, 6
Biostatistics, 289
Bone, Sen. Hugh, and National Cancer Act,
    33
Brecon Hospital, Wales, 352
British research, disquieting trends in, 336.
    See also Research
Brotherstone, Sir John, 342
Bush, Dr. Vannevar, and World War II
    research effort, 11

Canada, equality of access in, 328
  physicians in; acccess to and distribution
    of, 185, 370
Cancer, cause(s) of, 138-144
  characteristic types of, 138-139
  chemotherapy in, 93
  epidemiology in, 130
  lung; smoking in, 140
  metastasis in, 141, 144
  prevalence of, 108
  risk factors in, 139-142
  status of, 138
  See also Carcinogens, chemical
Carcinogenesis, factors in, 142
  "promoters" in, 143
Carcinogens, chemical, 143

Care, health, at large distances, 285. *See also* Health Care
Care, home, technologies for, 323
Care, primary, comprehensive and compassionate (Britain), 347-352
  expanding demand for, 268
  and family medicine, 263-270
  hospital for (Britain), 354-355
  provisions for, 275
  See also Family practice; Physicians; Nurses
Careers, professional, preparation for, 287
  spectrum of, 258
  see also individual health professions
Careers, research, preparation for, 290-295
Cause of diseases, *see* Etiology of disease
Carroll, Alexis, and vascular surgery, 105
Child Health and Human Development, National Institute for, forward plans, 75-76
Cholera, suspected causes of, 130
Christian Scientists, health of, 302
Churchill, Sir Winston, and National Health Service (Britain), 339
Clinical evaluation, 99. *See also* Health services research
Clinical investigation, 99, 137. *See also* Research, clinical
Clinical trials, mechanisms for, 241
  outcome evaluation, 222
Colds, common; interferon in, 159. *See also* Respiratory infections
Commissions, Royal (Britain), 359
Compensation, equitable; complications of (Britain), 344-345
Competence, characteristics of, 293
  definition of, 292
  in research, 291
Complaints, common; rational responses to, 311
Complications, avoidance of, 178
Concepts, generally accepted, 5
  subjective observations in, 8
Cooper, Theodore, 36
Counseling, health, 317-318
  scope of, 317
Counselors, health; categories of, 317
Creative ability, development of, 294
Creativity, for academic research, 292
  characteristics of, 293
  indicators or tests of, 294
Credibility, crisis in, 42
Curricula, core, 257
  medical; alternative careers, 258-259
  essentials of, 289

Data, laboratory patient tests, 260. *See also* Devices, diagnostic
Death rates, declines in; before 1875, 6
  from scarlet fever, 6

from tuberculosis, 6
from whooping cough, 6
Decision trees, 313-316
Dental Research, National Institute of; forward plan, 73-74
Department of Defense, budget, 18-19
Department of Health, Education and Welfare, forward plan for health, FY 1978-1982, 36
  table of organization, 60
Dependence, degree of; and severity of illness, 303
Deputizing services (Britain), 345
Design, experimental, 289
Developments, diffusion of, 103-106
  processes of, 100-102. *See also* Technology, transfer of
Devices, development of, lag times, 132
  diagnostic, 168-176
  see also Electronics, medical; Instruments, diagnostic
Diagnosis, dangers from, 227
  technologies for, 166-176
  overuse of, 180-181
  without therapy, value added in, 220
Dictionaries, medical, mathematical and physical terms in, 8-9
Disability, causes of, 106
Disease and disability, activity limitations in, 156-157
  causes of, 129-133, 155-160
  epidemic, 127
  microbial origins of, 5
  prevention of, value added, 219-220
  registries for, 239
  of unknown origin, medical management of, 129
  suspected causes of, 129
Diseases, chronic, conquest of, 127-131
  impact of, 109
  management of, 323
  mortality rates in, 132
Diseases, common, of respiratory system, 265
Drug reactions, adverse, 226, 281
  patient sensitivity and, 226

Echocardiography, 104. *See also* Ultrasound, diagnostic
Edison, Thomas, and x-ray machines, 104
Education, elementary, 291
  by example, 260
  medical, AMA Council on, 254
    common misconceptions of, 256-257
    deficiencies of, 10, 273-275
    impacts of research grants in, 255-256
  professional, 253-295
  see also individual health professions
Efficacy of care, assurance of, 233
Electronics, medical, 170-171

Engel, Arthur, and Regional Hospital
    System (Sweden), 363
Engineering, evolution of, 4-5
    quantitative concepts of, 5
England, hospital services in, 340
Environmental Health Sciences, National
    Institute of, 67
    forward plan for, 77-78
Environmental stresses, protection from, 12
Epidemics, 127
    control of, 12
Epidemiology, causal factors elicited by, 131
Etiology of disease, epidemiology in,
    130-132
    importance of, 129-134
Exposures, environmental, 12
Eye, National Institute; national plan for,
    72-73

Faculties, medical; specialized physicians
    in, 259
Family practice, 263-269. *See also* Care,
    primary
    presenting problems in, 265-267
Farmers, health of, 302
Fee-for-service, national health program
    (Canada), 368-373
Fibroplasia, retrolental; blindness in
    infants, 225
Fishermen, health of, 302
Flexner, Abraham, 10, 254
    philosophy, 11
    Report, 10
Fogarty, Rep. John, 15, 43
Forward plan for health (FY 1978-1982),
    tactical plan priorities, 36
Fountain, Rep. L. H., 30
    Committee, report of, 30
Frederickson, Donald S.; Director, NIH, 37,
    41
Fries, James, and self-care manual, 313
Functional research, 98. *See also* Research,
    categories, definitions
Funding, research, by NIH, 254

General Medical Sciences, National
    Institute of, forward plan, 75
General practice, decline in, 261
Goals, national, of health-related research,
    22
    public support for, 22
    research, 55
    see also Research support,
        rationalization of
Goldberger, Dr. Joseph, on pellagra, 128
Graduates, foreign, 260
Grants, research, extramural, 113
    and independence, 255
    number of, 85, 114
    output, 114

and professional prestige, 255
Great Britain, equality of access in, 328

Hammond Report, smoking and mortality
    in, 140-142
Hazards, health; resistance to, 301
Health, broadened definition of, 268
    deficiencies in, 12
    expanding horizons of, 269
    forward planning for (FY 1978-1982), 36
    hazards to, 268
    self-reliance in, 302
    without health care, 302
Health Advocates, 311-317
Health Aides, Village in Alaska, 284
Health Authorities, Area (Britain), 340
Health care, 298
    access to, emergency rooms, 186
        home calls, 186
    Canadian, cost-control mechanisms in,
        371
    comparative results, international, 190
    costs of, 188-189
        projected for year 2000, 190
        and third-party payments, 188
        fringe benefits in, 189
    equitable access to (Canada), 370-371
    standards for, 236
Health care teams, as a "nucleus"
    (Britain), 348
Health Centers (Britain), 348
Health Information Center, concept of,
    318-324
    scope of, 318-
Health legislation, coalition for, 15
Health maintenance, 298. *See also* Risk
    factors
Health professionals, specialization of,
    183-186
Health-related research, in academic
    institutions, 20
    in governmental agencies, 17
    national goals of, 22
Health Service Corps, National, 285
Health Service, National (Britain), 337. *See
    also* National Health Service
Health services, appraisal of, 200
    indicators for, 229-231
    assessment of, 202
        process evaluation, 202-203
        program evaluation, 202-203
        outcome evaluation, 202-203
    benefits from, by definitive therapy, 220
        by diagnosis, 220
        by "doing something" (placebo effect),
            221
        by prevention, 219
        by symptomatic management, 220
    in Britain and the United States, 359-361
    in Canada, 369

Canadian, fee-for-service, 368
evaluations of, alternate sites: clinical
    settings, pre-paid, 245
  departments of health, expanded roles,
    245
  medical schools, 245
  physicians in private practice, 245
  schools of public health, 245
extravagance in, 234
forces impelling, 204-206
home (Britain), 351
National, reorganization of (Britain),
    339-342
outcome assessment, clinical trials
    (NHLBI), 222-224
value-added, 217
perceived needs of, in Britain, 346
program evaluation; components of,
    207-211
  conceptual considerations, 211-217
  cost/benefit analysis, 211-217
  cost/effectiveness, 211-217
  demand, 203-204
  need, 203-204
  targets for, 223-225
  utilization, 203-224
provincial governments in (Canada), 369
research, definitions, 201
  evaluation of efficacy, 233
  examples of extravagance, 234-236
  health statistics, sources of, 237-241
  new mechanisms, requirements for,
    241-247
priorities (1976, 1979-1980), 201
process of evaluation, 206-211
programs, in Europe, 356
surgical operations, 204-205
Health Statistics, National Center for, 108,
    200, 301
  surveys of, ambulatory medical care
    survey, 241
  health examination survey, 240
  health interview survey, 240
  hospital discharge survey, 240-241
Health statistics, sources of, 237-241
  surveys of, 239
Health status, indicators of, 106
Health team, development of (Britain), 348
  integrated (Wales), 352-354
Health understanding, barriers to, 306-308
Heart, Lung and Blood, National Institute,
    forward plans, 69-72
Heart, performance of, 301
Heart disease, coronary, epidemiology of,
    130. See also Atherogenesis;
    Atherosclerosis
Hearts, artificial; implantable, 153-154,
    194-196
Highways, hazards of, 268
Hill, Sen. Lister, 15, 43

Hill-Burton Act (1946), and hospital
    construction, 15
Hindsight, Project; and Department of
    Defense, 103
Hodgkin, Keith, and general practice, 263
  and "trivial" ailments, 300
Home and Health Service (Scotland), 342
Home Helps (Britain), 351
Home Nursing (Britain), 351
Hospital resources, use of, 260
Hospital System, Regional (Sweden),
    361-368
Hospitals, academic (Sweden), 364
  community, "ideal model" of (Britain),
    354
  day (Britain), 351
  and emergency room use, 186
  general practice (Britain), 347
  new technologies in, 187
  physician benefits of, 187
  Swedish and American, contrast between,
    367
  teaching, and referred patients, 260
Hygiene, 311

Illness, burden of, relative rankings, 108,
    110
  mental, 265. See also Problems,
    behavioral, psychosocial
  see also Disease and Disability
Immunology, research on, distribution, 115
Indian Affairs, Bureau of, 284
Influenza, immunizations for, 158
  and pneumonia, 156-157
Injuries, 265
  emergency care of, 233
Innovations, nursing, inventory of, 279
Insight, flashes of, 132, 290
Instruments, diagnostic, 158-176
  energy probes in, infrared radiation,
    168-169
    radionuclides (isotopes), 168-169
    ultrasound, 168-169
    x-rays, 168-169
Interdependence, encouragement of, 307

Kay, Sir Andrew Watt, 342
Kidney disease, costs of dialysis in, 194
  dialysis machines for, 136
Knowles, Dr. John, 309

Laboratories, clinical, metamorphosis of, 169
Lasker, Mary, and lay lobby, 14, 16, 43
Library of Medicine, National, 226
  expanded roles of, 120
Life expectancy, and Breslow (1693), 6
  in Britain (1838), 6
  and living conditions, 7
  nutrition in, 7
  United States (1970), 6

Lumbermen, health of, 302

Magnuson, Rep. Warren, 13
Mahoney, Florence, and lay lobby, 14
Management, of data, 289
Mansfield Amendment (1970), and
    Department of Defense research, 19
Manuals, self-help, 313
Mathematics, as language of science, 3-5
Mavericks, education of, 295
    identification of, 294
McKeown, Thomas, and declining
    death rates, 6
MEDEX program, physicians assistants,
    283
Medical care, fragmentation of, 183
Medical Research Council (Britain), basic
    mechanisms of, 331
    counterpart for NIH, 331
    policies and priorities of, 333-334
Medical Service, Alaska Native, 284
Medicine, Board on (National Academy of
    Sciences), 284
Medicine, "holistic", 38
    metropolitan, maldistribution of
    (Britain), 345-347
Merit review, guidelines for, 28
Microscopes, electron, 166
Morbidity, statistics on, 239
Mortality, cause-specific rates of, 238
    data, 238
    major causes of, 107
Mutual Aid Groups, 324

National Cancer Act Amendments
    (1971, 1974), 44
National Cancer Institute, 44
    legislative mandate, 13
National Cancer Program, 66-67
    budget for, 45-47
    components of, 51-53
    development of, 48-54
    objectives, 48
    participation of scientific community in,
    51
    plans for, individual program plans, 48-51
    operational plan, 48-51
    strategic plan, 48-51
    planning prototype, 47
    research thrust, 51
National Center for Health Services
    Research, 200-204
    priorities of (1976, 1979-1980), 201
National Health Insurance Act, 1911
    (Britain), 338
National Health planning, goals and
    guidelines for (1974), 35
National Health Program (Canada), 368-373
National Health Service (Britain), budgets,
    358

defects in, 346
    and general practitioners, 342
    reorganized, 340
    Royal Commission on, 357-359
    taxation and, 344
National Heart Institute, budgets for
    (1950-1966), 24
National Institutes of Health, areas of
    responsibility, 81-82
    boundaries of, 79
    budgets for, 24-25, 60
    as bursar, 28, 35
    categories of, combined categories, 57-60
    disease or cause-oriented, 57-60
    organ-oriented, 57-60
    congressional intent, 31
    criticisms of, 30-32, 35
    developmental states, Fall from Favor,
    25-38
    Forward Planning Phase, 25-38
    Mobilization Phase, 25-38
    evolution of, 13-17, 22-30
    expansion of, 21
    forward plans, 22-25. See also individual
    Institutes
    Fountain Committee and, 30
    individual institutes of, Aging (NIA),
    76-77
    Arthritis, Metabolic and Digestive
    Diseases (NIAMDD), 22-23, 68-69
    Cancer (NCI), 22-23, 44-54
    Child Health and Human Development
    (NICHHD), 22-23
    Dental Research (NIDR), 22-23, 73-74
    Environmental Sciences (NIES), 77-78
    Eye (NEI), 72-73
    General Medical Sciences (NIGMS),
    22-23, 69-72
    Heart, Lung and Blood (NHLBI), 22-23,
    69-72
    Neural and Communicative Diseases
    (NINCD), 22-23, 74-75
    intent of Congress, 26
    legislative history, 22-23
    as management, 28, 35
    organizational framework of, 60-61
    three-tiered, 80
    policies, review of, report of Biomedical
    Research Panel, 35
    the Wooldridge Report, 31
    priorities, 137-143
    SATT system, 95
    and the Ransdell Act (1930), 13
    Reorganization Act (1970), 34
    territorial boundaries; ambiguity of,
    79-80
    three-dimensional view, 58-59
    see also individual Institutes
National Research Council (National
    Academy of Sciences, contracts, 12

382   Index

Neely, Sen. Matthew, and cancer
    legislation, 13
Neoplastic diseases, 138. *See also* Cancer
Neurological, Communicative Disorder and
    Stroke, National Institute of, forward
    plan, 74
Nomenclature, biomedical, 8
    mathematical and physical, in medical
        dictionaries, 8
"Noncompliance", 299
Normality, specifications of, 133
Northern Ireland, health services delivery
    in, 342
Nurse Consultants, 322-323
Nurses, community psychiatric (Britain),
    350
    functions of, 276-280
    as health visitors (Britain), 350
    number of, 276
    public health, 280
    roles of, 276
Nursing, diversification of, 276
    functions of (Britain), 349-351
    and "tender loving care", 279

Objectives, research, 55. *See also* Research
    support, rationalization of
Obstacles, technical and theoretical, 290.
    See also Technical problems,
    Theoretical problems
Optometry, 276, 283
Osborn, Alex, and development of
    creativity, 295

Pandemics, 127
Paraprofessionals, 282-283
Partnerships, participative, 298-324
    opportunities for, 308-311
Pathophysiology, *see* Research, targeted
Patient, role of, 300
Payoff for research, pressures for, 29-30
Pellagra, etiology of, 127
Penicillin, early observations of, 104
Pepper, Sen. Claude, 14
Personnel, health; numbers of, 182
    proliferating, 181-182
    professional; underutilization of, 275
Pharmacists, 276
    compliance and, 282
    role of, 316
    underutilization of, 316
    untapped talent of, 281
Pharmacy, curricula in, 281
    professional degrees in, 281
"Physicians' assistants", 283
Physicians, access to, 320
    apparent shortage of, 186
    British, emigration of, 345
    drain on world supply of, 260

in family practice, 258
family, responsibilities of, 262
    as an underdeveloped resource, 268
in inner cities, 185
maldistribution of, 185
    in Canada, 370
number of, expansion (Sweden), 366
as primary filters, 272
as professional purchasing agents, 272
research training of, 257
responsibilities of, 270-275
roles of, 257
in specialties, 183-185, 258
    numbers of, 261-263
training of, 253
See also Education, medical
Physics, quantitative concepts of, 5
Placebo, 135
Planning, forward, 41
    components of, 54-56
    criteria for, 106-110
    impacts of, 53-55
    obstacles to, 56
    long range, pressures for, 35
    See also Research, health-related, forward
        planning of
Pneumonia, risk factors in, 158
Podiatrists, 276, 283
Policies, payment, professional (Britain),
    342-345
Practice, family, as an expanding specialty,
    265
    presenting problems in, 265
    and residency training, 268
    general, and patients, 263
Practitioners, balance with specialists
    (Britain), 343
    family, problems presented to, 265
    general, group practice (Britain), 347
        need for, 263
        number of, 261
        "vocational" training of (Britain), 347
    health, parallel pathways for, 287
    nurse, 280
        and increased responsibility, 279
        in pediatrics, 280
        as women's health care specialists, 280
Preston, Thomas, and coronary surgery
    evaluation, 152
Priest, Rep. Percy, and mental health bill, 14
Primary care team, 349
    new hospital for (Britain), 354
Priorities, long-range planning, 356-359
    research, 55. *See also* Research support,
        rationalization of
    criteria, 106-110
    postwar, 12
    reappraisal of, 38
Problems, behavioral, "medicalizaiton" of,
    269

presenting, characteristics of, 316
psychosocial, 269-270
Products, new, orderly introduction of, 242
Professionals, dependence on, 302-308
health, education of, 275
Profiles, practice utilization, and
    computerized data systems (Canada),
    372
Programs, screening, and annual checkups,
    265
Progress, biomedical, concepts of, 89-90
obstacles to, technical and theoretical,
    90-93
pressures for, 43-44
research, monitoring of, 112-122
surges of, 290
toward cure and control, 132
Prototypes, in the world laboratory, 327-373
Pseudo-solutions, 133-136
Psychology, clinical, 282
Public Health Service, component agencies
    of, 36

Radioisotopes, applications of, 104
Radiology, diagnostic, overuse of, 235
Rationalization, Age of, 5
Regional Hospital System in Sweden,
    363-364
Research, applications of, 63-64
basic vs. applied, 32, 37, 87, 166-176
    definitions, 88, 93-94
    requirements for, 94-95
behavioral, 38
biomedical, criticisms of, 42
British, 330-337
categories of, 126-127
    operational definitions, 95-100
    clinical evaluation, 99
    clinical investigation, 99
    functional research, 98
    fundamental research, 96
    targeted research, 98
competence and creativity in, 291-295
continuum concept, 88
forward planning programs for,
    individual institutes of health, 65-79
    NIH directorate, 61-65
    priorities and strategies, 87-125
    fundamental (pure), 96-98
health-related, forward planning, 41-84
    among government agencies, 17-19
    relevance of, 33
    transition of, 42
Health Services, See Health Services,
    research
Health Services (Britain), 355-356
Health Services, National Center for,
    200-204
medical, laboratory facilities for, 27
and prestige, 256

priorities for, current, 137
productivity, monitoring of, 114-124
and professional advancement, 256
redundant or repetitive, 110-112
support of, 16-17
    by federal government, 257
    among government agencies, 17-19
    targeted, 98, 136-137
    during World War II, 12
Research careers in Britain, disincentives
    for, 336
Research grants, vs. contracts, 28
institute-initiated, 113
investigator-initiated, 115-119
monitoring of, 112-113
peer review of, 27-28
Research Grants, Division of, extended
    role for, 119
Research personnel, basic medical
    scientists, 26
clinical investigators, 26
recruitment of, 26
Research proposals, peer review of, 27
Research review, investigator intentions,
    115-119
Research support, and Department of
    Defense (Mansfield Amendment,
    1970), 19
governmental, 18
    distribution of, 19
    DOD, NASA, NSF, VA, DOT, HUD,
    DPA, 20
grants vs. contracts, 28
industrial, 18
NASA, 20
private, 18
rationalization of, 54-55
sources of, 17-20
Respiratory infections, influenza and
    pneumonia, 156. See also specific
    diseases
upper, 156-160
Reward system, 256
Risk, avoidance of, 308-310
Risk factors, 129, 139-142. See also Diseases
    and disability, of unknown origin
Rockefeller Foundation, and support of
    medical education, 11
Roentgen rays, initial application of, 104
Rothschild Report (Britain), 334-337
specific recommendations of, 335

Scheele, Leonard, 16
Scarlet fever, declining death rates from, 6-7
Schools, medical, and community service,
    256
departments of, 254
educational processes of, 257
family practice pathways in, 288
and the incentive structure, 256

metamorphosis of, 254-257
research in, 256
teaching in, 256
Science, progress in (World War II), 11
and technology, crisis in credibility, 42
Sciences, behavioral, interfaces, 269
Sciences, National Academy of, 284
Scientific merit, guidelines for review of, 28
Scientists, freedom of, 37
Scotland, health service delivery in, 342
Screening, laboratory, limiting factors in,
235-236
Sehnert, Dr. Keith, self-care manual, 313
Self-care, definition of, 298
education about, 310
as a health service, 298-324
kits for, 316
obstacles to, 303-308
as a predominant mode of health, 300
promotion of, 307
as a viable option, 310
Self-reliance, aided, 321-324
Service, nursing, rural, 280
Services, for the elderly (Britain),
351-352
health, in selected countries, 328
Shannon, James, 15
and basic medical sciences, 16
and NIH categorical Institutes, 57
Shapely, Willis, and zero-based budgeting,
34
Social work, 283
"Socialized medicine" (Britain), 328
Specialists, 183-185, excess numbers of, 261
growth in, 262
influence of, in medical schools, 253
in medical community, 253
nursing, for the seriously ill, 280
See also Physicians, in specialties
Statistics, National Center for Health, 108
Students, medical, 258
of diverse backgrounds, 259
Surgery, coronary bypass, 5, 152
mortality, post-operative variations in,
229
surplus, examples of, 228
Sweden, county councils in, 362
equality of access in, 328
National Health Insurance of, 362

Targeted research, 98. See also Research,
categories, operational definitions
Team Training, 286-287
Technical problems, 90-93
accomplishments, health benefits from, 6
Manhattan Project, 93
NASA, 91-92
triumphs, complications of, 180-184
Technicians, emergency, 285

Technology, assessment of, for artificial
implantable heart, 194
components of, 193
examples of, 193
for renal dialysis, 194
transfer of, 61-65, 100-104
Technologies, appropriate utilization of,
232
diffusion of, constraints on (Britain), 346
health, assessment of, 165-197
diffusion of, 103-106
personnel for, 181-185
research, conversion into diagnostic
devices, 166-170
Teeth, caries of, fluoride in, 131
Terms, physical, in medical dictionaries, 8
Tests, diversity of, 260
Theoretical problems, 90-93
cancer chemotherapy, 93
Therapy, for coronary heart disease, 150-154
deficiencies in, 176
definitive, 137
value-added in, 220
empirical, supportive and symptomatic,
134, 176-178
levels of, 176-179
management methods, supportive and
symptomatic, 134, 176-178
physical, 135
progress in, 176-180
Thomas, Lewis, 132, 301
Tomography, computerized axial (CAT
scanners), 172-174
Transfer for technology, 61-65, 100-104
Tuberculosis, declining death rates from,
6-7

Ultrasound, diagnostic, 174-175. See also
Instruments, diagnostic, energy
probes

Value-added, concept of, 217
by "doing something", the placebo effect,
221-222
supportive management, 220
Veterans Administration, budgets for, 20
Vickery, Donald, self-care manual, 313
Virchow, Rudolf, on atherogenesis, 146
Vital statistics, 238
Vitamin deficiencies, 130

Wales, hospital services in, 340, 352
National Health Service and, 340
Wallingford Hospital (Britain), 354
Welsh Scientific Committee, 341
Whooping cough, declining death rates
from, 6-7
Wooldridge, D. F., committee report (1965), 31

Yellow fever, causal factors, 130